THE MINIMAL
BRAIN DYSFUNCTIONS

THE MINIMAL BRAIN DYSFUNCTIONS

Diagnosis and Treatment

Leonard Small

THE FREE PRESS
A Division of Macmillan Publishing Co., Inc.
NEW YORK

Collier Macmillan Publishers
LONDON

The Free Press
A Division of Macmillan Publishing Co., Inc.
866 Third Avenue, New York, N.Y. 10022

Collier Macmillan Canada, Inc.

Library of Congress Catalog Card Number: 82-71471

Printed in the United States of America

printing number

1 2 3 4 5 6 7 8 9 10

Library of Congress Cataloging in Publication Data

Small, Leonard, 1913-1982
    The minimal brain dysfunctions.

    Bibliography: p.
    Includes index.
    1. Minimal brain dysfunction in children.
I. Title. [DNLM: 1. Hyperkinetic syndrome—Diagnosis.
2. Hyperkinetic syndrome—Therapy.   WS 340 S635m]
RJ496.B7S6   1982   618.92′8589   82-71471
ISBN 0-02-929300-6

To

those learning-disabled youths
whose valiance and perseverance
teach us so much.

"I was always in trouble when I was small.
Anything I wanted to do didn't turn out right."

Contents

III Treatment

Preface

THE PREVALENCE OF the minimal brain dysfunctions makes them a national problem. Estimates point to as many as ten percent of school-age children as their victims.

This serious problem is dangerously played-down by efforts to simplify the true complexities of the disorders. One influential group of specialists devalues the importance of etiology, even though its discovery often leads to the single most effective treatment. Others argue for a simplified diagnostic battery that sacrifices procedures which may provide the key insight into cause and thus treatment for a child. And other professionals—particularily psychiatrists— avoid the complex therapeutic considerations and possibilities by regarding this syndrome of syndromes as one disorder, to be treated by one method: stimulant medication.

Motivations for oversimplification can be understood. Simultaneous investigation of more than one variable and their interaction is difficult to design, even more so to execute, and the variables in MBD are many. Selecting one promising factor to study may eliminate from investigation the essential causal factors in many subjects. Few if any studies of complicated disorders have exhaustively examined one factor after another. For example, consider the decades of unresolved debate about the etiology of schizophrenia.

A wish to preserve optimism about prognosis may be operating. The simple disorder is easy to treat and thought to be more responsive. Expectation has been demonstrated to influence outcome in psychotherapy, as in many medical situations. But hope and positive expectation are likely to founder over the long haul if simplicity proves to be only denial of the facts. A successful search amidst complex factors for the significant ones contributes more realistically to positive expectation.

Fear of facing the cost in dollars and time may be another impetus to over-simplification. Complex disorders are more costly to diagnose and to treat. Parents or patients may not have the resources and/or the resilience for a lengthy treatment. But again, a false promise of lower economic and psychological costs based upon oversimplification may result in irreparable damage.

But understanding motivation is not acceptance of the resulting behavior. This book eschews oversimplification. It presents in clinical context the complexities of cause, diagnosis, and treatment of these multiple dysfunctions. A child may suffer one or several of them. He can be helped best, sometimes be helped only, by careful location of his individual key problem or problems.

No panacea exists for the minimal brain dynsfunctions. Remedial instruction, environmental manipulation, behavioral modification, medications, special diets, megavitamins, eye exercises, psychotherapies of several types— each benefits some people but not others. Some people respond well to single treatment interventions, others respond better to combinations of efforts provided concurrently, and still others respond to different interventions at succeeding life-stages. And some remain unbenefited by all methods. The clinician facing a patient must confront all these diagnostic and therapeutic possibilities. The approaches and insights which may have worked so well with one patient may be far off the mark with the next.

Personal competence in one special area of diagnosis or treatment should not seduce the responsible clinician into claims for the primacy of that area. Such claims prevent helping patients who are unresponsive to that particular intervention.

Expertise in all the methods of diagnosis and treatment is not to be expected of any clinician. But acquaintance with all of them—their content, practices, and appropriate applications—is possible. This book seeks to contribute this level of knowledge.

A willingness to use what is known is essential to the responsible clinician to whom this book is addressed. An understanding of the possibilities and limits is also useful to all others actively concerned for victims of the minimal brain dysfunctions: teachers, social workers, psychologists, pediatricians, psychiatrists, opthalmologists, audiologists, optometrists, nutritionists, counselors, and parents. I hope, too, that some victims of these dysfunctions may at some point in their lives find this work helpful in understanding their disorder and in overcoming its effects. The minimal brain dysfunctions have long arms that reach from childhood through adolescence into adulthood.

Acknowledgments

SEVERAL COLLEAGUES GENEROUSLY OFFERED suggestions for the improvement of the manuscript and encouraged its progression. For this I am grateful to Dr. Leonard Diller, Chief of Behavior Science, Institue of Physical Medicine and Rehabilitation, New York City; Dr. Harold Pass, Clinical Psychologist, University Hospital, State University of New York at Stony Brook; and Dr. Aaron Smith, Director, Neuropsychology Laboratory, University of Michigan at Ann Arbor.

My wife, Verna, has lent her writing and editing skills to the effort at directness and clarity on some very complicated issues. I have learned much from her in the past and continue now to learn from her about what I want to write and how to write it.

LEONARD SMALL

I

DIMENSIONS

Chapter 1

Concept and Definition

Is MINIMAL BRAIN DYSFUNCTION (MBD) a reality or a chimera? Most efforts to define and conceptualize MBD have evoked objections and negative criticisms: consensus is elusive and debate continues. The controversy reflects the ambiguity arising from the many symptoms and symptom clusters, or syndromes, identified with MBD, and from the near impossibility of establishing a simple etiology from the half dozen or more major causal factors hypothesized. This is not an empty war of words because the successful treatment of an individual depends upon ability to diagnose his disorder as accurately as possible, to identify the probable etiology, and then to select the appropriate intervention or interventions.

MBD is at best only a category, imprecisely defined, which encompasses many disorders: hyperkinesis, dyslexia, dysgraphia, dyscalculia, learning disabilities, and disorders of attention, conceptualization, language, and sensory and motor functions. The looseness has ominous potential for harm to the MBD sufferer. The therapist, Lewis (9) observes, may tend to overlook not only the specific and individual characteristics of a patient but also any phenomena that, while present in him, seem unsuited to the presumed diagnosis. When ambiguity, confusion, controversy, and imprecision are recognized, when the effort to erect an unassailable edifice on shifting sands is abandoned and the professional ceases to pontificate, an MBD diagnosis can be made useful to the patient. The professional who can review all the possibilities and ponder the probabilities can gradually narrow the range of alternatives and focus on the most likely ones for the individual.

Efforts to improve the focus and rigor of the concept itself have been hampered by the pursuit of single-dimension definitions that emphasize one major symptom (e.g., hyperactivity or letter-reversal) and ignore other symptom phenomena (14).

Sçhain (18) found eighteen diagnoses in frequent use, all equivalent to MBD. In addition to those that incorporate the words "brain," "organic," "cerebral," "disorder," "dysfunction," and "damage," he reports these in the literature:

> choreiform syndrome
> clumsy-child syndrome
> visual-motor disability
> hyperkinetic-behavior syndrome
> developmental Gerstmann's syndrome
> strephosymbolia
> specific dyslexia
> developmental dyslexia
> congenital word blindness
> perceptually handicapped
> primary reading retardation
> specific language disability

To these are now added the labels in the new *Diagnostic and Statistical Manual of Mental Disorders* provided by the American Psychiatric Association (7a):

> Attention Deficit Disorder *with* hyperkinesis
> Attention Deficit Disorder *without* hyperkinesis
> Residual Type (The person once showed symptoms of hyperkinesis, but no longer does. Other signs may persist: poor organization of work, difficulty completing tasks, impairment of social and vocational functioning)
> Developmental Arithmetic Disorder
> Developmental Reading Disorder
> Developmental Language Disorder—Expressive Type
> Developmental Language Disorder—Receptive Type
> Developmental Articulation Disorder
> Mixed Specific Developmental Disorder

In short, the vagueness of the syndrome and its variability are widely recognized as the major impediments to comprehending and treating this group of disorders (13). Slowly this confusion has given way to a more realistic, more encompassing multidimensional approach to the definition and diagnosis of MBD, one that recognizes the syndromes within the syndrome. Benton, in an appraisal (1) of the current knowledge of dyslexia gathered in a volume he edited with Pearl (2), concludes that while a satisfactory understanding of the nature of dyslexia is yet to be achieved, there have been improvements in its definitions. The definitions are more realistic, advancing from those that focus on single variables to those that encompass multiple syndromes. These latter differentiate dyslexia according to etiologies and types of dysfunctions, rather than assuming a single pure symptom. This progress in definition has been accompanied by advances in detection at an earlier stage of the child at risk for dyslexia. Early detection allows more time for interventions and for progress in the development of treatment and remediation.

Benton's observations on how progress can be achieved apply to all the other syndromes under the all-too-commodious MBD umbrella. MBD is a multiple-syndrome disorder in which the component syndromes are in turn conglomerates of subsyndromes. There is more than one kind of activity disorder, or attention deficit, or learning disability, just as there is more than one type of dyslexia. This concept of MBD as a syndrome of syndromes guides the approach of this book to its diagnosis and treatment.

Equally important is the concept that the patterns of symptoms constituting the syndrome indicate disorders in brain-behavior relationships. This is the case with the etiologies proposed, except where a purely emotional origin is advanced, as when a child's hyperactivity is seen as an effort to obtain the attention of a depressed, withdrawn mother, or where a purely cultural influence can be demonstrated. The connection of the symptoms to brain-behavior disorders underlies the use of "brain dysfunction" in the widely accepted term, "Minimal Brain Dysfunction" (7). While definitive, "hard," clear-cut neurological signs are rarely found in the MBD patient, so-called "soft" neurological signs are frequently seen upon careful examination, as are electroencephalographic abnormalities when pursued with painstaking methods. Also prominent among the signs suggestive of brain-behavior disorder are the patterns of neuropsychological test findings. And thus the adjective "minimal" in the term serves a cautionary, restraining role for the diagnostician: it reminds him that while the behavioral patterns in MBD resemble those observed in persons with established brain damage, a rigorously defined diagnosis of brain damage is elusive (6).

It is here, in the diagnostic designation "Minimal Brain Dysfunction," that much of the controversy centers and much of the confusion arises. The presumptions of brain damage as causal in MBD, originating with Werner and Strauss in 1941 (20), aroused vigorous objections that still continue (4, 5, 6), as discussed in Chapter 2, Etiology. The weight of these objections has led to moderation of the etiological assumption in the term used, with "dysfunction" substituted for "damage." This substitution was warranted by the reasoning that all learning and behavior reflects brain function, and that although the site of a slight brain dysfunction usually cannot be established, some brain dysfunction logically may be assumed as the cause of a learning or behavior disability, in the absence of more convincing explanation.

A striking feature of MBD is that its victims usually function less adequately than one would expect them to from intelligence test scores. Many children suspected of MBD produce overall intelligence test results that range from the near-Average to Above-Average levels (10, 18). Yet they fail to meet chronological and/or mental-age levels of expectancy in learning and behavior (11). The explanation appears to be that their performances on the different subtests that are averaged to arrive at an overall test score vary over wide extremes; a Borderline-Mental-Defective level in one subtest may be found along with a Very-Superior level in another subtest in the same person. A reasonable assumption is that without MBD these children would test and function even higher than the near-Average to Above-Average levels that have been observed in them. Presumably, children of lower than near-Average levels of endowment who have MBD are most usually diagnosed as Borderline Mental Defective or lower, an error with grave consequences for their lives. This diagnostic error continues to occur frequently and tragically, despite the differentiation of the syndrome from mental retardation by Werner and Strauss in 1942 (20).

A further important feature of the MBD syndrome is the presence of emotional disturbance. MBD symptoms are found more frequently among the emotionally disturbed, particularly children, than among individuals without such disturbance (8). Severe emotional reactions may be consequences of cognitive, sensory. memory, and other impairments, appearing as depression, aversiveness, delinquency, and, in later life, alcoholism.

A final feature of the syndrome is its usually unremitting course unless detected early and lengthily treated. Without these interventions most children with MBD will grow into adulthood with one or more apparently permanent impairments of cognition, attention, activity, and sensory and motor functions among a variety of other dysfunctions, along with concomitant emotional disorders usually varying with the severity of the MBD. There are, of course, exceptions to this rule. In a few individuals the impairments become progressively less marked, and sometimes disappear with time. But the exceptions are not frequent enough to allow parents of a child who shows MBD to rest assured by a pediatrician's confidence that this, too, will pass.

To summarize, the organization of this book derives from the following understanding of Minimal Brain Dysfunctions:

1. The symptoms constituting MBD are many; their combinations into syndromes are varied; their etiology is often ambiguous, yet always important to hypothesize, if not to establish. Thus proper diagnosis is most likely from a "team" of different specialists who coordinate their individual findings about a patient from each of their special disciplines.

2. Proper treatment may be as complex as the adequate diagnosis; it may require more than one type of intervention, applied either simultaneously, in tandem order, or at developmentally appropriate times. Treatment is usually of long duration, and may extend from early childhood into the adult years.

3. The complexity of both diagnosis and treatment requires coordination of the findings and services of diagnosticians and therapists. Parents cannot be expected to have enough knowledge of the disorder to select and designate

priorities among the many options, or the power and/or diplomatic skills to coordinate several professionals. An adequate program thus requires a coordinator, of necessity one of the diagnostic or treatment team members accepted by the others (12).

4. The earliest possible diagnosis of MBD and prompt initiation of indicated treatment interventions has great value. The earlier this process is begun, the longer the time for treatment to facilitate gains from maturation and the greater the response to these efforts. MBD, unidentified and untreated, certainly handicaps the victim to some extent, and may result in major and irreversible detriments to his life. Moreover, the syndrome is not a rare one. A conservative estimate of the federal government is that hyperkinesis, just one of the MBD disorders, occurs in about 3 percent of the children in this country (15). Other estimates variously place the incidence of MBD in some form between 5 and 10 percent. MBD is reported by one worker to be the most frequent psychiatric diagnosis (found in 10 percent of grade-school children) in child psychiatry (17). Benton (3) comments that the wide range of estimates of the occurence of dyslexia, for example, is due to the lack of a consensus definition of the disorder.

5. The daily anguish and frequent psychopathological consequences of MBD cannot be safely minimized, as is made all too clear in numerous personal accounts, among them the story of an artistic, verbally fluent adult male who can neither read nor write (19). A young woman, also artistic, intelligent, personally attractive, but with self esteem vulnerable to quick damage, recalled that in the first grade, "I couldn't tell left from right; I couldn't tie my shoelaces. I couldn't read. I wanted to die." This suffering can be reduced.

Chapter 2

Etiology

A SURVEY OF THE MAJOR hypotheses about the causes of MBD, staggering in number, suggests its multiple and diverse origins, and the probability that the cause in one child differs from the cause in another, or is multidetermined. While a clear distinction may be sought between intrinsic and extrinsic causes (61), it is not always found.

Hyperkinesis provides an excellent illustration of this confusing multiplicity of possible determinants. Walker (134A), speculating on the increased incidence of observed hyperkinesis during the past several decades, attributes it to five causes (some of them compound): increased ingestion of brain-harming substances, car and skateboard accidents, more schooling for all children, anoxia, and larger numbers of single parents less able to care for their children medically and psychologically. Zrull et al. (149) find hyperkinesis determined by a number of co-existing etiological forces involving the interplay of organic and psychological components: structural damage to the brain, changes in the physiological substances of the brain, the psychological reactions of both the child and his family.

Dyslexia, dyscalculia, and other learning disabilities have also been attributed to etiologies that include perceptual disorders, genetics, and family and cultural influences, among many (12, 14, 52, 82, 101).

Is value for the patient, the parent, the therapist, to be found in any attempt to identify etiology? If a reversible, remediable condition can be identified for which a predictably favorable treatment is available, the answer obviously is yes. One commentator, more serious than his tongue-in-cheek account would suggest, told of the rapid cure of hyperkinesis that was found to be caused by excessively tight underwear (70). Differential diagnosis has significance, argue Kinsbourne and Caplan (61), only when it leads to differential treatment. This, of course, is why diagnosis is pursued in any matter.

Naturally, the search for reversible causes requires that *all* possibilities be considered. Finding a single reversible cause in a patient does not guarantee that another condition more difficult to treat is not also operating.

Underlying etiology in all cases directs proper treatment. Nonetheless diagnosis alone, however helpful, is inadequate as a basis for a therapy program. Beyond description, beyond allocation to syndrome or subsyndrome, the cause must be found wherever possible (13). Establishment of etiologies encourages accumulation of the data needed to guide the initiation of measures to prevent more harm to children: for example, the elimination of lead from paint; the modification of obstetrical practices; the assurance of adequate nutrition for all mothers and children. Some preventive measure can probably be sought by parents, therapists, and legislators for most of the etiologies that can be established.

This chapter organizes into *four* major categories the nearly forty etiologies of MBD reported in the literature as identified in individual cases or as having guided treatment or research. These are neurological dysfunctions, genetics, emotional disorder, and cultural influences.

Neurological Dysfunctions

In neurological dysfunctions, the causes reside in the brain. They range from permanent damage to brain tissue to transient, temporary conditions modifiable by changes in diet, other physiological processes, or time. Any brain area presumably may be involved, but usually these etiologies are understood to be focused either in the cerebrum, especially the cortex, or in the connecting mechanisms, anatomical and physiological, that integrate cortical activities with each other or with other neural functions.

Sensorimotor Dysfunctions

Support for a hypothesis of general neurological dysfunction is obtained from the observation of higher-cortical dysfunctions in patients manifesting the subsyndromes of MBD but no demonstrable brain damage. Sensorimotor dysfunctions are prominent among those reported, and have led some single-syndrome advocates to assert that they are *the* cause of MBD. Dysfunctions of all the senses have been implicated, but vision has been emphasized because of its role in reading skill. Some professionals, usually optometrists, maintain that the dysfunction is peripheral, in the eye itself (visual acuity, oculomotor control), and is correctable by refraction, or special eye exercises (77).

Specific color-blindness has been implicated as an etiological factor in dyslexia. The Orton Society *Newsletter* reports the finding of blue-blindness among some nonreaders. Tests duplicated in blue, blue-lined writing paper, even yellow chalk on green "blackboards" are suggested culprits in this specific dysfunction. A contrary view appears in a series of reports by Leisman (64, 65, 66) of findings indicating that dyslexics do not differ from normal readers in scaccadic (jerky) eye-movement control or perceptual localization.

Opthalmologists usually oppose the view that peripheral vision is crucial in dyslexia. While agreeing that ability of the eye to see clearly is imperative and that poor vision must be corrected, they also stress that the dyslexic child cannot read properly even when his vision is corrected. Goldberg and Schiffman conceptualize (48) visual perception as the entire process, from the reception of a stimulus by the eye through its transmittal to the brain, where the stimulus is comprehended and interpreted. It is thus a *brain dysfunction* that limits reading ability where vision is normal or returned to normal. In short, they separate visual *perception* from visual *acuity*. They refer to studies indicating that poor comprehension of the written or printed statement produces abnormal eye mobility that is eliminated when comprehension is corrected. A related finding (38) suggests that abnormalities in the eye movements of dyslexics while reading result from a left-hemisphere dysfunction in processing visual information. In any case, peripheral-visual deficits in perception should be corrected, and only thereafter ruled out as the cause of any learning disability after which dysfunctions in higher-level cognitive process (49) may be postulated.

The acquisition of reading ability is even more complex than this schema suggests. Auditory comprehension is basic to this skill, and dysfunctions in ability to differentiate and compare the sounds of speech are associated with dyslexia. Some dyslexic children have difficulty processing auditory stimuli; the faster the stimuli come, the more difficulty they have in handling the rapidly changing acoustic input. This difficulty affects the ability to process more advanced linguistic material which should develop later. Middle-ear pathology occurred with significantly more frequency in learning-disabled children than in normal ones, although "general" language abilities were similar in the two groups (72). Significantly more learning-disabled hyperactive children were found to have otitis media than normal children (58).

The pioneering work of Quiros and Schrager (95) on the central role of the vestibular apparatus (the inner ear) leads to an interesting hypothesis that links dyslexia and dyspraxia with disturbed equilibrium of sensorimotor and spatial-temporal sequencing and processing, induced by a dysfunction of the cerebellar-vestibular apparatus. Frank and Levinson (40, 41) hypothesize that the sequencing of input and output is "scrambled, blurred, or uncoordinated." They liken the phenomenon to reading a signboard from a moving train; as the speed increases, tracking ability is lost, and the visual sequence becomes blurred. Tracking ability is dependent upon ability to maintain an *optical fixation point,* and when that in turn is lost the cerebral cortex finds it increasingly difficult to interpret rapidly moving or changing sensory input. The normal cerebellum, they suggest, is able to modulate the rate of transmission of sensory data to the cerebral cortex for interpretation. This presumed dysfunction in the pathways between the cerebellum and the inner ear results in reading difficulties. It also correlates with the balance difficulties observed in some dyslexic children. They claim that they identified inner-ear dysfunction in 98 percent of 115 dyslexic children.

To these hypothesized etiological factors are added dysfunctions in the haptic and kinesthetic senses, intersensory or bisensory integration (2, 17), attention, memory, discrimination (89), dichotic auditory fusion (these may indicate temporal-lobe disorder) (52), retrieval (143), sequencing, cortical arousal (148), figure-ground differentiation, inter-hemispheric communication (129), and apraxia.

Increasingly, as research has become more extensive and sophisticated, a language disorder is suspected as the basic cause of dyslexia. Velluntino (133), reviewing the large body of research on psychological factors related to dyslexia, identified the following dysfunctions as implicated, in descending order of frequency: visual perception and memory, intersensory integration, temporal-order recall, and verbal processing (semantic, syntactic, and phonological processing). Recent findings, he reports, dispute the perceptual-deficit theory, despite the fact that the cause of dyslexia most frequently cited was a deficiency in visual perception and memory. These recent findings suggest deficiencies in verbal processing rather than perception, deficiencies that "possibly" are in turn related to basic language problems. He concludes that the language deficit could be an "extrinsic experiental factor" or an "intrinsic developmental disorder of neurological origin," and warns that these are not mutually exclusive and through interaction may obscure the basic cause.

Brain Damage

Damage to brain tissue, with its effects in producing cognitive deficits, has been and remains a major cause postulated for MBD. This hypothesis, introduced by Werner and Strauss in 1941 (141) and specifically using the term "Minimal Brain Damage," persists despite the rarity of "hard" neuropathological signs readily found associated with the disorder. A key question is: can the human brain be damaged so subtly that no convincing evidence of such damage can be detected by procedures conducted and interpreted by a competent neurologist? This question is central to the present enigma of MBD. Professionals and researchers are divided on the issue.

Benton (16), for example, cites evidence that in infants and children brain damage must be extensive, not minor, to produce significant behavioral deviations. He objects, therefore, to the word *minimal* as well as *dysfunction.* More specifically, in dyslexics, Benton (15) finds the evidence for a neurological etiology so "sparse and circumstantial," albeit strongly suggestive, that he would substitute for "developmental dyslexia" the term "reading failure of unknown origin." Block (19) objects to the term "minimal brain damage," because in the children to whom the term is applied no "unequivocal, objective evidence that the brain is anatomically damaged" is found. Cantwell (24, 25) has come to prefer the designation "minimal deficiency syndrome." Birch (18) earlier suggested that brain injury as a "fact" be differentiated from brain injury as a "concept." In the former there is pathological alteration of brain tissue. In the latter, he suggests, there is behavioral disturbance, with or without the fact of brain damage.

The willingness to assume a predominantly organic etiology without clear supporting evidence is contested by Dubey (37). Hyperkinesis may be present without corollary brain damage, and a child may be brain-damaged without being hyperkinetic.

The role of brain damage in hyperkinesis is questioned by Werry *et al.* (142). Their follow-up of children with known histories of traumas (e.g., anoxia) indicated that the incidence of hyperkinesis among them was not remarkable, but similar to that in the general population. Obviously, this finding does not rule out brain injury as one cause of hyperkinesis in some children. The damage may be or may not be correlated with hyperkinesis, and hyperkinesis may be caused by factors other than those discerned by the investigators.

Conversely, observers are impressed by the similarity in behavioral and cognitive expression of children with known brain damage and those diagnosed as having MBD. Moreover, comparison of the neuropsychological test patterns of the two groups reveals pronounced similarities (106), particularly when the test profiles of the brain-damaged are those obtained after a lengthy recovery period (100). And careful examination of these children with methods beyond the usual neurological and electroencephalographic procedures yields a strongly suggestive array of "soft" signs and abnormalities (91). (These are described in Chapter 9.) Equally careful interviewing and history-taking frequently uncover events—a head injury, a severe febrile episode, a toxemia—that correlate with signs suggestive of brain damage. Learning-disabled children were found to have a greater number of pregnancy and birth complications on their records than the norm. This datum correlated positively with lower intelligence-test scores and academic achievement (29).

The brain is vulnerable to injury from many sources. Early brain injury is associated with MBD by many studies and observations (4, 9, 43, 53, 78, 94). These injuries may occur during gestation, the birth process, or during the years of critical maturation of the nervous system. The history of MBD children often produces, as just stated, evidence of pregnancy and birth conditions exposing the infant to brain damage, including malnutrition or toxemia in the mother, anoxia in the fetus, mechanical injury to the infant, prematurity, and low birth weight. Cognitive deficits, language delay, and hyperactivity have been associated with asphyxia and apnea, in turn associated with premature birth (117, 131). An injury to the brain may be disease-caused—as by infection, tumors, fevers, circulatory disorders—or associated with a seizure disorder (90, 112). One example: 90 percent of the children who contract bacterial meningitis now survive, but 18 percent of these suffer disabling sequelae (136). The brain may be injured by harmful substances: anesthesia and other drugs used during pregnancy or birth; lead and other toxic agents ingested as a result of pica; or exposure to environmental pollutants, such as mercury, cadmium, or lead (32, 93). There is reported evidence that nontoxic blood-serum levels of lead may be correlated with hyperkinesis without indication of brain damage (21, 26). Low serum-lead levels, below those producing clinically recognizable symptoms, have been associated with deficits on neuropsychological testing that in turn are associated with learning deficits (84). And of course, the brain can be damaged by trauma during the birth process, or any time afterwards. "A blow to the head and a subsequent deficit in mentation have been associated since antiquity" (92).

Most recently, a single-case histological study of the brain of a 20-year-old accident victim who had been early-diagnosed as having a developmental dyslexia, revealed abnormalities of cellular organization in the brain usually associated with language functions. The abnormality was not likely to have been produced by any of the factors cited above and was attributed to early malformation of fetal brain tissue, an embryological anomaly (44).

One unusual hypothesis, centering on anatomy, postulates a faulty coupling of the brain stem to the cortex, thus accounting for the longer reaction time and the difficulty in making rapid intentional motor responses observed in these children. Their distractability and inflexibility is attributed to their decreased autonomic reactivity (126). The site of the assumed defect is located by some in the brain stem, particularly the reticular activating system. Such a locus is considered by them to be a logical necessity to account for the high incidence of negative EEG findings in this group. One result of this anatomical reasoning is to favor use of the term "*brain* dysfunction" rather than "*cerebral* dysfunction."

Early temporal-lobe damage resulting from fevers during infancy and producing symptoms similar to some of those found in epilepsy (e.g., attentional and motor deficits) has also been hypothesized (71).

Cerebral Hemispheric Asymmetry and Maturational Lag

In most right-handed people and in many left-handed ones, the left hemisphere is dominant for language functions while the right hemisphere is dominant for nonverbal ones. Discovery of cerebral hemispheric specialization through study of stroke, trauma, commissurotomized, and hemispherectomized patients (20, 122) has led to hypotheses that dyslexia reflects an "incomplete" cerebral dominance, due in turn to a lag in maturation of the left hemisphere, or that the learning-disabled child may be trying to use a right, minor hemisphere, nonverbal information-processing mode to do academic tasks and acquire verbal skills (20, 56, 122). Goldberg and Schiffman (48), however, citing evidence that dyslexia may be associated with dysfunction in either the dominant or the minor hemisphere, argue that cerebral dominance itself is not related to reading and learning abilities and their disorders.

Lateral preference in the use of the hand, eye, visual field, ear, and foot has been widely used in the study of cerebral dominance, a link being well established between the preferred use (as in the hand) and the dominance of the contralateral hemisphere; that is, right-handed persons are usually left-hemisphere dominant for speech. Left-handedness and ambidexterity are assumed to be indicative of weak or incomplete lateral dominance. Harris (55) in 1957 reported an association between left-handedness, ambidexterity, and reading disability. His observation has been repeatedly confirmed, with a greater frequency of left-handedness and ambidexterity among dyslexics than among normal readers. In turn, more parents of learning-disabled children were found to be bilateral in performance modes than those of normal children (114). A number of factors have been associated with bilateral asymmetry and in turn with learning disabilities: dysfunctional processing of linguistic information (50, 83), distractability, and poor selective attention (34).

But there is disagreement about whether these deviant hand preferences indicate incomplete or weak lateralization of hemispheric dominance. Zangwill, once a vigorous advocate of the "anomalies of handedness," has modified his emphasis somewhat, although he is reluctant to abandon the likelihood of an association (146). He reasons that since a sizeable number of dyslexics are right-handed and many left-handed persons are not dyslexic, left-handedness and ambidexterity do not in themselves indicate incomplete lateralization of the hemispheres (147). Spreen (123) also doubts that hand, eye, ear, and foot preferences are valid indicators of cerebral dominance. But he, too, is unwilling to abandon the hypothesis that poorly developed or mixed dominance indicates brain dysfunction that may predispose to learning disabilities; variant hand preference, he agrees, is significantly greater among dyslexic children.

Less equivocal are studies of visual fields, dichotic listening, temporal processing of auditory stimuli, and their transformation into spatially arranged visual stimuli. These studies suggest that left-lateral dominance for language is not as firmly established in right-handed dyslexics as in right-handed readers (125, 144, 150). Rourke (106) finds support for this idea in his neuro-psychological-test study of three groups of children with different learning disabilities: (1) those whose arithmetic ability was good compared to their performance with reading and spelling; (2) those sharing deficits in all three subjects; and (3) those whose arithmetic was poor while their reading and spelling were average or above. He reports that the children with good verbal skills relative to arithmetic ability produced neuropsychological-test patterns similar to those of persons with a "relatively dysfunctional right hemisphere." Those good in arithmetic but poor in spelling and reading and those poor in all subjects produced test patterns identifiable with a "relatively dysfunctional left hemisphere."

An emerging hypothesis gaining credence from the neuropsychological study of the effects of commissurotomy—surgical severance of the major connecting pathways between the two hemispheres—postulates an abnormality or deficiency in the integrity of these pathways. Gazzaniga (46), a pre-eminent student of the effects of commissurotomy, reports that surgical separation of the commissure impairs the processing of information between various centers of the brain, and so sheds light upon the major capabilities or dominant functions of each hemisphere. Recent studies suggest that the dominant hemisphere is the site of *central* processing. If dominance is not established, there is no central point to which stimuli requiring cognitive acts are channeled, appraised, and responded to, and confusion results. He cites studies indicating that the right hemisphere is superior to the left in some word-classifying tasks, but not in semantic comprehension, so that the ability to shift data between the hemispheres is important to cognitive skill. These impairments, he believes, may produce some of the symptoms of MBD. The MBD child, he suggests, may resemble the commissurotomized patient in suffering from inability to synthesize multiple cognitive processes. Conflicting pathways or systems operate in the MBD child to confuse his ability to control and to make decisions (45). Again, other studies supply supporting findings (7) and contradictory ones (132).

Another major hypothesis is that the higher-level cognitive processes develop out of, and only after, the acquisition of motor and perceptual skills, and that when maturation of the latter lags the cognitive processes are impeded (47). Thompson (130) bases his support for this view upon his long clinical experience; he states that the cause of reading difficulties is not brain damage or environmental influence but maturational lag. Weinstein (137), in a carefully reasoned presentation, suggests that dyscalculia is a result of maturational lag, a delay in the normal sequence of acquiring arithmetic concepts and processes. The errors made by dyscalculic children are similar to those made by younger average-level math students, and the dyscalculic children also show delay in achieving the progressively higher stages of logical thought development described in Piaget's system. Consolidating these observations, she hypothesizes that normally both logical operations and arithmetic skills are acquired at or about the same time, and that this development marks a shift in cognitive emphasis from right- to left-hemisphere processing.

We are warned by Lieberman (67) not to rush into the diagnosis of neurological immaturity, which may be within the norm until the age of 12. Normally, neurological maturation occurs by the eighth year, with a four-year lag not unusual. There are many accounts of sudden changes toward better cognitive integration around the age of 12. Thereafter in a 14-year-old with only second grade reading skill, for example, factors other than immaturity merit consideration.

A non-neurological but related study of maturational lag has been made by Oettinger *et al.* (86) in their X-ray examination of the wrist bones of 53 MBD children. Three skilled judges, reading the X-rays without identifying data, found their ''bone age'' significantly retarded. The authors believe this finding indicates that the MBD child is physiologically immature, a factor that should be considered in their education. Lag in skeletal maturation (bone age) is also reported for both male and female MBD children (113).

Biochemical-Physiological Dysfunctions

Receptor sites are present at neuronal synapses; when electrical nerve impulses reach the synapse, they stimulate the production of a specific chemical, the neurotransmitter. This chemical crosses the synapse to stimulate receptors in the next nerve to produce an electrical impulse that travels to the next synapse. Neurophysiologists are studying the behavioral effects of increasing and depleting the quantities of these neurotransmitters, enhancing or limiting their action. Among the principal biochemicals being investigated are dopamine, serontonin, norepinephrine, and copamine.

Biochemical malfunction at receptor sites in the brain is hypothesized as the rationale for the treatment of hyperkinesis by stimulants. The paradoxical effect of the stimulant drugs is believed to increase synaptic resistance at the diencephalic level, thereby returning the diencephalon to normal function and thus preventing the over-stimulation of the cortex (121). But on the other hand, there is some evidence that the child who responds best to stimulant medication is in a state of *low* central-nervous-system arousal before treatment, as determined by EEG and skin-conduction levels (110). The hypothesis is a complicated one. Buckley (23) proposes a model in which he likens hyperkinesis to temporal-lobe seizure activity. A physiological dysfunction in the temporal lobe is presumed to *increase* activity in the amygdaloid nucleus, which has the effect of *decreasing* activity in the ventromedial nucleus. This leads to *increased* activity in the lateral and medial posterior areas, which then appears as hyperactive behavior. The amphetamines are presumed to activate or arouse the ventromedial nucleus when it has been inhibited by temporal-lobe activity.

Some hyperactive children have been shown to have a low arousal level in the central nervous system (CNS). Animal and human studies (109) suggest that this low level of arousal is correlated with a low level of inhibitory ability in the CNS.

The prescription of stimulant drugs, first introduced on an empirical basis because of their observed paradoxical effect, is now explained by these hypotheses concerning their effect upon receptor sites and upon the neurotransmitters themselves. Wender, a leading proponent of the use of the stimulant drugs, believes that MBD is caused by inadequately metabolized monamines, the neurotransmitters, and that the drugs improve the metabolic action (138, 139, 140). Silver (120) holds that the activating drugs stimulate the release of norepinephrine. Knobel's (61A) model postulates decreased cortical control of subcortical impulses in hyperkinesis; he reasons that the methylphenidates stimulate the cortex to increased resistance to or control over these lower-level impulses.

A flurry of contesting hypotheses about the role of dopamine depletion in hyperkinesis, based on studies in neonatal rats, suggests that we are at a very early stage in the understanding of neurophysiological brain-behavior relationships. Shaywitz *et al.* (116) report that dopamine depletion in these rats produced a time pattern of increased, then declining activity rate; this they hold is similar to the pattern observed in the life span of hyperkinetic children. Pappas *et al.* (88) criticize Shaywitz *et al.* because the agent they used to deplete dopamine is not selective but depletes the other neurotransmitters as well. Kalat (60) also contests the Shaywitz findings, claiming that hyperkinesis results from a predominance of norepinephrine relative to other transmitters. McLean *et al.* (cited by May, 75) report that their investigations obtained raised activity levels with the depletion of norepinephrine. At least three case studies with adults in whom hyperkinesis and other MBD symptoms persist have demonstrated improvement when levodopa and/or carbidopa was introduced (51, 98, 111). The investigators suggest that the symptoms resulted from reduced activity of the dopaminergic system in the brain.

These current biochemical hypotheses are related in a general way to earlier conjectures about the cause of hyperkinesis. Hyperactivity was long regarded to be the result of over-stimulation or susceptibility to CNS hyperarousal. Strauss and his colleagues, Kephart and Lehtinen (128), pioneers in MBD, reasoned that hyperkinesis originated in brain damage that affects perception and leads to difficulty in filtering sensory input and in ignoring irrelevant or distracting stimuli. The resultant "flooding" of stimuli produces a "flooding" of response. This hypothesis was translated into a recommendation for a therapy regimen of reduced environmental stimuli.

A more recent theory—Optimal Stimulation—is based upon the opposite view, that hyperactivity is actually an effort to increase stimulation, visual, kinesthetic, and motor; that it is a response to understimulation, or sensory deprivation. Zentall (148) has reviewed available evidence and finds support for the Optimal-Stimulation theory, rather than Strauss's overstimulation hypothesis. This evidence, he reasons, favors a treatment that provides designed stimulation, not avoidance or reduction of stimulus input. The hyperactive child, he concludes, needs more stimulation than the normal child to maintain the same level of concentration, performance, and achievement. As support, he points to the suggestion that the hyperactive child who responds well to amphetamines is in a state of under-arousal. Corollary findings are that sedative barbiturates increase hyperactivity instead of decreasing it, and that behavior modification, when successful in reducing hyperactivity, does so by increasing stimulation through its reinforcement procedures.

A quite different genre of biochemical hypotheses involves nutrition and allergic reactions. In the allergy hypothesis, some children, as a result of their sensitivity to chemical elements in food, manifest hyperkinesis that makes learning more difficult but is not a fundamental cause of their disability (22). According to another study, the mechanism does not produce the usual allergic symptoms, but causes disturbances in behavior that intensify, even possibly initiate, learning disabilities (96).

Feingold's work (39) with the link between food additives, learning disabilities, and hyperkinesis originally implicated the chemistry of food additives and coloring with an allergic reaction, either in utero as a result of the mother's diet or in infancy and childhood as a result of the child's diet. Later he came to hypothesize a nonallergic reaction, in which the chemistry of the ingested material (a salicylate) causes blocking of receptor sites in the brain. Feingold believes this blocking causes inhibition of a series of chemical productions that leads to behavior change. He reports that the effect is reversible, treatable by a strict diet that rigidly eliminates the salicylates. As with all etiological hypotheses, there is some support (31) and some contradiction. Spring and Sandoval (124), for example, argue that the placebo effect has been insufficiently controlled in determining the effect of Feingold's diet, a finding countered in a two-case study by Rose (102). And an intensive dose-ranging and crossover study of a ten-year-old boy failed to find artificial food coloring causal in producing significant changes in hyperactivity (73). Conners (30) sought to examine popular claims about diet and behavior as they have or have not been supported by controlled investigation. He concludes that the food additives do not cause hyperkinesis, but acknowledges that some—less than 5 percent of hyperkinetic children—may improve after following the Feingold diet.

Other nutritional hypotheses lean heavily upon Pauling's advocacy of treating illness by providing the brain with its optimum molecular composition. Cott (32), a prominent practitioner of efforts to improve the biochemical processes in the MBD child, prescribes the elimination of "offending" foods and the addition of vitamins and minerals, the former in large doses. He also directs attention to the general health of the child, specifically to the possible presences of diseases such as hypoglycemia and diabetes that may affect brain chemistry.

Genetics as Determinant

The evidence implicating genetic transmission in MBD is largely suggestive. Population sizes in these studies are relatively small, there are no significant longitudinal studies, and no chromosomal abnormalities in children with MBD have been demonstrated (135). But the weight of repeatedly suggestive findings is nonetheless considerable, and the clinician must consider a genetic factor in history-taking. One example of a puzzling fact: dyslexia occurs more frequently in boys than in girls, and the correlation increases as I.Q. and age increase (15).

One suggestion is that MBD derives from an autosomal mode of inheritance; another is that a genetically determined predisposition to the syndrome produces vulnerability to the consequences of perinatal distress, manifest in vicissitudes of later cerebral development. More support exists for the latter hypothesis: if a genetic transmission operates, it does not directly transmit a MBD condition, but rather a vulnerability to trauma, toxemia, and anoxia. A child without that heritage of vulnerability is not affected so adversely by them. Or, it is postulated, what is transmitted is sensory dysfunction, a maturational lag tendency, or a biochemical disorder that results in the MBD symptoms.

The clinical experience of Rossi (104) is that 80 percent of slow learning or disturbed children have diadochokinesis which is likely to augment seizure activity of the Purkinge cells of the cerebellar cortex; this, he states is caused by a genetically determined biochemical transducer—GABA.

The monamine disorder that Wender (138) postulates in MBD is believed by him to be based on a genetic factor. His belief is founded upon observation of the frequent occurrence of MBD in siblings and/or a history of MBD or "other psychiatric disorder" in the parents. He cites Hallgren's (54) findings: 90 percent of 112 cases of dyslexia had parents and/or siblings with similar disorders, compared to 10 percent for controls; 50 percent of foster-care placed siblings of hyperkinetic children were independently diagnosed as hyperkinetic, while only 15 percent of their half-siblings were so diagnosed. The full siblings of MBD children were found by Safer (108) to have significantly more clinical evidence of MBD, shorter attention span, and more repeated antisocial behavior than their half-siblings, findings supported by Siggers (118). Patterns of reading disability in dyslexic children were similar to those of siblings and parents in a large-scale test study by De Fries *et al.*(35). And the mothers of hyperactive children with learning disorders made significantly more spelling errors than did a matched control group (57). The older age of both father and mother was found to be associated with a greater incidence of dyslexia, in a pattern similar to the age distributions of both chromosomal aberrations and mutation defects (59).

Mixed dominance, without any kind of brain or eye damage, transmitted genetically, is widely believed to be the neurological basis of dyslexia (99). A "vulnerable family" syndrome for dyslexia is postulated by McGlannan (69) on finding higher rates of left-handedness and ambidexterity in a three-generation study of 65 families with dyslexia. An eminent pediatric neuropsychiatrist wrote of a young adolescent that he manifested a lag in development of the cerebral functions that support language, and that the lag is *believed* to result from an inherited lack of definitive cerebral dominance. Silver (120) believes that the MBD child has probably inherited a tendency toward maturation lags.

A genetic linkage between MBD symptoms and psychiatric disorders is favored by some investigators and clinicians. Cantwell (25) suggests that hyperactivity is genetically passed from generation to generation and portends psychiatric illness in adulthood, a view based on family, twin, and adoption studies. These, while small in population size, consistently suggest genetic rather than environmental transmission. He finds that the data favor a polygenic inheritance model rather than a chromosomal anomaly, either simple autosomal dominant or recessive, or a sex-linked transmission (24).

Hysteria, sociopathy, and alcoholism were found by Morrison and Stewart (80, 81) to occur more frequently in the natural parents of hyperkinetic children than in their adoptive parents. They believe the finding is consistent with a genetic transmission of the syndrome. Satterfield *et al.* (110) found in a survey of studies a suggestion that hyperactive children who do not respond to stimulant medication tend to come from families with alcoholism and mental illness. The finding would support either a genetic or environmental etiology, or both. They favor the genetic hypothesis, but their reasoning is not made explicit.

A broad-ranging survey of genetic findings in dyslexia leads Owen (87) to prefer the view that certain types of dyslexia may be transmitted through multifactorial inheritance. The severity and expression of the disability in this scheme is the outcome of an interaction between genetics, environmental forces, and the effectiveness of treatment. The case cannot be allowed to rest on genetics alone. Where the genetic factor is strong, the effect of controlling environmental forces and of treatment interventions may be to *mitigate* the disability; when the genetic factor is weak, the influence of these other variables may *prevent* the disability.

The hypotheses favoring a genetic etiology, when grouped, illustrate an effort to encompass other possible etiologies within the genetic-transmission concept. The MBD child is believed to have inherited a special vulnerability or sensitivity to traumas that do not affect other children, or do not affect them as severely. Or he inherits biochemical dysfunctions, a tendency to maturational lags, or vulnerability to emotional stress. Or he responds to familial cultural forces.

This inconclusiveness reinforces the importance of a careful differential diagnosis (63) of each MBD child, in which consideration is given to the multiple and diverse etiologies possible, leading to a specific individual therapy for him. Certainly there is more than one kind of dyslexia, or hyperkinesis, or learning disability. As Owen (87) concludes, our knowledge of the genetic variable is equivocal and indecisive. A major research problem is defining the disability and designing the conditions necessary to test the genetic hypothesis.

Cultural Determinants

As with other etiological hypotheses, the findings about culture are contradictory: Perplexed by conflicting reports that MBD occurs predominantly in low socio-economic classes or is more common in upper classes, Alley *et al.* (3) studied the records of 230 children diagnosed as MBD, and compared them with 93 normal control children. No significant differences in the incidence of MBD were found in the five Hollingshead social classes used as a structure for comparison. They conclude that both MBD and normal children are distributed proportionately across all five social levels.

In their conceptualization of hyperkinesis, Lambert *et al.* (62) see the child's behavior as defined by the child's social environment, so that often behavior deviant in his social group is labeled hyperactive rather than viewed as the result of the child's internal state. The lack of clear diagnostic standards is perhaps related to the confusion about social class and MBD prevalence.

Behaviorists (28, 103) reject all etiological variables in MBD except a deficient learning experience; MBD is seen as correctable by an adequate learning experience. Putting aside organic, emotional, and cultural factors, Ross (103) flatly attributes learning disabilities to the "unspecialized instruction" he observes to be prevalent in most classrooms. The problem, he concludes, is educational, not psychological nor medical; children differ in the manner of instruction each needs in order to learn, and such individualized instruction is not generally provided.

Emotional Determinants

The emotional disruption and psychopathology observed in MBD children are viewed as primary causes of the symptoms of hyperactivity and learning disabilities by some observers; by others they are regarded as interacting phenomena with the MBD symptoms, reactions to them that intensify them. Lambert *et al.* (63) suggest that hyperactivity, for example, may be a sign of emotional instability caused by stress in the child's environment, particularly the home. Meacham (76) studied three children with reading problems. All were normal by physical, neurological, and psychological examination. In each case the like-sexed parent had dropped out of school before the twelfth grade. Meacham conjectures that the parent denigrated school activity and achievement, so that the child's dyslexia was induced by identification. Two cases are reported by Ravenette (97) that indicate that a child's living situation can contribute to reading disability.

Environmental factors are of equal importance to organic variables according to Bax (11), who sees hyperactivity as a *defense* of the child who is unwilling or unable to admit his true learning difficulties and seeks to divert attention from them. A similar proposal suggests that academic failure resulting from a variety of etiological factors is the cause of hyperkinesis and related behavioral patterns (33).

In a related hypothesis, Zrull (149) sees cerebral pathology interacting with both the child's emotional response to its effects and the family's feelings, attitudes, expectations, and frustrations. Depression and withdrawal lead to avoidance of learning efforts and the MBD symptoms intensify or become fixed.

Just as the psychodynamically oriented clinician has been warned not to forget the brain, Anthony (5) warns the biologically oriented not to forget the mind. He proposes that the structural model of the personality—ego, id, and superego—interacts with the contributions of the cerebral cortex and the limbic and reticular systems. His model emphasizes the child's discovery of his body, the effects of any damage to or deficiency in it, and his evolving concept of it.

Loney et al. (68) see hyperactivity as a sign of a poorly developed ego in a child with poor impulse control and high hostility levels, and with an intense need for control and affection. Specifically, the hyperactivity is viewed as an effort both to gain attention and release tension.

An ego-function model of MBD is advanced by Bauer and Kenny (10). Comparing levels of strength and weakness of various ego functions in MBD children with those in schizophrenic and brain-damaged children, they found that the MBD group shows mild impairment of autonomous function, cognitive focusing, and concept formation. Reasoning, reality testing, and the synthetic function are normal. They propose that in diagnosis an effort be made to identify the pattern of ego-function impairment and that therapy focus on that pattern. A cogent schema is suggested by Rubenstein and Levitt (107): in an early traumatic infant-mother relationship, ego energy is diverted from the task of developing cognition needed to adapt to the environment, toward the compelling task of managing affect.

Difficulties in the separation-individuation process are suggested as a cause of learning disabilities (1). These separation difficulties may arise at any time from infancy to adolescence, and their causes are many. One example cites placement of the child away from the parents as disrupting the normal development of narcissism and thereby causing learning disabilities (119), an hypothesis that appears to overlook the family conditions mandating placement.

Two types of emotional determinants of hyperkinesis are identified by Ney (85). In one, conditioned hyperkinesis, the parents are depressed. Usually a single mother makes the child the scapegoat for her feelings about her lost spouse. Withdrawn, the mother reacts to the child only when he is "bad," hyperactive. In the other type, chaotic hyperkinesis, the child's environment is marked by intense conflict, usually between the parents. The child defends by staying "on the move." The child's restlessness arouses anxiety in the parents about their own impulse control and they may abuse the child, who reacts with his own anxiety and hostility, and so a cycle of pathological interaction is perpetuated. Depressed, disinterested, and angry mothers are also cited by Bannatyne (8) as causing dyslexia in their children. A review of emotional factors in etiology is a strong reminder that the subsyndromes of MBD occur in a context that requires understanding as much as do the symptoms.

Emotional factors as both causes and consequences of MBD symptoms are discussed further in Chapter 17.

Multiple-Factor Etiology

A study of children suspected of MBD (145) could not establish a relationship among abnormal history, neurological, electroencephalographic, intellectual, or behavioral findings. The investigators suggest that the clinical picture in a given child is probably the result of a unique combination of causes, which could include innate, traumatic, psychological, and social factors. The MBD syndrome, they hold, is not homogeneous and does not reflect a single cause.

Consensus for this view is growing. Genetics, developmental lag, biochemical factors, and neonatal differences are offered as possible explanations of the greater number of boys over girls frequently observed among the learning disabled (79).

The increasing incidence of hyperactivity is attributed by Arnold (6) to improved diagnostic methods, increased survival rates among birth-damaged infants, increased use of offensive chemicals in food processing, and tolerance for acting out in a more permissive society. In another view of the causes of hyperactivity, Marceca (71) stresses temporal-lobe damage caused by fevers and resembling epilepsy, disorientation and locomotion difficulties, anxiety, serotonin-catecholamine imbalance, allergies, social disapproval for immaturity, and various home and school factors. Widely different outcomes in different samples of hyperkinetic children suggest to Shaffer and Greenhill that the symptom alone tells little if anything about its etiology (115).

The search for etiology in dyslexia shows that there is more than one kind of dyslexia, and more than one cause for each kind. Spreen (123) observes a grouping of types and associated causes in studies of dyslexia: (1) symptomatic dyslexia resulting from early brain damage; (2) primary dyslexia having a genetic etiology without brain damage; (3) secondary dyslexia caused by emotional, environmental, and health factors. Mattis (74) offers a model of dyslexia, poor reading skill, or "atypical reading development," in which dysfunction in any of several "independent clusters of higher cortical functions" may be causal. While he sees no need to determine if brain damage is present, he does stress the need to include brain-damaged groups in etiological studies.

The suggested causes of dyslexia are "extrinsic experiential" factors or an "intrinsic, developmental disorder of neurological origin," according to Velluntino (133), a vigorous advocate of the hypothesis that the disorder is one of deficiency in verbal processing rather than of visual perception.

Doehring (36) concludes that "...no workable definition of dyslexia as a unitary disorder is possible." Dyslexia, he reasons, has many dimensions; it is a complex disorder, a multiple syndrome, in which many of the factors may be antecedents of the disorder, as well as, or in addition to, consequences: home life, socio-economic factors, educational opportunity, intelligence, personality, perception, memory, language ability. In a careful, comprehensive review of the etiological data in dyslexia, Rourke (105) agrees with Doehring's multiple-syndrome concept. His examination of the following major etiological factors, while omitting biochemical, physiological, and genetic studies, provides an informative guide to this complex matter:

1. Pregnancy and birth complications (PBCs) occur more often in the perinatal experience of dyslexics than in that of normal readers, but some normal readers have experienced these potential adverse vissisitudes.

2. Finger agnosia in children (associated with Gertsmann's Syndrome) is highly correlated with right-left discrimination difficulties, and indicates a high risk for dyslexia.

3. Little relationship has been demonstrated between the Choreiform Syndrome, MBD, and positive neurological-examination findings.

4. Only a small proportion of dyslexics show more abnormal EEG findings than do normal readers.

5. Binocular dyscoordination, faulty visual scanning, and/or other ocular-motor deficiencies seldom play a critical role. Visual-perceptual and visual-spatial factors appear to be somewhat more important, but ambiguously so.

6. Disorders of temporal sequencing and serial positioning are frequent in dyslexics, but with such marked individual differences that an association is tenuous.

7. Associating disorders of auditory-visual integration with dyslexia requires a large group of readers and dyslexics, and a need remains to identify for study the subgroups of dyslexics who do and do not have this problem.

8. The data illuminating the role of cerebral dominance is not clear-cut. No clearly significant relationship with hand and eye preference has been established. This is true also of studies of ear advantage, cerebral asymmetry and dyslexia, and those involving separate tachistoscopic presentation to the right and left visual fields. Haptic studies suggest a hypothesis that dyslexics have a greater right-hemisphere involvement with more dependence on spatial-holistic strategies, while readers show more left-hemisphere reliance, with more use of linguistic-analytic strategies. Reversals and mirror imagery occur in most normal readers, and not all dyslexics manifest the disorder. Much evidence correlates left-hemisphere dysfunction and language disturbance in adults. Among dyslexic children some similar evidence appears that they are deficient in many psycholinguistic abilities. But subgroups of such deficiencies

exist among these children. A small but significant group of dyslexics do not show these linguistic deficiencies. Some dyslexics show both linguistic and visual-spatial defects, thus implicating both cerebral hemispheres.

Overall, Rourke finds a significant correlation between dyslexia and many brain-related factors. A child dysfunctional in either right- or left-hemispheric skills is likely to be dyslexic. Dyslexic children of the same age with the same degree of reading dysfunction may show quite different neuropsychological deficits that must be evaluated against other variables, such as the socio-economic, for example.

The implications of this review of the etiological factors in MBD and its subsyndromes—hyperactivity, dyslexia, learning disabilities—are evident: the cause or causes can not be assumed; they must be pursued carefully and individually; alleviation of secondary causes are likely to ameliorate the disorder, but not eliminate it; much remains unresolved, but what is known should be meticulously applied for each victim. Establishing the probability of an etiology or of etiologies influences the proper selection of treatment interventions and therefore the prognosis for a child.

Chapter 3

Prognosis

"THE SYNDROME APPEARS to be self-limited, since many of the characteristics fade during early adolescence" (21).

"Achieving independence is not a realistic goal for the minimally brain damaged" (2).

These conflicting statements reflect the contradictions among the conclusions of present investigations into the prognosis of MBD.

After an extensive 1972 survey of the literature, Wender (41, 42) found little reason to anticipate that MBD symptoms will disappear with age. He held unwarranted the widespread belief that the MBD child outgrew his disorder. On the contrary, he concluded that the disorder could be an early precursor of serious psychiatric disturbances in adolescence and adulthood, including the infantile and impulsive character disorders, sociopathy, and schizophrenia. His view finds considerable corroboration (36, 43). Later (40) he was to modify this ominous outlook to the slightly more reassuring conclusion that a "fraction" (its size not stated) of MBD children do not outgrow their disorder with age, but require medication for indefinite periods of time, during which the drugs are suppressive but not curative. These later conclusions also find some support. Katz *et al.* (14) caution that there is a group of MBD children who retain significant symptoms beyond puberty, a possibility of which parents should be made aware. Safer and Allen (27), in a study of the ages at which medications were introduced to different children, found that while aggressivity decreased, hyperactivity and inattentiveness remained problems. A follow-up intelligence-quotient study (10) of learning-disabled children, originally seen between the ages of 8 and 12, recorded that two to six years later one-third of these children decreased 10 points in Verbal I.Q., while one-half of the controls increased Verbal I.Q. by 10 points. The disabled children remained several years behind in reading, spelling, and arithmetic, and had significant difficulties with conceptual, sequencing, and symbolic abilities.

More optimistic prospects are often offered by pediatricians who assure parents that their children will outgrow disturbing symptoms. Optimism is also encouraged by reminders, usually in newspaper accounts, that many accomplished and famous people overcame learning disabilities: Albert Einstein, Woodrow Wilson, General George S. Patton, Niels Bohr, Leonardo da Vinci, Thomas Alva Edison, Nelson Rockefeller (18). Louise Clarke (7) provides a moving, realistic account of the painful, often discouraging progress of her dyslexic son, from an early diagnosis of mental retardation by an outstanding private school to a Ph.D. in mathematics. A personal account of triumph over dyslexia and its traumatic effects in exposure to ridicule is offered by Eileen Simpson (31). And Rawson (25A) reported highly favorable outcomes among 20 boys from a private school. Highly intelligent at the outset (Mean I.Q. = 131), the lads also received unusually intensive remedial instruction. Their educational attainment at follow-up was higher than that of controls. Their life adjustment was described as superb, although they continued to have difficulties in reading and spelling.

What is the truth about prognosis in MBD? Is there one outlook or several? Can it, or they, be gleaned from among conflicting research outcomes and attitudes? A review of some of the major research must follow a tortuous path through a maze of research designs that somehow seems never to engage the complexity of the problem.

A five-year follow-up of untreated MBD and hyperkinetic children found no change in either neurological or behavioral maturity (24). And while another study found that hyperkinesis subsided spontaneously in about 50 percent of those observed by the twelfth to thirteenth year, the educational and emotional handicaps are acknowledged to persist (8).

A more favorable view of the modification of some MBD symptoms over time—presumably as the result of maturation and learning—has been demonstrated by Menkes et al. (19A). They located 14 former patients of a children's psychiatric clinic who had been treated a mean of 24 years earlier. All originally had I.Q.'s over 70; they had exhibited hyperkinesis, impaired attention span, and "soft" neurological abnormalities (visual-motor dysfunctions, poor coordination, impaired speech). Eleven of the 14 were accessible for complete re-examination; information about the others was collected. Two of the former patients were neurologically normal; definite abnormalities were identified in eight and suspected in one. Hyperactivity was observed in three (now aged 22–23), but in the others had disappeared between the ages of 8 and 21. Eight were self-supporting; two, mentally retarded, were supported by their families; four were institutionalized as psychotic. I.Q. was established as a major prognostic factor: seven of the eight self-supporting subjects had scored an I.Q. above 90 at their initial contact with the clinic. Low I.Q. and clearly diagnosed damage were found to be prognostically unfavorable.

The findings in this now classic study, neither optimistic nor pessimistic, are prototypical of what is most generally reported: some symptoms in some children improve. Even the optimistic estimate of the *Merck Manual* (21) which heads this chapter (and which, incidentally, describes MBD as a psychiatric disorder of childhood) acknowledges that "some" of the learning or emotional difficulties associated with MBD may continue beyond childhood in high levels of anxiety, low self-esteem, and school problems.

Hyperkinesis

Hyperkinesis, probably because it is a symptom extremely troubling and emotionally costly to the patient and to all around him, as well as being the symptom or syndrome most readily available to psychiatry for medication, has received the most research attention. This research effort persists, despite evidence that lasting benefits are not seen in children chronically medicated (25).

A two-year follow-up (26) of 72 hyperkinetic boys (mean age = 10.2 years) and a control group found 65 percent still on medication. Classroom and home behavior had improved, but improvements in academic achievement, peer status, or depressive symptoms were not observed. A similar short-term follow-up period in another study (32) used a placebo control period. Of 42 hyperkinetic subjects, 40 percent remained sufficiently stabilized so that they could be taken off medication.

A longer follow-up (two to five years) is reported by Mendelson *et al.* (19). Fifty-five percent of 83 patients formerly treated for hyperkinesis were judged to be improved, while 35 percent were the same or worse, according to interviews with their mothers. These interviews inquired into behavioral symptoms, school records, family history, police records, and the mother's opinion of the effectiveness of the treatment. The study highlights the design defects that distort research results in this complex problem. No uniform criteria for selection are reported; while 92 percent of the children had been on drug treatment, neither the length of such therapy nor its congruence with psychotherapy are reported, except for the notation that most of the children still attending psychiatric clinics were those who had improved on drugs. The authors make a cogent point which merits emphasis: low self-esteem and defeatism are, and tend to remain, serious aspects of MBD, and have a crucial affect on prognosis.

A similar observation of Weiss *et al.* (38, 39) after a five-year follow-up of hyperactive children is that low self-esteem characterizes hyperactive children in adolescence. They are aware that their parents and teachers resent them and feel frustrated by them. While the hyperactivity diminishes with age, other dysfunctions and handicaps persist: disorders of attention and concentration, academic underachievement, emotional immaturity, low self-esteem, and pessimism. Antisocial behavior is reported in a significant minority; members of this smaller group tended initially to have been the more restless and aggressive.

Five years later, at the end of a ten-year follow-up of the same subjects, Weiss and her associates (37) report continuing low self-esteem, although the patients do not regard themselves as more psychopathological than their peers. About 25 percent of the 75 hyperactive subjects in the study were exhibiting antisocial behavior, were failing more grades than controls, and were unpopular with teachers and peers. An encouraging finding was the reaction of employers, who saw no significant differences between the hyperactive subjects and the controls, although their high school teachers did find such differences.

A twelve-year follow-up of 100 hyperkinetic patients treated with amphetamine or methylphenidate drugs, reported by Laufer (16), sought to answer more questions than the number usually addressed in such research. The former patients were asked to complete a wide-ranging questionnaire; 66 responded. At the time of treatment their mean age was 8 years, with a range from 3 to 18; at follow-up the mean was 19.8, the range 15 to 26.

Drug use and abuse followed this pattern. Twenty-four took medication for less than six months, 31 for six months to five years; of 57 reporting, 10 were continuing on medications that included anticonvulsants, minor and major tranquilizers; none were taking stimulants or antidepressants; two had had an overdose experience, 96.5 percent had not; five acknowledged using marijuana or LSD, 91.2 percent had not; no addictions were reported; three of 56 had used Benzedrine or Dexedrine, 94.6 percent had not; four of 50 responding were excessive drinkers, 92 percent were not.

Hyperactivity was no longer present in 27 respondents; most of these, 61 percent, reported cessation of the symptom between the twelfth and sixteenth year. Seventeen percent acknowledged that they were reckless drivers; 82 percent stated that they were not. Sixteen (30 percent) had had encounters with the police; none were jailed.

Five of 56 respondents to the question stated that they had been hospitalized for psychiatric reasons; one person had been hospitalized more than once. None of these 56 had made a suicide attempt. Twenty (35 percent) received psychiatric treatment after the early period of medication, most of these during adolescence. Five (9 percent) were currently receiving psychiatric treatment.

Eighteen of 37 respondents 19 years or older were employed, 14 were attending colleges or universities, one was in graduate school. Of ten who were or had been in military service, one had a bad-conduct record.

Most of the formerly hyperactive patients now responding (no figures given) were described as pleasant, meticulous, and having friends. The minority were moody, aversive, and loners, given to outbursts of violence, and suffering feelings of persecution.

Agreement is general that, while hyperkinetic behavior can be mitigated or aborted by medication and that the behavior may subside spontaneously in about 50 percent of hyperkinetic children as they enter adolescence, profound ongoing effects upon the emotional, social, and personality structure are likely into adulthood. Some diagnoses of schizophrenia in adults are believed to result from MBD rather than psychosis (13). Clinical experience suggests a possible connection between MBD in childhood and some borderline personality manifestations in adulthood: the dysfunctions of MBD are believed by one investigator to distort object relations and so lead to borderline ego organization (23). Both hyperactive and hypoactive children grown to age 14 had more conflicts with authority and more behavioral problems than controls (1). A psychomotric and psychophysiological study of hyperkinesis indicated that symptom correlates (short attention span, distractibility, and impulsivity) persisted into adolescence and adulthood (6). Adult psychiatric patients who had been hyperactive showed significantly more personality disorder than did matched patients who had not been hyperactive; especially differentiating were sociopathy and alcoholism (22).

A survey of the long-range follow-up findings of leading researchers of hyperkinesis, Loney, Rapaport, Sprague, and Weiss, indicates some reasonably general agreement (33):

1. Few differences in adulthood between those who had received medication and those who did not are recorded.
2. The basic problems correlated with hyperkinesis remain more often than not after medication is stopped: lifelong difficulty with attention, problems in forming and keeping close relations, impulsivity, and low self-esteem (12).
3. Early initiated and consistently maintained family and educational support has a positive effect on outcome.
4. Drug abuse, delinquency, and undue aggression in adolescence and adulthood are not likely to be problems. Loney has found that selection of vocational and social pursuits that do not aggravate symptoms has positive prognostic value. She also reports that hyperkinesis has little connection with delinquency or aggression (17), while aggressivity (considered a secondary symptom) in childhood has more prediction value than the primary symptoms of hyperactivity and inattention (20).

Dyslexia and Learning Disabilities

In an extensive survey of the literature on prognosis in dyslexia, Benton (4) observed these major typical patterns:

1. Most improve only gradually over time; the dyslexic child grown into early adulthood reads slowly, spells poorly, and has great difficulty learning foreign languages.

2. Some make a "remarkable spurt" for a year or two, usually at about age 13 or 14, with modest improvement thereafter.
3. A few make only slight improvements over time; in adulthood they remain seriously disabled readers.

In long-range studies Satz (28) finds that dyslexia is the most frequent cause of school dropouts, that it is a major problem in referral to clinics and courts, and leads to emotional problems and criminality in adolescence and adulthood. Unless treated, he contends, the severity of dyslexia increases with age, a situation that may evolve from attendant emotional problems or an inadequate educational system. Satz finds that when dyslexia is diagnosed in the first and second grades, treatment can develop normal reading skill in 82 percent; when diagnosis is made and treatment begins in the third grade, normal reading results in 46 percent, and in only 10 to 15 percent when help begins in the fifth to seventh grades.

Similar findings are reported by Schiffman and Clemmens (29). If potential learning disability is diagnosed in the second grade, 82 percent can be brought up to grade level within two years by special intervention. If not identified and treated until the fourth grade, only 15 percent can be brought up, and if delayed until the ninth grade, only 6 percent can be advanced through intervention. But there is also some evidence that many learning-disabled children may never be without the need for remedial, special education specifically designed for their dysfunctions (11, 15).

Overview

The more or less obvious design faults in prognostic studies apart, it is clear that a general prognostic statement about children with any of the subsyndromes of MBD cannot be made. The major factors for this seeming ambiguity should be understood by all concerned with these children. The symptoms and behavioral sequelae of MBD, as of brain damage, can be most diverse. They range from little or none, through neurotic disorders of various degrees of severity, to serious disruptions of social, intellectual, and personal functioning (35). It can be seen, however, that all symptoms do not disappear, either with time and/or treatment. Spontaneous remission is not to be expected in most cases. No data tell us what symptoms are most likely to remit with time, with treatment, or with both. Degrees of remission cannot be predicted.

Patterns of change are as diverse as those of symptomatology. A few general trends are observed, as in Benton's study of dyslexia (4) which indicated "slow-steady," "sudden-spurts," and "very-little-change" patterns of improvement. In most studies of hyperkinesis, medications suppress hyperactivity and improve attention in some children without assured concomitant improvements in academic achievement, peer relations, and self-esteem in these same children. Personal reports (7, 18) verify that outstanding capabilities may develop in the adulthood of some MBD children. In other children, dysfunction may appear only as increasing age confronts them with types of tasks or levels of difficulty or abstraction not required of them earlier, or that they had been able to escape. It is as if "chronological age" catches up with and passes a fixed "mental age" in a specific function and a deficit is thus fully revealed for the first time. An interesting account of a related process is presented by Shelley and Riester (30). A group of Air Force soldiers were referred because of difficulty in coping with "basic tasks" in their training, primarily motor and spatial, such as folding and arranging clothing or equipment in required ways. Ability to learn and develop speed in new motor tasks such as judo and formation drills were inferior to that of peers. Comprehensive examinations revealed "soft" neurological signs. Performance I.Q.s were lower on the average by 22 points than Verbal I.Q.s. Bender reproductions were characterized by rotation, distortion, and fragmentation. Psychiatric histories indicated that they had been able with the aid of their families to minimize their difficulties until the Air Force compelled them into motor-spatial activities not encountered before.

Gender appears to influence prognosis to some extent, in some measure because of a difference in social reaction to the appearance of the same behavioral characteristics in boys and girls. Battle and Lacey (3) found that three-to-six-year-old hyperactive boys were significantly less striving and persistent in mastering an intellectual task than hyperactive girls of the same age. The girls attacked these problems in a socially accepted way, striving for achievement; the boys avoided them. These forces of social interaction and their potential influence on outcome are not sufficiently understood.

The effects of various treatment interventions, singly or in combination, are obscure. Most studies of the treatment of hyperkinesis, for example, focus on the use of medication, yet we know little about the comparative outcomes of medication alone, or medication in various combinations with psychotherapy, behavioral modification, environmental manipulation, special education, vocational training, teacher counseling and parent counseling, or psychotherapy. We are equally ignorant about the effects of length and timing of treatment.

Prognosis is clearly improved by inputs of concern, time, and determination, a point made by Benton in his survey of dyslexia (4). And Clarke is moved to attribute the successful outcome for her son to the family's refusal to accept the verdict of the educational system, to his opportunity to get the kind of schooling that proved effective, and to his indomitable personality (7).

The personality of the child and the family's treatment of him are major influences upon prognosis. The nature of parental input and interaction are, of course, enormously significant in the personality formation of the MBD child, as of any child. Consistency, acceptance, and support allow favorable temperament to emerge; denial, rejection, and excessive demands erode the constructive aspects of temperament. Findings from work with children with clearly established brain damage contribute to reasonable prognostic hypotheses in MBD. Birch *et al.* (4A) found that temperamental organization was to have the greatest prognostic value. Favorable temperamental organization is manifest in ease of adaptability, ready modifiability, predominantly positive mood, and predictable rhythmicity. A less favorable prognosis faces the arhythmic child, negative in mood, markedly unadaptive, with low response threshold, and short attention span.

Three brain-damaged patients were followed by Chess (6A) from early infancy into their school years. Brain damage in early life influenced each child's developmental course differently. Chess concluded that temperamental organization of the child in each case was prognostic of the developmental course, and that the nature of interaction between the child's temperament and the environment was crucial to the outcome, conclusions reaffirmed by subsequent follow-up of the same patients (35).

These hypotheses imply that the child with MBD reared in social, cultural, and economic disadvantage carries an enormous negative prognostic burden. If many MBD children of the middle and upper social classes pass unnoticed and neglected from year to year, grade to grade, to emerge later with severe personality, emotional, and behavioral pathologies, one can only imagine with horror the numbers of such children in deprived groups. There seems no escape from this conclusion or from society's responsibility.

The dysfunctions of the MBD child modify slowly. Beneficial developmental and maturational changes are enhanced by all the fostering conditions cited. Parents, educators, treating professionals, and government, all concerned with and for the MBD child must be aware that prognosis can be improved by multiple services over a long period of time to meet his multiple needs. "Wait and see" prescribes only denial and neglect.

Given all the factors that make for a favorable prognosis, the earliest and most comprehensive diagnosis possible becomes essential. Early identification and early treatment finds the child most responsive, and, of course, assures the longest possible treatment span. Equally important, the subtle development of negative expectations for the child by parents, school, and the child himself, a pernicious process, is interrupted and reversed.

That we are a long way from attaining this ideal goal for all is evidenced by the recent change in name of the Association for Children with Learning Disabilities (ACLD) to the Association for Children and Adults with Learning Disabilities.

II

DIAGNOSIS

Chapter 4

Diagnosis of MBD:
A Syndrome of Syndromes

THE MBD POPULATION HAS no single definition, and such multiple definitions as are offered lack rigorous criteria for inclusion and exclusion, a confusion that clouds the diagnosis of the disorder. Many symptoms associated with MBD are also found in children with clear-cut emotional problems, compelling these questions: Does such a child have both MBD and emotional problems? Are his emotional problems caused by the MBD? Or could the reverse be true? Emotional instability, mood swings, impulsivity, and aversiveness with or without hyperactivity may coexist with either "soft" or "hard" neurological signs. Some workers find fruitless any attempt to separate children with learning disabilities from those with social and emotional problems (8). Hyperactivity appeared only rarely in one survey of 60 learning-disabled children, but attention difficulties and easy discouragement were noted in about 50 percent (13). MBD is often criticized as a catch-all diagnosis that diverts attention from the need for work with the individual's personality (28).

Diagnostic estimate of the severity of MBD in a child is seldom ventured, even though the evaluation may be of the greatest significance. A slight degree of dysfunction early detected and treated usually has the best prognosis. But a mild limitation may escape detection, only to appear when the difficulty level of cognitive demand increases to a point where the dysfunction is unmistakable, a point in development at which the prognosis is less favorable. A severe degree of MBD, however, may approach the symptomatic picture of frank brain damage, although rigorous match with criteria is lacking.

In part the ambiguity confusing the diagnosis of MBD results from inconsistent screening and diagnostic practices. Methods for early recognition of the child with learning difficulties are still relatively primitive; they must be elaborated, tested, and standardized. Even when learning difficulties are recognized, characterization of a child's deficits is too often superficial, and all too often determined by theoretical bias in the diagnostician. And despite the vigorous growth of neuropsychology and the proliferation of tests batteries, universally accepted diagnostic procedures are still lacking. Those used vary markedly from examiner to examiner, from investigation to investigation, to the detriment of both patients and research.

Clinical neurological-examination procedures also contribute to the confusion; most were designed to evaluate the adult whose nervous system is established and presumably once was normal. In many instances of MBD, a reasonable presumption is that the child's nervous system was damaged at or before birth. The major neurologic question in these cases is "What has not been gained?" rather than "What has been lost?" Techniques, criteria, and norms that follow a developmental gradient are much needed.

A major difficulty in establishing MBD criteria has been the absence of clear correspondence between the syndrome and unequivocal evidence of damage to the brain. Diagnosis of MBD is obscured both by this elusiveness of the neurological evidence, and by the heterogeneous elements grouped in the syndrome. Paine *et al.* (29A), among others, stress that a variety of *unrelated* minor dysfunctions are subsumed, some neurological, some behavioral, and others cognitive. Some workers (29A, 36) are seeking procedures that will result in firmer neurological corroboration of behavioral manifestations, short of the "hard" signs upon which some insist. They report that increasing the precision of the clinical neurological examination produces definitive evidence of neurological abnormality in almost all children diagnosed as having MBD on the basis of behavioral criteria. These neurological abnormalities include tremor of the hands, disarthria, hyperreflexia, and mild choreoathetosis. Indeed, the diversity and number of symptoms associated with the diagnosis are striking. Not all occur, of course, in any single child, and not all occur with the same frequency.

Diversity of symptoms in a range of dysfunctions of the brain is not unexpected in light of the complex brain-behavior relationship. But the diversity can be overwhelming, as a study of the literature reveals. At least eighteen different terms are in wide use as equivalents of "minimal brain dysfunction" (33). Some of the terms are held to be incompatible with each other under a single rubric. Erickson (12) suggests that we do not have sufficient data to equate reading disabilities with MBD. Lahey *et al.* (20) believe that separation of the two conditions, learning disabilities and hyperactivity, must be sought through an analysis of the independent dimensions of behavior identifiable with each. And Farnham-Diggory (14) argues that learning disability is not a scientific diagnosis but a political one, intended to obtain special funds for children with otherwise unclassifiable disorders. And we are reminded that the debate over dyslexia, its definitions, and diagnosis has now spanned more than 50 years (32).

MBD obviously is not a single disorder. MBD has been compartmentalized and the divisions have been further subdivided. Nor does it appear to be a single syndrome but rather a syndrome of syndromes. A review of the major diagnostic-taxonomic efforts follows, to illustrate this point and perhaps to illuminate the confusion for the wary traveler.

The MBD Syndromes

The two major symptoms of MBD are seen by Wender (39) to be: (1) increased arousal accompanied by decreased ability for concentration, focusing attention, and inhibiting response to the irrelevant; and (2) a diminished capacity for positive affects, for experiencing pain and pleasure, and for sensitivity to positive and negative reinforcement. He hypothesizes that the attention deficit accounts for learning disabilities and social noncompliance, since what is not heard cannot be acted upon, and that the lowered affect makes the child harder to satiate, so that seeking of sensation and pleasure leads to delinquency and other socialization difficulties. Wender carefully observes the diversity of etiologies and symptoms among MBD children and cautions that they are heterogeneous both for behavior and for their responses to stimulant medication, indicating that not all are under-aroused. Wender incorporates learning disabilities and hyperkinesis within his view of the syndrome.

An effort to separate the two is made by Peters (30) who defines "pure" hyperkinesis and "pure" learning disabilities, but finds necessary a "mixed" category displaying qualities of both "pure" types. He identifies many symptoms that may appear in varied combinations: rapid decay of attention, distractibility that makes maintainance of a plan or position difficult, faulty pattern perception in identifying the pertinent cues of a situation (the fulcrum of a fork, or the weight of a door in slamming it shut), hyperactivity, impulsivity, labile emotionality, disorders in language development, poor motor coordination, and disturbances in identifying direction (right/left, up/down). A child with MBD may manifest as few as three of these signs, or all of them, according to Peters.

The designation *Minimal* Brain Dysfunction is rejected by Block (5), who renames it the *Vague* Cerebral Dysfunction. He urges that the group be diagnostically separated from those children identified as suffering from: (1) organic brain damage; (2) the Hyperkinetic Behavior Syndrome; (3) specific learning disabilities, of which dyslexia would be considered a distinct subgroup; and (4) maturational lags. A variety of schemes has emerged from both individual and conference efforts (2, 18, 25, 29, 38).

The Hyperkinesis Syndrome

Four types of hyperkinesis are distinguished by Ney (27) according to their presumed etiology: (1) constitutional hyperkinesis, a sex-linked, genetically transmitted syndrome; (2) conditioned hyperkinesis, resulting when a depressed parent, usually the mother, makes the child the scapegoat for her feelings about the lost spouse, and reacts to the child only when he forces her attention by "badness"; (3) chemical hyperkinesis, produced by a biochemical disorder; and (4) chaotic hyperkinesis, arising when the child's environment is marked by intense conflict, usually between the parents, against which the child defends himself by keeping on the move; the child's restlessness provokes anxiety in the parents about their own control, so that they may abuse the child, who reacts in turn with anxiety and hostility.

Children diagnosed as hyperkinetic obviously do not constitute a homogeneous group; the selection of treatment interventions requires recognition of their individual differences. Katz *et al.* (17) note at least three groups: (1) those who function well in quiet settings generally, but not in the classroom; (2) those in whom hyperactivity combines with a strong emotional overlay, in whom stress may interact with deviant psychology; and (3) those whose behavior is antisocial and aggressive. Convincing data are presented by Loney *et al.* (22) to separate aggressivity from hyperactivity. These, they propose, are relatively separate and independent symptoms with different prognoses (35). And, finally, hyperkinesis has been regarded not as a diagnostic category but as an aspect of a number of disorders, each of different etiology (10). Anorexia, with hyperkinesis, is one example unrelated to MBD (19). Another study finds hyperactivity often dependent upon the situation in which it occurs (21).

The Learning-Disability and Dyslexia Syndromes

The learning disabilities are many and varied, and a major focus for disagreement has been their etiology. Cruickshank (9) traces the adoption of the label to the year 1963, when there was a general orientation among professionals toward a neuropsychological basis for the problems. Following this momentary general agreement, a flood of other disorders was attached to the designation. These included any disturbances, even emotional ones, that impeded educational progress, apparently an effort to minimize the implications of emphasizing organicity. This effort created more partisanship than knowledge and insight.

Dyslexia and dyscalculia are the most prominent of the specific learning disorders identified. Dyslexia has received the most attention from all the disciplines. Comparatively neglected are the other language disorders, those of speech and writing, dysphasia and dysgraphia. One evidence of this comparative neglect is the fact that in this country we regularly test for grade levels in reading and mathematics but not those in speech or writing.

The concentration of effort upon dyslexia has produced much convincing evidence that it, too, is a multiple, not a single syndrome. Dyslexia, states Brown (6), is a "multi-faceted, interdisciplinarian" disorder that requires the cooperative efforts of psychology, psychiatry, education, neurology, and genetics. To these we may add opthalmology, audiology, and neurophysiology. Doehring (11) finds no single reading disorder and no single cause. His experience is that many factors associated with dyslexia are either antecedents of the disorder, consequences of the disorder, or both. He and his colleagues (15) speculate that a limited number of learning-disability patterns exist, most of which, but not all, involve reading deficits.

The disorder is placed within the context of retarded language development by Zangwill (41), and seen as varying in manifestation from person to person. Among its most typical features are slowness in early language learning, a relatively poor level of verbal intelligence in comparison to nonverbal intelligence, and retarded verbal learning. The contrast between verbal and nonverbal intelligence is also emphasized by Bannatyne (1), who calls attention to the "spatially competent learning-disabled child." An optical-acoustical model is proposed by Bruschek (7), who tests for four transformational steps in information processing: (1) optic stimulus—optic response, (2) optic stimulus—acoustic response, (3) acoustic stimulus—optic response, (4) acoustic stimulus—acoustic response.

An extensive and penetrating analysis of the literature on the neurology of developmental dyslexia was made in 1975 by Benton (3). He evaluates the role of seven neurological factors in the disorder in his "state of the knowledge" overview:

General language dysfunction. The evidence (although in some studies derived from questionable procedures) substantially associates some oral language dysfunction with dyslexic children, relative to their levels of general intelligence, a dysfunction antedating the emergence of dyslexia. This point is also made by Zentall (42).

Sequencing. Dysfunction in perception and retention of temporally organized patterns of stimuli in both auditory and visual modalities are associated with dyslexia.

Directional orientation. Benton cites Orton as first to observe reversal in dyslexia while visuo-perception functions other than reading (e.g., in games, recognition of objects, interpretation of pictures and diagrams) were normal, so that the dysfunction appeared limited to symbolic material. Later workers related the symbolic dysfunction to a right/left body-schema disorientation that affects lateral orientation primarily, and in turn all directional sense, up/down as well as right/left. Benton reports that earlier (1962) he had found right/left disorientation associated with dyslexic children in grades 1—3, but not in older dyslexics.

Visuo-perception. The evidence of an association of visuo-perceptual disorders with dyslexia is judged by Benton ambiguous and conflicted. Some dyslexics are found to be inferior to normal readers in these functions, others are not. And where positive findings are reported, the numbers of visuo-perceptual disorders in dyslexics are small. Also, children with congenital or acquired disorders of eye movement generally do not have the features characteristic of dyslexia even though they are poor readers. Myklebust (26) agrees, in a report of negative opthalmological findings in an interdisciplinary study of 2,704 under-achieving children.

Intersensory integration. Studies both supporting and questioning the findings of Birch and Belmont associating cross-modal (audio-visual) dysfunction with reading disability are cited. Factors advanced but not established are attenuation of short-term memory, and the matching of disparate types of stimuli, those temporally sequential with those spatially disturbed. Benton questions the mechanism, but acknowledges that cross-modal difficulties have been found in some dyslexics.

Finger localization. Again, Benton finds the evidence equivocal, not firm enough, for example, to identify developmental dyslexia with either congenital or hereditary Gerstmann's Syndrome. Other investigators, moreover, have remarked the presence of the Gerstmann's Syndrome in normal readers, and the present writer has examined such a case. The syndrome illustrates all too vividly the controversy and confusion that surrounds the diagnosis of MBD and its subsyndromes. Gerstmann in the 1920s had identified a post-traumatic syndrome that included four specific symptoms: finger agnosia, right/left disorientation, acalculia, and agraphia. More recently, other observers have added difficulties with constructional activities to the syndrome. Ascribing the syndrome to damage in the left parietal area (37) is challenged by the argument that such damage can exist without all of the syndrome's symptoms being present, or the argument that the syndrome is actually a manifestation of aphasia (4, 31). Counter arguments point to the presence of the syndrome without aphasia (31, 37). The syndrome has also been associated with dyslexia, but as indicated above, dyslexia may occur without the Gerstmann symptoms; some children with the symptoms are fine readers, while some are markedly dyslexic.

Cerebral dominance. Although Benton finds evidence associating "deviant lateral organization" with reading disability inconsistent and equivocal, he recognizes that the data trend suggests such an association. Left unanswered is the question of what comes first, poor language development or hemispheric immaturity.

Benton believes that the findings are best described as equivocal, sparse, and inconsistent, a situation due to an inadequate definition, first of dyslexia, and then of established and recognized subtypes of reading disability. These, he suggests, could be more firmly identified with specific patterns of neurological dysfunction.

Mattis *et al.* (23), publishing in the same year as Benton (1975), made a significant contribution to the understanding of dyslexia as a neuropsychological disorder and the classification of its varieties. They have identified three, possibly four, dyslexic syndromes. Their review of the literature demonstrated that every disorder of higher cortical functioning is found more often in dyslexic children than in normal controls. No single dyslexic child, however, shows all of these deficits. Neuropsychological findings generally indicated that children with similarly severe reading problems had significantly different patterns of higher corical dysfunctions, a fact of major significance for diagnosis and treatment. They concluded that the likelihood of finding brain dysfunctions in the dyslexic child that are not directly causal to his reading disability required their effort to exclude as etiological any cerebral dysfunction that was also found in the brain-damaged child who can read.

To pursue their neuropsychological model, they used the *WAIS* or *WISC*, the *Benton Visual Retention Test*, the *Ravens Progressive Matrices (Coloured* or *Standard)*, the *Illinois Test of Psycholinguistic Abilities (ITPA)*, the *Sound Blending Test*, the *Spreen-Benton Token Test*, the *Benton Sentence Repetition Test*, the *Wide-Range Achievement Test (WRAT)*, the *Purdue Pegboard,* and tests of graphomotor coordination, speech-sound discrimination, and verbal labeling ability (naming).

Their study population was 113 children selected from among 252 referred for evaluation of learning and behavior disorders. They had Verbal or Performance I.Q.s greater than 80, ages between 8 and 18, normal visual and auditory acuity, "adequate" academic exposure, and no evidence of psychosis or thought disorder. Neurological diagnosis of 84 of the children as brain damaged enabled the investigators to establish three diagnostic groups for neuropsychological study: (1) dyslexic children without brain damage; (2) dyslexic children with brain damage; and (3) brain-damaged children who could read. Three dysfunctional neuropsychological patterns were identified among the dyslexic children without brain damage:

1. Language Disorder. Anomia is prominent in this group; they produced 20 percent or more errors on the verbal-labeling test. They also showed one of the following: (a) disorder of comprehension evidenced in a − 1 Standard Deviation (S.D.) level on the *Token Test;* (b) disorder of imitative speech manifested in a performance level more than − 1 S.D. on the *Sentence Repetition Test;* or (c) disorder of speech-sound discrimination evident in 10 percent or more errors in discriminating letters rhyming with "e."

2. Articulatory and Graphomotor Dyscoordination. This group produced levels more than − 1 S.D. on the *ITPA Sound Blending* subtest, and graphomotor test performances also more than − 1 S.D. Acousto-sensory and receptive-language processes were within normal limits in this group.

3. Visuo-Spatial Perceptual Disorder. Members of this group had Verbal I.Q.s and percentile ratings on the *Ravens Coloured Progressive Matrices* less than their equivalent Performance I.Q.s would imply, and a score on the *Benton Visual Retention Test* on 10-second exposure at or below the borderline level.

The Language-Disorder group had the most severe reading problems. The Visuo-Spatial Perceptual Disorder group were the least significant in frequency, contrary to general assumptions about the role of perceptual dysfunction in dyslexia.

A simpler neuropsychological approach to dyslexia is reported by Fuller and Friedrich (16). They sought to elaborate the neuropsychological patterns identifiable with Rabinovitch's three diagnostic groups for children with reading disabilities, first using the *Minnesota Percepto-Diagnostic Test* to place each child in a group. They then administered the following tests to identify the distinctive neuropsychological pattern of each group: *WISC, Illinois Test of Psycholinguistic Abilities, Hawthorn Concepts Symbolization Test, Wide-Range Achievement Test,* and the *Durrell Analysis of Reading Difficulty.* Three patterns were identified:

1. Primary Reading Retardation, in which an auditory deficit and associational difficulties combine into a verbal-expressive dysfunction. The Performance I.Q. *(WISC)* here is usually higher than the Verbal I.Q.

2. Secondary Reading Retardation, with fewer and less severe deficits on most variables. Members of this group are subject to tension and anxiety that affect verbal expression and motor performance. They are able to see mistakes and correct them when given cues.

3. Reading Retardation Associated with Brain Damage, where deficits are more pervasive. Those in this group exhibit both auditory and visual problems and more deficits on manual tasks. Verbal expression is poorer, and problems in right/left orientation and identification are distinct.

A "cybernetic" model is proposed by L. B. Silver (34) based upon logically assumed brain processes in learning: (1) Input, recording data in the brain; (2) Integration, comprehending and organizing the information; (3) Memory, storage and retrieval of the information; and (4) Output, communication of information from the brain to another person. Disorders may be present in any or all of these brain processes.

The first category, Input Disorders, is manifest confusion in left/right and top/bottom orientation and identification, with difficulties in distinguishing between geometric figures, certain letters (p and d) and words (*was* perceived as *saw*), the right and left sides of the self or others, depth perception, eye-body coordination in use of the hands (throwing, hitting, kicking), and in figure-ground discrimination. Also present are auditory problems in confusion of phonemes, figure-ground discrimination, and a lag in the recording of sounds. These, of course, are essentially sensory-perceptual processes. Integration Disorders encompass difficulties in abstraction, comprehending the general connotations of data, and particularly the sequencing of input data (visual, auditory, haptic, and intrasensory). Considering Memory Disorders, both short-term and long-term, Silver notes that the child with a long-term memory disorder is most likely to be seen as mentally retarded. In Output Disorders, with spontaneous language usually intact, "demand" language may be impaired. Also present may be disorders of motor behavior, fine and gross. Secondary to these disorders is the presence of hyperkinesis or distractibility in about 40 percent of learning-disabled children.

L. B. Silver emphasizes the organic etiology in learning disabilities, maintaining that the emotional problems present are reactions to the primary and secondary disorders. He emphasizes danger in the recognition of emotional problems to the exclusion of organic ones, thereby concentrating treatment upon the former, while the latter, more basic problems, go undetected and untreated. Silver's system, which appears related to Mark's Systems-Analysis procedure (24), is useful in calling attention to the presumable brain-behavior stage in the learning process for each child and in identifying the focus for treatment.

Clearly, we are far from a working set of definitions for MBD, hyperkinesis, and learning disabilities. While more and more syndromes and subsyndromes are being identified and defined, the clinician in a one-to-one relationship, working diagnostically and therapeutically with a population of one, is not likely to facilitate his work by an effort to identify a single syndrome or subsyndrome in his patient. Rather, he is well advised to scrutinize each person suspected of MBD for *all* of the symptoms that have come to be associated with it, and to establish as precisely as possible the dysfunction or, more likely, the several dysfunctions that limit that person. Efforts at diagnostic definitions are enormously helpful in this venture; they remind the worker of the many diverse symptoms possible in MBD, their manifold possible sources, and their manifold implications for treatment. The six following chapters review the signs and symptoms of the MBD syndrome and discuss methods for their diagnostic investigation.

Chapter 5

Signs and Symptoms in MBD

THE SYMPTOM, not the syndrome, is the key to treatment of a person suspected of MBD. Attempts to identify a set of symptoms in him that correspond even loosely with one of the syndromes or subsyndromes recognized in this disorder are as likely to fail as to succeed. More realistic is to identify the symptoms to be found in the patient, and to describe each one as clearly as possible to guide selection of treatment interventions for his particular limitations. In MBD the symptom clusters vary widely from patient to patient, in both type and degree.

Increasingly, and happily, diagnostic scrutiny is being applied earlier and earlier in life, in efforts to identify the child or even the infant at risk. Crow (9) has listed 100 of the most frequently observed symptoms in children five to eight. The first year of life has recently received careful attention from the Collaborative Perinatal Project, under the National Institute of Neurological and Communicative Disorders and Stroke (16). Pediatric examinations, histories, the Bayley Scales of Infant Development, and the Apgar Scale were studied as predictors. These are welcome efforts. Medical procedures developed to save the lives of infants and children unfortunately contribute to the number of children with physical and cognitive disabilities that escape recognition or fail to impress as serious because their signs are ''soft'' or ''vague.''

This chapter reviews eight sets of major symptoms associated with MBD in one grouping or another, from person to person. Alertness to these signs, although the list is not all-inclusive, enables the observer to recognize early most of the children in difficulty, and so to initiate helpful interventions. The worker must keep in mind that these signs and symptoms occur with varying severity, as do all symptoms, and that the degree of dysfunction as well as its nature should guide the treatment and influence the prognosis.

Intellectual Deficits

Frequently, the MBD child is defined as one of average or better intellectual endowment who functions below his level. Lower than average test levels lead usually to a diagnosis of mild to severe mental retardation, an unfortunate tendency because it would seem to imply that any child of Below Average I.Q. is not a victim of MBD. Also it may consign a child of average or better endowment to a mentally-retarded diagnosis because his Full Scale I.Q. falls in the Below-Average category. Yet Superior-level I.Q.s in some cognitive functions may be observed in a child whose Full-Scale I.Q. is in the Borderline to Mentally-Retarded range.

A distinctive feature of the intelligence-test profile of the person with Minimal Brain Dysfunction is scatter, a marked or moderate variation from one subtest to another, from one group of subtests to another. This variation is helpful in identifying the child's cognitive deficits in a general way: verbal, arithmetical, attention, memory, spatial, and constructional. (Chapter 10 discusses the use of the intelligence test as a diagnostic method.) More careful examination of responses in each subtest may reveal more specific dysfunctions, such as a verbal-expressive, or a verbal-comprehension, difficulty.

Specific Learning Deficits

Dysfunction in reading, writing, speech, or arithmetic may be observed. The dysfunction is usually relative to other learning skills. The child may read well but be poor in arithmetic, or do arithmetic easily while stumbling in reading, or may write or speak poorly. He may spell correctly while reading well, or both may be dysfunctional. Silent reading may be performed better than oral reading by one child, the opposite may operate in another child. In arithmetic tasks one child may do better on written tasks than on oral ones, while another presents the reverse condition. The modalities of perception and response must be considered in evaluating the learning disability.

In reading dysfunctions the child may fail to read at grade or age level. His reading may be marked by persistent reversals of letters and words, omissions of words, stumbling over pronunciation or punctuation, slow pace. He may read from right to left, be unable to detect similarities and differences in forms, shapes, and words. He may not be able to pronounce a word that is strange to him, or to differentiate the sound of words. He may substitute an unprinted word for a printed one. He may be able to speak what he reads but not understand what he has read and spoken. He may be unable to keep his place in a sentence as he reads. Spelling may be poor and similarly characterized by reversals, omissions, and slow pace. Any or all arithmetic processes may present difficulties, as may abstract concepts. Letters, numbers, decimal positions, and punctuation marks may be persistently misplaced. Insight into the relationship of parts-to-whole may be impaired in spatial visualization tasks, confusion about time, distance, weight, volume, speed, and other measurements may be observed. The dyslexic child of normal intelligence is likely to be deficient in either the analytic-sequential processing of selected features *or* the holistic perception of the significant feature of the whole word. Deficient in one, he usually is normal in the other (1).

Any or all of these may be manifest. Along with age and grade norms, estimates of the child's innate capacity and his motivation are important in the diagnosis. The quality or adequacy of his instruction must also be considered in the diagnosis. A child may perceive his learning difficulties before his teachers or parents do. Indeed this is often the case, and causes anxiety, guilt, and depression. These emotional reactions may be the first signs observed in the presenting picture, when in fact they are secondary to the learning difficulty.

In many children the deficit may be so slight that difficulty will be experienced only when a confounding complexity is reached on attaining higher grade levels. On the other hand, the deficits may decrease slowly and progressively as maturation proceeds.

Learning deficits often persist into adulthood, along with the reactive emotional problems of anxiety, guilt, and depression. An adult presenting himself for psychotherapy and offering a history of persistent learning difficulties should be scrutinized diagnostically for evidence of MBD.

Motor Impairments

As indicated earlier, the motor abnormalities observed in MBD, except for manifest hyperkinesis, are usually of slight degree, constituting so-called "soft" neurological signs, as discussed in Chapter 9. Some of those signs are the following:

Graphic activities—writing, printing, drawing—may be poor, with the pencil held in an awkward and unusual position between the fingers and poorly controlled.

Tremor of the fingers when extended, or when intentional movements are requested, may be observed. Movements may become inaccurate when their rapid execution is required. Clumsiness may generally characterize motor behavior. Balance may be poor when visual cues are withheld. Slight asymmetrical gait abnormalities may be observed. Tics, grimaces, and apraxias of lips and tongue may be present. At rest, muscle tone, position, and posture may be abnormal. During acts of vigilance (concentration), body movements are likely to increase (34).

Choreiform activity—slight jerky movements appearing suddenly and of short duration—has been noted among MBD children (37), but the diagnostic import is questioned (35). Differentiation from a psychogenic tic is necessary.

Hyperkinesis—high activity level—is the most frequently cited motor sign in MBD. High activity level and impaired coordination are viewed by Wender (48) as the principal motor abnormalities of the syndrome. But underactivity and listlessness also have been observed in MBD children (2, 48), although far less frequently than hyperactivity. Thomas (47) warns that hyperactivity may be a sign of conditions other than MBD, such as encephalitis or emotional disturbance. Brain-damaged children spend more time in locomotion and engage in more motor activity when required to do a difficult task, as compared with controls.

Motor abnormalities tend to disappear with maturation, so that signs of them are not usually evident in the adult suspected of MBD. Ozer (32A) finds that the pattern of complex responses and associated movements provides the most discrimination in detecting "neurological immaturity," but notes that such measures are less useful after the age of nine, by which time the child is likely to have matured through his lag. There may, however, be some connection between hyperactivity in the child and some cases of so-called hypomanic or agitated behavior in the adult.

Sensory Impairments

Perception in all modalities—visual, auditory, haptic, gustatory, olfactory, and kinesthetic—is the beginning point of learning, and disorders of perception or of the entire perceptual process are considered by many to be the most likely factor making for learning disabilities (50).

Visual-perceptual dysfunctions have received much attention because of their direct association with dyslexia. Reversals of left and right and top and bottom, difficulty distinguishing between figure and ground, and between geometric shapes, are among the disorders noted. Errors in depth perception and in spatial orientation of self, others, and objects are observed. Nystagmus, pupillary inequality, and extraocular movement have been associated with MBD (24, 37). Other visual dysfunctions correlated with learning disabilities are faulty binocular fusion, accommodation, and eye aiming, which decrease the efficiency of reading, and make for poor word-recognition skill. Some visual-perceptual defects become apparent through motor-expressive tasks, as in copying figures (in the *Bender Gestalt Test*), in block-design constructions (*WISC, WAIS*), or in the *Benton Visual Retention Test* and constructional tasks requiring the assembly of parts into wholes (*WISC, WAIS*).

Visual stimulation is only the beginning point in learning through the visual modality. The stimulus must be differentiated from other visual stimuli, which requires memory, processed and organized into a perception in the brain, where it is interpreted and comprehended, acquiring meaning to the perceiver, termed visual acuity. While end-organ integrity is essential to learning to read, often reading remains dysfunctional after the eyes are corrected, implicating a cerebral disorder (14).

Equally important in the genesis of learning disabilities are disorders of hearing. Kennard (19) reported auditory deficits with associated "soft" neurological signs in 25 percent of emotionally disturbed children, suggesting that the sensory impairment may be primary in this proportion of the study population.

The ephemeral quality of the auditory stimulus is well described by Zentall (50). He notes its rapid transitory quality, the fact that the observer cannot scan the auditory stimulus as he scans the printed page, except from memory, nor can he skip ahead "to see what is coming." The spaces between spoken words, sentences, and paragraphs are far less structured and distinguishable than they are in printed material. Separating figure from ground is more difficult in auditory than in visual perception.

As with visual perceptions, central processing of auditory stimuli is necessary for their comprehension. Temporal-lobe dysfunctions have been suggested in dichotic auditory fusion difficulties, for example (15). Middle-ear and vestibular processing dysfunctions have also been implicated (22, 32). Dichotic listening asymmetry (related hypothetically to problems of cerebral dominance) has been proposed, and also contested, as a sign associated with learning disabilities (13, 17).

The importance of hearing in language and speech development is obvious, but the complexity of the process is often neglected, states Sabatino (36). The auditory-perceptual function involves: (1) recognition of sound as meaningful; (2) retention of the sounds as informative; (3) integration of the symbols into syntactical units; and (4) comprehension of the units. Effective audition therefore consists of recognition, retention, integration, and comprehension. Sabatino has incorporated these measures into a *Test of Auditory Perception,* so that each area may be assessed differentially. His study emphasizes the necessity to test audition as well as vision to avoid overlooking bright under-achievers.

Reading ability also requires integration of both visual and auditory perception. Investigating the ability to integrate two or more stimulus modalities simultaneously is more productive of accurate diagnosis than is the testing of single sensory modes. Birch and Belmont (5), using an ingeniously simple test (*Auditory-Visual Pattern Integration*) demonstrated that learning to read "requires the ability to transform temporally distributed auditory patterns into spatially distributed visual ones." Disturbance of ability to integrate these two sensory modalities was at the root of reading problems among their population of children, none of whom were found to have a significant hearing impairment or an uncorrected visual defect.

Comprehension of incoming data often requires abstracting and/or sequencing of the data. Disorders in these processes may be intrasensory or limited to a single sensory modality (42).

A related process requires the ability to recognize the presence of two haptic stimuli presented simultaneously. With the child's eyes shut, he is touched simultaneously upon, successively, both hands, right hand and right cheek, right hand and left cheek, left hand and right cheek, left hand and left cheek, both cheeks. Another sensory-integration process requires ability to rule out an irrelevant stimulus (sound) while identifying the simultaneous relevant stimulus (touch).

Attention-Memory Impairments

Learning disabilities are believed by some observers (11) to be caused by impairment of ability to attend and recall, rather than by a deficit specific to the material or process to be learned. Certainly limited concentration span, easy distractibility, and poor memory are characteristics of many MBD children. Parents will report, and in the playroom it will be observed, that the child does not stay with one task or play for very long, that he cannot sustain concentration in opposition to an intruding stimulus. While such symptoms tend to diminish with age, they may be discerned in the formal psychological testing of adults.

Despite the frequency of attention problems in MBD and the development of many measurement and treatment devices for improving concentration, we actually know very little about the nature of attention, its neurological base, or its relationship to memory, to the retrieval of data stored in the brain after it is acquired by whatever degree of concentrated perception necessary. For example, we don't know if memory is impaired by limited capacity for attention or by a central processing deficit involving inability to integrate and comprehend. Is attention secondary to the hyperactivity that causes easy distractability along with impulsivity (29)? Or to some unknown brain condition that may or may not be linked with hyperactivity, as the inadequate functioning of the corpus callosum to inhibit transmission between the cerebral hemispheres of data irrelevant to the current cognitive focus (12)?

We do know that attention is necessary for learning and for the storage of what is learned. But we know little about how long concentration must be sustained for learning or memory to take place. We know that the person must be conscious, alert, able to focus (7), and able to exclude extraneous data, to inhibit consciousness of the unrelated. But we do not know how completely inhibited such consciousness of the irrelevant must be to permit learning. Psychoanalysis has taught us, as has research of the subliminal process, that awareness or consciousness has more than one level, that denial as a defensive mechanism may preclude from awareness that which has all too vividly been perceived and registered.

In any event, degrees of impaired attention and memory are among the major characteristics of the MBD disorders. In some children they are all too apparent and require no special procedures to identify. In others they may be detected only through a sustained testing procedure demanding an extended period of attention (7). And the examiner must compare one modality of attention with another in the same person. Does he sustain visual attention better than auditory concentration? Or vice versa? How does he function with bimodal, intersensory attention, and memory tasks?

Other Maturational Lags

In effect, any symptom in MBD may represent a maturational lag. One child may not begin to read effectively until age seven or eight, another may reflect his early maturation in spontaneous reading at age four that appears self-motivated. Sensory or motor dysfunction, or poor attention span, may diminish or be resolved as the child gets older.

Deficits of right-left differentiation may continue beyond the age of seven or eight when they usually disappear. This pattern may be related to a persistent mixed cerebral dominance or to a delay in emergence of a relatively clear-cut lateral dominance. Dysfunctional right-left discrimination may be associated with dyslexia, with clumsiness in moving about or dressing, with ambidexterity, mixed or inconsistent preference in eye, foot, and ear use, or with contrasting patterns of dominance for the hand, eye, ear, and foot. These conflicting patterns are hypothesized by some workers (41) to represent a lag in the maturational development of hemispheric dominance for language.

A major problem for the diagnostician—one of grave importance for the MBD child and his parents—is the degree of confidence that can be placed in the assumption that any dysfunction observed is due to a maturational lag. The degree of such confidence may determine whether treatment is recommended, or the child and parents are assured that "he'll grow out of it." Such assurance is tempting to offer. It stills troubled feelings, lifts clouds of depression, and allays anxiety. But it all too often only delays the time when confrontation with a persistent dysfunction becomes necessary, a time by which the child has become an adolescent or adult, and when years of possible remediation have been lost, when the emotional and social damage surrounding MBD have severely and adversely affected the personality.

Sometimes confidence in a maturational-lag diagnosis is reinforced when the individual has a history of earlier dysfunctions that moderated with age. The parents may report a history of generally slow development, or of different rates of development: "He didn't walk until he was two, but spoke at an early age." Bowel and bladder control may have been delayed beyond the norm, as may have ability to focus the eyes, button a shirt, or tie shoelaces. There may be a family history that favors the maturational lag diagnosis: the father and his father showed a pattern of dysfunction followed by gain, for example.

But even where such contributory evidence is available, the diagnostician should offer the lag hypothesis cautiously, and should couple it with recommendations for either immediate intervention to facilitate the hoped-for maturation, or monitoring of the child's development for a certain period, with treatment to be started should the expected maturation not evolve.

Impairments of Speech and Writing

With much diagnostic and remedial attention focused on the dyslexic manifestation of MBD, comparatively little has been directed to the other important language functions. Speaking and writing should also command our attention and investment. Speech has crucial social consequences. The character, quality, and content of language productions influence the response of others to the speaker. They may even seriously influence the judgment of the diagnostician, who can miss a moderate dysphasia, and perhaps diagnose instead a nonexistent schizophrenia or mental retardation (43). Dysfunctions of either expressive or receptive language or both may be so mild as to escape detection because they do not resemble a clear-cut aphasia. Or because they are moderate, the auditor's comprehension may not be affected because he spontaneously applies closure to the slightly stumbling, slightly illogical-sounding speech of the MBD victim, and grasps its meaning. Or the speech dysfunction may be severe enough to make communication with others so difficult that withdrawal and social isolation results.

Impairment of ability for the abstract verbal conceptualization expected for I.Q. and age has been observed. "Demand" speech, in contrast to spontaneous speech, à la Jackson, may be dysfunctional. The child may spontaneously respond appropriately in a structured situation ("Bless you" when someone sneezes) but be bewildered and unable to respond when questioned about the identical situation "What do you say when someone sneezes?" Naming difficulties may be detected. Extended speech involving the interrelating of two or more ideas into a conclusion or propositional statement may be impaired, but noticeable only in contrast to much better functioning with speech tasks that require responses of few words or concern single ideas.

Usually in MBD, writing dysfunctions become apparent more readily than do speech deficits. In writing the dysfunction is made concrete and visible. Zentall (50) observes also that teachers place more emphasis upon written language as a reflection of learning than they do upon spoken language. Omissions, reversals, or errors of grammar and syntax may be present in speech, but go unnoted.

Motor impairments associated with speech or writing may appear alone or in relationship to content dysfunctions. A high frequency of mild to moderate speech apraxias have been observed in MBD (19). These included lisping, stammering, and stuttering. Poor graphomotor control of a pencil may be reflected in distorted writing and drawing. Lags in speech and writing and in drawing skills may be early and sensitive indicators of an MBD disability (24).

Psychological and neuropsychological tests are helpful in identifying and evaluating disorders of speech and writing. Slight to moderate speech and writing deficits may escape detection by standard tests of aphasia, but these tests as well as a comparative analysis of responses to the Wechsler scales can provide insightful clues to anomia, semantic uncertainty, and to expressive and receptive difficulties (see Chapter 10).

Behavioral and Emotional Concomitants

The effects of brain damage can be most diverse; no single sign or cluster of several signs appear in all brain-damaged persons in the same way or in similar degree. The emotional and psychological consequences vary from almost undetectable behavioral disturbance to disruption of social, interpersonal, and intellectual organization so severe as to be indistinguishable from psychotic conditions. Brain damage may initiate a series of behavioral changes, each begetting the next, so that in relatively short order the original etiological factor is obscured by emotional and behavioral problems. Distortions of sensory data may cause body-image disturbances and misperception of body boundaries and of external reality, leading to alienation and maladaption to a degree that resembles the functional psychoses.

The same set of emotional disturbances have been observed in MBD patients, in hyperkinetic and hypoactive children, and in learning-disabled ones. Kline (20) writes of the "emotional carnage" resulting from untreated dyslexia. Because structural brain damage is seldom identifiable in the child suspected of MBD, some workers tend to rule out neurological dysfunction as an etiological base and to regard the emotional symptoms as primary, in themselves causing the activity disorders and learning impairments. And indeed this is often the case: the child of a depressed, withdrawn mother may plead for attention through misbehavior and intensified activity; another child, burdened with abandonment anxiety, may seek to perpetuate dependency ties through learning and social difficulties. But the possibility of these purely psychodynamic causes does not obviate the direct role of minimal neurological dysfunctions. These dysfunctions often cause personality and emotional disruption, as well as adverse parental, familial, and social interactions that reinforce the psychopathological process.

An invaluable review of the major sources of anxiety and personality distortion in children with central nervous system dysfunction is provided by Silver (40). He cites three such major sources inherent in CNS dysfunction.

First, distortions of perception create frustration and confusion; difficulties in learning develop that evoke pressures upon the child at school and at home. The child's emotional reaction to repeated failure varies with the nature of his dysfunction, his personal resources, and the quality of understanding and support he receives from home and school. Here, three major groups of emotional consequences are discernible: (1) At best, some children develop a pervasive, unrelenting sense of inadequacy; they feel the world is harsh and unreasonably demanding, asking the impossible of them. (2) Others "stagger" along academically; at school they adopt a defensive clowning role, but at home they are depressed, demanding, rigid. (3) The most unfortunate ones give up early; they withdraw to the point where they may appear autistic.

Secondly, the child with a dysfunction of the central nervous system is subject to ongoing psychopathological consequences of the startle, or Moro, reaction. This reaction may be evoked by any sudden, unexpected stimulus. The infant reacts with abduction and extension followed by adduction and flexion of the arms and legs. The normal CNS system allows the person to react and quickly restore homeostasis. But where CNS pathology exists, persisting waves of physiological reactions (heart-rate increases, sweating, gastrointestinal disturbances, dilation of pupils, muscle tension, metabolic upsets) continue and progress into anxiety states. This reaction and progression may be initiated by either internal or external stimuli, ranging from the reflexive and autonomic to more complex psychic stimuli. Maintenance and restoration of homeostasis is difficult. Impulse control is poor, leading to inevitable conflicts with superego pressures. Anxiety and guilt result, generating phobias, often hypochondriasis; obsessive-compulsive behaviors are likely to develop in an effort to mitigate the guilt and anxiety.

The third source of personality distortion inherent in CNS dysfunction is the child's reaction to anti-gravity play. The child does not experience the normal delight in being held upside-down in swinging, bouncing, and tossing because of his impaired ability to maintain spatial orientation and muscle tone in relation to posture. Responding to enormous "survival" anxiety, he becomes physically clinging and then emotionally dependent. His dependency needs may become so great that they can not be gratified. Remaining always reactive in this way to all kinds of stress, he may always need available support and guidance.

Silver illuminates for us the emotional consequences inherent in CNS dysfunction itself. He touches upon the responses these emotional pathologies evoke at home and school, and within the child himself. These psychopathological responses deserve even more extensive discussion.

Difficulties in mothering the child with an activity disorder are noted by Schildkrout (39). Postnatal vegetative difficulties cause irritability and either lethargy or hyperactivity, and, in turn, feeding disruptions. The mother may become anxious and inconsistent in her response to the child. Fatigue sets in and makes her unresponsive to the infant, her husband, and other children.

She feels guilt about her withdrawal, or even possible death wishes for her infant.

These problems in developing maternal relations are further complicated by the other dysfunctions of MBD; limitations in drive level, perception, the basic language structure, and cognition may distort early object relations upon which personality structure is built. One consequence, among others, may be a borderline ego organization (28). Mordoch (25) believes that this difficulty in progressing through the early developmental stages is more pathological in its consequences than poor parental management. But certainly the child's pathology evokes related reactions from parents. Early ego disruption inevitably impedes the achievement of separation and individuation. The child, burdened with abandonment anxiety and already clinging out of what Silver has called ''survival'' anxiety, is afraid to grow up. Some mothers, particularly where the child is hyperactive, develop an intrusive relationship with the child, seeking to move the child to individuation by suggesting, then imposing social, play, and work activities (10). Their approach becomes less positive and accepting, more critical; the anxiety of the dependent child mounts out of fear of rejection, and he clings more desperately. The vagueness of symptoms associated with MBD may puzzle parents and suggest malingering. Lacking a definitive diagnosis that they can understand and with which they can empathize, parents become questioning, doubting, and rejecting. Children with a definite diagnosis of epilepsy were found to regard their parents as protective and having positive feelings for them to a greater extent than did MBD children (30).

These, then are some of the psychopathological processes evoked, first by the dysfunction itself, then by the response of parents—the mother particularly—to the child's perplexing symptoms.

As the child grows, his self-awareness increases, touching off further emotional complications. The pathological interaction with the parents may continue and may even intensify. To this strain will be added the interaction with adults outside the home, as in school, and with peers both in school and neighborhood. This expanding web of interaction tends to highlight the child's impairment, his cognitive, emotional, and social problems, to increase his sense of inadequacy, and decrease his motivation to continue working with material that represents prior failure. The complicated interaction of endogenous and exogenous forces defies adequate description.

Consider the child with an activity disorder. Impulsivity and emotional lability are frequently observed in MBD children. With their ability to inhibit decreased, they cannot restrain themselves from touching and handling objects; gratifications cannot be delayed. New environments, therefore, are frequently overstimulating. Aggressive outbursts, sexual displays, and antisocial behavior—lying, stealing, fire-setting, destructiveness, verbal outbursts—are frequent. Difficulty in inhibiting leads to poor judgment and inadequate foresight; the press of impulse obscures the consequences of behavior for the child. He becomes reckless. Rapid changes of mood and affect occur. The child easily cries or becomes irritable, sweetly appealing, or angry. He may appear high-strung, overly sensitive. Anxiety may escalate to panic with slight provocation. His negative self-image, poor impulse control, and high hostility level are in sharp conflict with his intense need for control and affection.

The *hypoactive* child by contrast is more likely to be even tempered, coopera-tive, and less likely to react to failure and frustration with blatant disturbance. Some such children nevertheless have been recognized as belonging within the MBD diagnosis (8, 48).

Children with MBD are also impaired in some measure in the basic developmental task of establishing a sense of competency. Exposed to repeated frustrations and failures, they experience intense anxiety while having little ability to tolerate anxiety. As we have seen, they are largely unable to elicit positive rewards from parents, teachers, or peers (38). Interaction between child and parent all too readily becomes pathological. Impulsivity, hostility, anger, and depression threaten the withdrawal of the very love and support they so much need. Poorly developed egos are a likely consequence. Clumsi-ness and lagging speech development further impair ego development (39). Ex-tremely negative self-concepts are an inevitable consequence; the children often feel that any successes they have are due only to luck or to the intervention of others, that their difficulties are insurmountable, their failures irreversible. One more argument for early diagnosis and treatment is the likelihood that these attitudes become firmly established by age nine, and thereafter become increasingly negative (6), as may the reactions of parents, teachers, and peers, in the vicious cycle described above. Low and increasingly fragile self-esteem is an all-too-painful hallmark of MBD.

Increased pathology of defenses is to be expected, and it is virtually impossi-ble to sort out the secondary from the direct, primary emotional and behavioral consequences of MBD. The MBD child has been likened by Reitan (33) to a person hanging on for dear life by the finger tips. When someone "pounds on those finger tips," that is, makes a demand for performance, achievement, suc-cess, the person goes to pieces, loses his grip, and falls.

Decathexis may be resorted to, in an effort to defend against the pain of humiliation from failure following failure. The child rationalizes: "I could do it if I wanted to, but I don't want to." Or projection becomes likely as the child moves through latency into adolescence. Others are to blame! "If only I had different parents, teachers, playmates." Application and effort are withheld, fulfillment is pursued in daydreaming. Withdrawal and aversion become habitual, and a schizoid personality may develop, marked by masochistic fea-tures. Masochism may increase to the point where it is difficult to separate from mild paranoid ideas: "I am inadequate, a failure" becomes "You hate me."

Denial is the ultimate and major defense of the child who has not been able to surmount or find his way around the obstacles imposed by MBD. Among its most serious consequences, denial may lead to a refusal to accept help. The child may become grandiose, refusing to cooperate in diagnostic appraisal or remedial efforts; he may see the diagnostic testing only as humiliating revelation.

A most serious "conspiracy of denial" may develop between child and parents. Parents, seeking to allay their own anxiety and pessimism as well as their child's, may support, even initiate, unrealistic grandiose fantasies of future success, thus delaying intervention and assuring the rigidification of pathology. Or they may join the child in projecting blame onto others (teachers, the "system") rather than pursuing diagnostic clarification. The "conspiracy," by fostering grandiosity, may encourage a tendency to narcissism inherent in the borderline ego organization. The effort to enhance the child's self-esteem is likely only to decrease whatever real sense of self-confidence is there. Driven underground by denial, the pain of low self-evaluation is kept in check by repeated expression of exaggerated self-worth, by fantasies of prominence and notoriety, a process maintained by increasing aversiveness and schizoid detachment. But with denial come also, predictably, the qualities of emotional chilling and brittleness, the fragile presentation of cheerfulness and unconcern coupled with now inexplicable troughs of depression, loneliness, aimlessness, and pessimism.

Some may seek to control by being bossy and demanding, while at the same time they are stubborn and unyielding; they tend to resist control by adults and so are hard to socialize or acculturate. Wender (48) describes them as "obstinate, stubborn, negativistic, bossy, disobedient, sassy, and imperious."

The child may assert his independence in efforts to mask his disability by antisocial acts that increase his anxiety and in turn increase his dependency. This is a frequent and painful dilemma for the MBD child and his parents; its negotiation becomes the central task of the child's upbringing.

The MBD child may make friends easily in an outgoing mood, but lose them quickly as he becomes irascible, or as his deficits alarm his peers so that they reject him, or he withdraws to hide depression or protect his self-esteem.

Wender (48) associates four qualities of dysphoria with the MBD child: anhedonia (diminished pleasure in things, activities, relationships), depression, low self-esteem, and anxiety. Long after maturation has overcome some of the lags, socialization has improved, and skills have developed around assets that serve to mask deficits, these dysphoric qualities may persist. Some investigators believe that the frequently observed depression in MBD children may be the actual underlying cause of hyperkinesis (31). Others regard it as reactive to the hyperkinesis, reflecting the child's poor self-image because of his inability to live up to parental expectations that he be able to control himself (51).

Depression and anxiety are found more prominent than impulsivity among adults who had been diagnosed as MBD when children. Mann and Greenspan (21) attribute this to the acquisition over the years of sufficient ego maturation to develop internalized impulse control. However, confrontation with their self-perception of inadequacy continues as the demands of adulthood accompany their maturation: separation from parents, vocational development and identification, financial responsibility, sexual intimacy.

Other workers are impressed by the continued effects of childhood hyperkinesis and dyslexia upon adult behavior characterized by explosiveness, delinquency, alcoholism, and general sociopathy. Dyslexia is regarded by Taglianetti (44) as a predictor of delinquency; Tarnpol (45) associates delinquency with visual-motor deficits on the *Bender*. Mauser (23) notes an association between learning disabilities and delinquency, although he finds the causal aspects obscure. Fifty-seven percent of a delinquent population produced brain-damaged levels on the *Halstead-Reitan Test Battery* in an investigation by Berman (4).

Suggestive evidence that early hyperkinesis may evolve into an explosive personality in adulthood is offered by Morrison and Minkoff (26). In a related study (27), childhood hyperkinesis is correlated with adulthood alcoholism, hysteria, and sociopathy. A greater incidence of retrospectively reported symptoms of MBD in childhood has been correlated with the more severe degrees of alcoholism among adults (46).

While many symptoms of MBD are to be found among adolescent and adult delinquents, alcoholics, and probably schizophrenics, these findings must not be misread as predictive for the individual MBD child, or for the bulk of the MBD child population. They tell us little or nothing about the possibilities of early detection and treatment, or the effects of various support systems. As in so many clinical areas with equivocal diagnoses and hypothesized etiologies, small-population, cross-sectional study is inadequate; large-population, multivariable, longitudinal studies do not yet exist.

In the absence of "hard" scientific fact, the clinician must rely upon his experience in evaluating the individual. We know that the MBD child grown into young adulthood may have trouble with those age-specific tasks that then confront him: vocational choice and development, and peer, social, and sexual relationships. These difficulties are likely to evoke the major emotional symptoms of anxiety, depression, lowered self-esteem, and anhedonia, although without the symptoms of motor, sensory, and attentional impairments that characterized his childhood. For these states the MBD adult may seek psychotherapy, but for him the pursuit of essential psychodynamic causality, in masochism or inward deflection of rage, for example, may well lead to failure of the therapeutic effort because the dysfunctions are part of the picture.

Perhaps more than any other syndrome of an equivocal neurological nature, MBD justifies—more strongly, demands—an attitude of diagnostic skepticism and thorough scrutiny with all persons who present themselves for psychotherapy, because of the psychological disturbances derivative from it. Of course, due care must be given to the possibility that the cognitive, perceptual, motor, attention, memory, speech, writing, and other learning difficulties are caused by rather than cause the emotional problems observed (3, 14). Consideration of this possibility helps the diagnostician select treatment interventions. The most exhaustive diagnostic inquiry is crucial to prevent the flood tide of personality disorganization that may flow from MBD unrecognized and untreated.

Chapter 6

Diagnostic Methods in MBD: An Overview

THE CLINICAL UTILITY of diagnosis is not only to specify disorders and to differentiate between them but also to guide the selection, even the course, of treatment. Diagnosis limited to labeling and classification may be a mystery-solving game interesting to the diagnostician, but it is an empty one for the patient. Where MBD is suspected, the valuable diagnostic process is a search, to identify and differentiate the origins and the nature of the symptoms, to separate out the roles of various influences (neurological, intellectual, familial-cultural, genetic), and to establish the level of language development achieved. In the process, specification takes place. Areas of strength and of weakness are identified. Areas of weakness are scrutinized minutely in an effort to identify the specific nature of the deficit. Specification is the best guide to treatment, suggesting the most promising combination among the many possibilities: remediation, family therapy, behavior modification, medication, habilitation, psychotherapy. Analysis of weaknesses guides and concentrates the remedial treatment efforts. Analysis of the strengths suggests support systems and cognitive procedures to circumvent the deficits, and to emphasize any realistic basis for encouragement.

The best cure, obviously, for any disorder is to prevent its occurrence. Next best is the earliest possible detection and treatment. Early detection is increasingly emphasized. White (14) reports new techniques by developmental psychologists who have established measures of development and maturation in some major processes during the first three years of life, and sometimes as early as the first three months. White and his colleagues have been studying one-to-three-year-olds for the development of competence in receptive language abilities, social skills, sensori-motor abilities, and abstract abilities. These, White ruefully comments, would appear promising for the early detection of any tendencies to learning handicaps, but few psychologists seem interested in using the measures to develop tests. The scales of Gesell, Bayley, Cattell, and Griffiths, although lacking the sought-for precision for the earliest months, are still those in widest use.

Clinicians have urged early observation in nursery, kindergarten, and early primary grades to spot MBD. Shrier (10) emphasizes the role of day-care personnel in this scrutiny and directs their attention to behavior that bespeaks hyperactivity, distractibility, impulsivity, frequency and severity of temper tantrums, a variety of learning disabilities, and to major secondary emotional reactions of withdrawal, fearfulness, babyishness, aggressiveness, clowning, anger, and destructiveness.

In similar fashion, L. B. Silver (12) urges the use of the playroom for an early-detection effort, with these manifestations to be looked for: inconsistencies of performance, delays in language or motor development, continuous increased motor activity, short attention span, seeming overuse of one sensory modality that may suggest difficulty in another, difficulty in organizing play activities, unusual expressive difficulties, difficulty in expressing abstract concepts, and memory difficulties. He also calls special attention to behavioral problems that emerge during the first years of school.

One experimental effort to detect MBD at an early age is reported by Eaves *et al.* (4). They enlarged the *Predictive Index* of deHirsch *et al.* (3) which includes *Pencil Use,* the *Bender,* the *Wepman Auditory Discrimination Test, Number of Words Used in a Story, Categories, Hoist's Reversal Test, Gates Word Matching Subtests, Word Recognition I and II,* and *Word Reproduction,* by adding *Draw-A-Person* and *Name Printing,* which they then labeled the *Modified Predictive Index (MPI).* This test battery was administered to 228 children in twelve kindergarten classes selected to represent all social levels. From among the 49 children who "failed" the *MPI* (scores of 0 to 1), 25 were randomly selected and matched with 25 who "passed" (scores of 2 or more). Of the 25 failures, 44 percent were then found to have MBD on the basis of extensive neurological and psychological examinations. Another 44 percent were diagnosed as "immature"; these children showed signs of MBD that were judged likely to improve in a few months. The "failures" were significantly distinguishable from the "passers" on all subtests of the *MPI.* The *MPI,* they therefore state, identifies children at high risk for subsequent school failure.

A study of major significance for early detection and preventive treatment is that of A. A. Silver and R. A. Hagin (11), who sought to avert the "destructive influence of cognitive disability on emotional development," to identify children at risk and treat them "before their symptoms harden into learning failures and emotional decompensation." They examined every child in the first grade of a New York City Public School during two years, 168 children in all, almost equal numbers of girls and boys. Each child received individual psychiatric, neurological, perceptual, psychological, and educational evaluations. Of the total number examined, 29 were selected for reading "intervention," presumably remediation; 27 were judged to be psychiatrically impaired; 25 were diagnosed as having mild to severe neurological deviation.

The children selected for reading intervention consisted of three subgroups: (1) Developmental language disability (N = 13). These children were characterized by specific perceptual deviations in spatial and temporal organization, unestablished cerebral dominance for language, praxic immaturity of some degree, no CNS deficit, no peripheral sensory deficit, I.Q. and educational experience adequate for learning. (2) Developmental language disability plus organic features (N = 12). These children manifested the first pattern, and also deviation in one or more neurological areas. (3) Non-specific type of immaturity (N = 6).

Training was directed to the specific disabilities identified in the child. In the fall of 1969 when the training started, the reading scores of the "intervention" children clustered in the lowest segment of the total class scores. In the spring of 1970 their scores resembled those of the entire class, except for the children still below first-grade reading level. By the spring of 1971 their scores were distributed identically with those of the entire class.

Obviously, care must be exercised to differentiate between the regressive emotional aspects of separation anxiety (a widespread phenomenon in nursery and early school) and MBD symptomatology, or between such symptomatology and differential developmental rates, as in reading, for example.

Factors in the Diagnosis of MBD

Again, a major factor complicating the diagnosis of MBD is the diversity of the numerous symptomatic behaviors that may be involved, and the different etiological sources possible for those behaviors. Assessment may be required of the processing and sequencing of sensory data (visual, auditory, and haptic), the integration of that sensory data, memory, symbolic operations, auditory language, reading, writing, qualitative concepts, motor behavior, personality, motivation, emotional state, and peer and family relationships.

The diversity, the extensive permutations of symptoms, and the numerous etiological possibilities suggest the kinds of professional scrutiny that may be needed for complete diagnosis of an individual case of MBD. An adequate team may require several specialists, as appropriate—remedial teacher, pediatrician, neurologist, psychologist, psychiatrist, electroencephalographer, social worker, audiologist, opthalmologist, and/or nutritionist.

In one expert's (8) experience, adequate diagnostic procedures must include a history, physical examination, neurological examination with appropriate assessment of "soft" signs, psychological evaluation of intellectual and emotional functioning, assessment of fine motor coordination, visual-motor coordination, auditory and tactile perception and discrimination, and establishment of baselines for the physiological functioning of kidneys, liver, and blood-forming organs against which to check if medication is used in the treatment.

Thorough history taking is central to the diagnostic process, especially in determining cause or causes. Benoit (2) emphasizes the medical, social, and personal history for the essential ''longitudinal view of the biological, psychological and social development and functioning of the child,'' the history combined with direct observation being the cornerstone of a careful evaluation. Appelbaum (1) maintains that no single method of identification is reliable, and that the history is superior to neurological, psychological, and psychiatric examinations.

Diagnostic considerations are so extensive in MBD that clinics not geared to the complexity of the task quickly become overburdened. The task is time consuming, and, if sufficiently comprehensive, usually requires integration of data from several professional disciplines. The Sinai Hospital in Baltimore, for example, found it necessary to establish a special multidisciplinary clinic for the diagnosis of learning disabilities, as a special service of their Pediatrics Department (5).

Yet the importance of total diagnostic procedures is inescapable if these ubiquitous and often elusive disorders are to be identified and properly treated. The great difficulty does not justify abandoning the attempt. Because of the complex relationships between various professionals, the early choice of a coordinator or case manager for each patient is now recognized to be desirable (7). The coordinator assumes central responsibility for overseeing both diagnosis and therapy, for collating the full range of diagnostic data and interpreting them to the parents and as necessary to the patient. The coordinator then continues to collate the different aspects of progress and interprets new needs as they emerge. The coordinator becomes the channel to relay information between diagnosticians and therapists, essentially serving as the control center for efforts on the child's behalf.

While the coordinator may belong to any of the professions involved, he should have ongoing responsibility, so that he is with the patient to the end of treatment. When the patient is a child, this necessity poses no transference problems. As that child moves into adolescence, the coordinator's relationship to the parents is likely to become somewhat limited, resting upon a continuing diagnostic survey and occasional progress reports given with the patient's permission. If the patient enters the diagnostic and treatment process as an adolescent or adult, the same limits hold.

The coordinator must combine knowledge of the disorder and its diverse possibilities with respect for all the various professions that cooperate and willingness to serve in a sometimes difficult role. We may hope that this real need will affect clinical training in some of the professions to include exposure to the coordination of teamwork. While this emphasis does not now exist, unfortunately, families of patients nonetheless should ask for coordination as they discuss the help they need. Where the idea has not already occured to a professional, the parent's or patient's request may strike a responsive chord.

Obstacles and Aids to Diagnosis

Elsewhere (13), I have attempted a "diagnosis of diagnosis" in an effort to emphasize, for psychotherapists particularly, the values of the diagnostic process. Some of the attitudes I have found to block a full appreciation of diagnosis bear repetition here, since MBD patients especially benefit from an expanded use of the diagnostic process by the professionals who treat them. Chief among the deterrents has been the view that diagnosis is limited chiefly to nosology, to labeling. However carefully used, taxonomy does not identify etiology, relate it to the choice of intervention, or yield an estimate of individual prognosis. Nor does the label, however accurate, illuminate the human drama of each patient, so different from any other. Nosological labeling can actually threaten the quest for individual meanings; it promotes only categorical understanding. Merely placing a patient in a category can blunt the effort to identify the all-important particular, the individual, in him.

In psychotherapy, and in other fields touching on MBD, some practitioners maintain that diagnosis becomes clarified only as treatment proceeds, not that the goal of diagnosis is to clarify treatment. This attitude begets a sense of timelessness. It may even invite lassitude, despite the therapist's wish to maintain a sensitive, individually humanistic contact with each patient, which the practitioner may consider damaged by the analytic-inferential-deductive process of history taking in energetic diagnosis. This argument may be the most serious impediment to insistence upon diagnosis as guide to treatment. But it need not be so. Not the method but the examiner using a method is responsible for a dehumanizing effect. The objection seems to argue that a diagnostician cannot be empathic while thinking. In fact, these simultaneous activities, seeing the person while searching for the disorder, make up his essential task.

Bias as to etiology can be another powerful deterrent to adequate diagnosis. Dyslexia, we have seen, may be caused by neurophysiological dysfunction, sensory, motor, or attention impairments, genetic factors, social-cultural influences, or by psychogenic forces. Bias can predetermine the choice of etiology found, or emphasized, and in turn the choice of treatment, with unfortunate consequences for many dyslexics assigned to a particular intervention or to a few that do not address all his limitations.

Still another major obstacle is the very mass and variety of data that a careful individual diagnosis produces, and the attendant necessity to collate data from several specialties. The diagnostician in the brief period usually available for sampling behavior allows little time for the "thinking through" that Ozer (9) identifies as the essential part of diagnosis, preliminary to categorization.

In an effort to "know," to "think through" the enormous data bank that may collect for each MBD patient, writers have sought to develop systematic, deductive approaches. Mark (6) offers systems analysis as the only rational approach to the complexity of diagnosis. The diagnostic examination, in this procedure a neuropsychodiagnostic battery, must be sensitive to each of the major systems of communication, learning, memory, localization, and perception. It must be sensitive to proper functioning and to disorders in these systems. The "organic learning disabilities" that Mark investigates are many: acalculias, dyslexias, aphasias, and disorders of concept formation, conditioning (agnosias and apraxias), resolution, discrimination, arousal, and habituation. Diagnosis of a disorder within an area of potential disability must have "adequate resolution." By this phrase, Mark apparently means that the procedure used must point to and test the next higher level of skill in the hierarchy of a particular channel of learning. For example, a language test administered with pantomime instructions is likely to fail to identify central language disorders of a major nature (agnosias or aphasias).

Mark cites difficulties with standard test batteries. Rote memory may imitate success in the processing of new information of which the patient is in fact incapable. Limitations of time and testing conditions may cause a failing score in skills which are less than optimal in a patient, but which may nonetheless be useful in teaching him to solve new problems as they arise in his life. Teachability can be important, as well as mastery. The diagnostic examination, therefore, should always include limit testing, to determine how far up in a ranked list of systems in any channel a person can be taught to achieve success.

Hearing and vision are the major channels of learning, of course; the haptic, olfactory, and kinesthetic channels are also important and facilitate learning. To simplify the complexity as much as possible, this example may serve. An auditory stimulus may require a gross or fine motor response, or specifically a verbal motor response, that is, speech. The speech in turn may or may not involve mathematics. This elementary complication increases the number of required inquiries.

Mark estimates 132 potential learning disabilities, and holds that diagnosis of them must be pursued at least to the point which identifies those responsive to teaching interventions and separates them from those which appear irreversible.

Mark's systems-analysis approach identifies a total of 42,432 data points in a set of hierarchal systems. To operate most efficiently, he begins with the "most complex system" in a test channel. If success is achieved there, minimal-level success is presumed in all the underlying subskill data points. If failure occurs, the system next below in level of complexity is tested. Mark developed a formal systems-analysis approach to both diagnosis and treatment. He trains technicians in the use of a digital paper-and-pencil computer system.

They start with the administration of standard tests in the standard fashion, and move to "channel-specific, system-specific, limit-testing techniques" when a "significantly deviant score" appears in the standard testing.

Such a systems-analysis approach is not now standard in any professional discipline. But it is through these disciplines that the patient must seek diagnosis and treatment. The careful diagnostician probably uses an informal, relatively crude systems-analysis approach. His investigation covers as many processing systems as possible. He interprets a response or performance in terms of age specificity. And he seeks to integrate all the data in its many varieties—sensory, motor, learning, attentional, maturational, behavioral, emotional, and social—into a statement of probable etiology and an estimate of potential response to appropriate treatment.

The four following chapters survey the diagnostic methods most frequently useful in MBD: (1) observational examinations at home and in the playroom and classroom; (2) inquiring examinations (the interview and history); (3) neurological examinations (standard and extended); (4) psychological testing (intelligence, psychoeducational, lateral hemispheric, spatial-constructional, neuropsychological).

The diagnostician should also be receptive to obtaining thorough medical, visual, and auditory examinations if these examinations are likely to illuminate the causes and most promising treatments.

Chapter 7

Direct Observation

DIRECT OBSERVATION of the child's developmental progress from infancy provides the earliest possible identification of a dysfunctional process. In this crucial scrutiny the parents, the mother especially, the playroom staff, and classroom teachers have the most important roles.

Observation at Home

With few exceptions, mothers normally observe and evaluate the development of their children from birth onward. How does the infant suck? How does he react to the sometimes difficult digestive and elimination processes? Do his eyes follow the mother as she moves about? Does he begin to show recognition in a smile? Or a sense of strangeness by crying? How does the child sleep? When does he walk? Talk? When and how are bladder and bowel control mastered? These are some of the concerns of mothers during the infancy of their children. They are vital concerns to many mothers, who may seek guidelines in reading authorities on child development (Spock, Gesell, even Apgar), in talking to other mothers more experienced than they, and in consulting pediatricians.

As her child successfully negotiates these early developmental tasks, the mother's intense concern about them abates and is shifted to the next important task for the child—socialization. How her child plays with and relates to other children, and how other children interact with her child becomes a focus of the mother's observation. Is the child assertive enough? Yet cooperative and giving? Is the child hostile and/or aggressive? Fearful? Difficult? Aversive? Do other children want to play with or visit her child? Do other mothers seem to like her child?

Simultaneous with these social observations comes judgment of the child's learning and skill development in play activities. Fine and gross motor coordination, visual and auditory tracking, eye-hand coordination are among these developmental tasks the mother can observe (without using those terms). How does the child throw a ball? Catch it? Climb a ladder and come down the slide? Jump off a step? Now, and earlier too, she can note the child's reaction to antigravity play, to being held upside down, to being swung, tossed.

Another ongoing observation to be noted is the child's capacity for attention and concentration. How long can these be sustained? Is the child unduly distracted by manifest intrusions? Or by what appears to be some stimulus from within himself? Closely related to this, of course, are the child's energy and activity levels. Does the child play, then tire appropriately and rest? Or is the child sluggish, lethargic, unresponsive to the stimuli of play situation? Is the child restless, constantly moving, jerking as it sits or rests? Constantly asking questions? Moving on to the next question before the preceding one is answered?

Cognitive development can be another major focus of ongoing child observation from the earliest months. Differential response to family members, then to visitors, shows the acquisition of facial recognition. Skills in coordinating shapes (the round object into the round receptacle, for example), comprehending the difference between in and out, up and down, and different sides of an object, all reflect the acquisition of some spatial visualization skill. Remembering where articles are placed in the home, where they are to be found when needed, where different articles of clothing go on one's body, all can be indices to the mother of her child's developing cognition and memory.

Language development is a major concern. Does the child show increasing understanding of words directed to him? Does he begin using words appropriately and continue into expressive speech? Does he begin to associate visual images with spoken words? And then later the visual image and the spoken word with the printed? Concepts of body-image, time, distance, speed, volume, size, color, shading, shape, and elementary arithmetical notions are among the many cognitive skills the mother hopes the child will show he is acquiring. Piaget's investigations of developmental cognitive stages guide many educated mothers in these evaluations.

The observation of motor, social, and cognitive development does not cease as the infant moves through childhood, latency, early, middle, and later adolescence. Does motor coordination develop into competent handling of the body? Into independent handling of clothing? Biking? Skating? Into athletic skills? Does word recognition develop into reading ability? Does grasp of elementary arithmetical concepts expand through the basic processes into more advanced ones? Do the child's good social interactions and acceptance continue? Is the child able to separate from the mother in order to play away from home? To attend school?

The mother's concern decreases or vanishes as the child masters each stage or task and moves on to the next in the hierarchal progression. Or her concern intensifies into anxiety if the child's development in some area falters or stops. Should this happen, the mother needs help in assessing her child's situation. Most often the mother will seek that help from the pediatrician or the school teacher. The pediatrician or family doctor is usually consulted if the developmental problem is a physical or social one, the teacher if the problem is educational or involves peer relations.

The point to be emphasized here is that the mother can make the earliest possible discovery of a potential MBD problem. But she needs help in carrying through to a diagnosis and ultimate treatment. Her observations are invaluable in this process; they should be respectfully received when volunteered and carefully sought if not fully expressed. Pediatrician and teacher should not seek to allay the mother's anxiety with glib assurances about maturational lag, although this possibility should always be considered. Both professionals should respond to the mother's concern by adding their diagnostic scrutiny to her observations. As part of this, they must evaluate the mother's emotional state. Does her concern have a realistic basis in the child's behavior? To what extent is her concern inflated by her own neurotic processes? They, like all professionals involved in MBD diagnosis, should take a careful history including the mother's observations with their own.

If a problem is strongly suspected, consultation with other diagnostic specialists, such as a neurologist or a school psychologist, may be indicated. If the existence of a problem is somewhat ambiguous, the recommendation should be continued observation by the mother and periodic consultation. A developmental dysfunction that has been present for years, of course, favors certainty of diagnosis. But many dysfunctions surface only as the child grows older and confronts increasingly complex tasks. When consultation is sought at such a point, ongoing observation and evaluation are also indicated if it can be established by psychological exploration that the emergent dysfunction is not a symptom of an emotional disturbance in the child.

Day Care and Nursery School

A child's participation in playroom activities at day-care centers and nursery schools allows observation by professionals with a broader population base for comparison than the mother has. They also should have more objectivity and less anxiety in their evaluations. Since MBD often is difficult to diagnose in early childhood except by careful comparison of the individual child with groups of peers, these settings can be most important in early detection if their personnel are trained to make meaningful observations. Essentially, they must evaluate the same factors that mothers instinctively look for. Because of their emotional distance from the child and his training, their observations can be more sophisticated and their queries more diagnostic. How does the child handle the separation from the mother? Does the interaction with other children produce stress in the child? What is the child's activity level? Normal or excessive? With or without focus? Is the child impulsive? Unable to control acts and emotional expressions? Do relatively minor demands evoke relatively extreme reactions of withdrawal, anger, sadness, aggressiveness? A combination of disturbed activity and emotionality is often the first clue to MBD.

The trained observer scans carefully for attention span, motor and perceptual levels. Is the child easily distractible? Clumsy? Responsive to visual, auditory, haptic, and kinesthetic cues? Secondary defensive reactions may be observed (2). Is the child aversive, avoiding interaction, regressed into infantile behavior? Or does the child cover with swaggering, bragging, aggressiveness, clowning?

The child's response to training efforts provides insight into cognitive levels and abilities. Does the child readily comprehend instructions, concepts, and abstractions geared to his age? Or do instructional efforts produce stress and evoke emotional defensive reactions?

The child's social interactions may first impel the staff to watch more carefully. In addition to the emotional manifestations already listed, how do other children react to the child? Do they ridicule, scorn, avoid, tease, mock, attack him? Normal children are likely to react to the dysfunctional child either with avoidance or attack.

Personnel of child centers must, of course, remember that these behaviors are not conclusively diagnostic of MBD. Children with primary emotional problems may exhibit the same behaviors. The behaviors are, however, signals of disturbance or dysfunction that should not be overlooked. Consultation with a pediatrician, psychiatrist, or psychologist trained to diagnose differentially between primary MBD and emotional disorders can guide the observer to the next steps—perhaps continued observation directed to specific behaviors, or a conference with the parents. Where such consultations are not available, the parents should be told of the behaviors observed and their possible meanings, and then informed of how to obtain further consultation.

Ideally, the training of personnel in child centers would always include the recognition and evaluation of significant behaviors. Some of the structured observational techniques that teachers use, discussed below, can be helpful to playroom personnel in guiding, recording, and evaluating their observations.

Classroom Observation

In the early elementary grades, the child moves from play activities to more structured learning tasks. Teachers are concerned with all of the categories of behaviors that draw the attention of mothers and playroom personnel. Cognitive and social skills are now more at the forefront, but motor and emotional behaviors are inextricably intertwined with these. Teachers are trained, of course, to recognize difficulties, to apply early remedial efforts, and to evaluate the child's need for more specialized instruction. Most teachers also have available to them consultation with school psychologists, social workers, and psychiatrists, as well as learning-disability specialists. Because the child in a classroom must sit in one place and attend to the task at hand, sustaining visual, auditory, or motor concentration, teachers are especially aware of hyperkinesis. Emotional and social disturbances also become evident to them.

Numerous guides are available to make the behavioral assessments of teachers more objective. One example of these is the *Pupil Rating Scale* by Myklebust (1) that screens for learning disabilities. The teacher rates auditory comprehension (comprehension of word meaning, following instructions, comprehension of class discussions, retention of information), spoken language (vocabulary, grammar, word recall, story telling, formulating ideas), orientation (judging time, spatial orientation, judging spatial relationships, sense of direction), motor coordination (general coordination, balance, manual dexterity), and personal-social behavior (cooperation, attention, organization, reaction to new situations, social acceptance, responsibility, completion of assignments, tact).

Similar instruments have been developed by Valett (4). The *Developmental Task Analysis* rates 100 behavioral tasks considered essential for success in learning normally mastered by children by the time they are in the middle elementary grades. The instrument lists 23 social and personal skills (e.g., "Shares and cooperates in play"), 20 motor skills (e.g., "Ties shoes"), 22 perceptual skills (e.g., "Does not make reversals or write backwards"), 15 language skills (e.g., "Talks in sentences"), and 20 thinking skills (e.g., "Understands *in* and *out* of a bag"). Considerable deviation from these normally anticipated skills in children in middle elementary school signals the teacher to refer a child for consultation.

A related device by Valett (3) focuses more directly on the behaviors in a child that make the teacher suspect a learning or behavioral disability. The instrument first helps the teacher formulate a statement of the child's problem and a brief history. The teacher then reviews additional lists: social-personal behavior difficulties (e.g., "Cannot predict consequences of personal behavior"), conceptual-cognitive behavior difficulties ("Poor number concepts"), language behavior difficulties ("Limited reading comprehension"), perceptual-motor behavior difficulties—visual-motor, visual, and auditory ("Tracing and drawing difficulties," "Cannot match pictures or symbols," "Cannot imitate specific sound patterns or noises"), sensory-motor behavior difficulties ("Poor balance, rhythm, agility"), and gross motor behavior difficulties ("Trouble skipping"). There follows an important section in which the teacher administers work tasks to the child that reflect each of the categories of difficulties already highlighted in the statement. In this way the teacher's judgment is checked against objective evidence in a work sample performed by the child.

Objectification of the teacher's own evaluations helps the teacher control any bias against a child for disturbing or "bad" behavior, before referral to psychiatrist, psychologist, or social worker. Valid data, carefully collected, documented, and reviewed, provide the essential basis for describing and interpreting the behavior to the child's parents. And, to repeat, the detailed description of learning and behavior difficulties structures and guides the remedial instruction.

Chapter 8

The Case History

THE HISTORY IS primary in the diagnosis of MBD and in substantiating that diagnosis when made. The patient's history is the key to establishing both his impairments and possibilities.

The Goals and Role of the History

Exactly because MBD is a *minimal* situation, the history must be especially detailed and thorough, spanning all the person's past and present. To repeat Benoit (4), a good history provides "a longitudinal view of the biological, psychological, and social development and functioning." It scans the entire life experience for any event suggesting a cause for investigation of the mother's pregnancy, the birth, and the patient's infancy and childhood, noting evidences of MBD in maturational lags, behavioral abnormalities, and educational impairment.

A history is an effort to document the extent to which the patient's functioning deviates from what is expected of him cognitively, physically, socially, and emotionally by those around him: his parents, peers, teachers, employers, spouse. It is the cornerstone of appropriate treatment. A poor history jeopardizes the diagnostic evaluation and with it the patient's future (6). Yet important as the history is, care must be exercised lest a pro-history bias overshadow the contributions of other investigations: the neurological, psychological, neuropsychological, educational, psychiatric, opthalmological, and nutritional examinations. A pro-history bias, usually coming from psychiatry, can be intense and politically powerful. Wender (12), for example, has an enthusiasm for the history not shared by many others concerned with the diagnosis of MBD: "The history is the most important diagnostic tool....." This comes after a derogation of psychological testing and neurological evaluation: "Most extra-historical information is of limited value." His put-down is based in large part upon the inability of nonhistorical methods either to confirm or to rule out the presence of the neurological, but Wender does not apply the same rigorous demands to the historical method. The history, too, often fails to uncover the facts to diagnose MBD definitively. An example is the work of Menkes *et al.* (10), who demonstrated the diagnostic efficacy of the *extended* neurological examination; they found that for only one-third of 83 children showing some neurological abnormality could the history produce evidence suggestive of MBD.

A more realistic view of the value of the history is provided by DeLeo (5). The history, in his view, directs and focuses the attention of a good clinician as he develops a diagnostic conclusion or "impression." The history in itself does not make the diagnosis, but it is an essential part of the diagnostic process. In many cases the cause of dysfunction cannot be located, even with a clear-cut neurological deficit, as in cerebral palsy. DeLeo is impressed by the frequency in the histories of impaired children of complicated pregnancy, bleeding from the womb, long or interrupted labor, difficult birth, instruments employed in birth, premature birth, underweight at birth, the use of resuscitation methods, visible damage to the head, convulsions, twitching, and restlessness. To these may be added incubation, signs of cyanosis and jaundice in the first ten days of life, or surgery for corrective or lifesaving reasons. Yet, as DeLeo points out, many children with histories including potential influences for pathology are normal in every way. The clinician must understand that the history may or may not support a diagnosis. Such is the lot of every element in the process. Each one, if used alone, can be ambiguous when equivocal neurological conditions are being examined.

The Case History Evaluator

The careful history may be done by any professional qualified to take and evaluate it and willing to assume responsibility for diagnosis and treatment planning. However, the contact of many of the contributing professionals with the patient is usually relatively brief, being confined to one specialized examination. And the part of the history of concern to each usually is confined to his special type of inquiry: pediatric, neurological, neuropsychological, educational. The comprehensive history stressed here is more often approached, if not reached, by the psychotherapeutic professions—social work, psychiatry, and psychology. To diagnose this complex disorder adequately, the professional should develop to an unusual degree the ability to incorporate data and concepts from other disciplines. The biologically trained professional must accustom himself to working with social, emotional, educational, and psychological data, for example. And even the different psychotherapeutic professionals must each further expand his specific professional range of inquiry and conceptualization, if these professions are to do justice to the requirements of the many afflicted with MBD.

Content of the History

How a disorder is viewed in one cultural milieu, or family context, may differ. ''Symptoms'' reported in one family and culture may be accepted as normal in another family-culture setting. What appear to be symptoms to the family may be insignificant to the examiner, and vice versa. A major objective of the history is to identify the levels of function and dysfunction in an individual in specific relation to the particular ambiance in which that person has grown and presently lives.

Identifying the Symptoms

Symptoms are usually presented first to the examiner as the concerns of the patient about himself or as the concerns about the patient from other individuals: parents, siblings, teachers, physicians. A first task is to identify these concerns. When the patient is adolescent or adult, the identification of concerns is best sought briefly from the patient. Even if the patient is a child, he may be given an opportunity to identify in his own words what concerns him about himself. The fact that few children are able to respond fully to this inquiry does not preclude its use. But usually the inquiry is directed to the parents, with teachers possibly recruited as informants. Teachers are likely to furnish more accurate data: usually they are less involved emotionally, their observations are current, and they have some comparative norms in a classroom of children. However, some teachers show a bias against learning disabilities; some are ignorant of hyperactivity, and of emotional reactions to dysfunctions. The reports of parents may be distorted by memory attenuation, shame, denial, and over-protectiveness. They may recall only symptoms that were important to them, but which throw little light upon the probability of MBD. Physicians may have protected the parents from a candid discussion of a critical illness or of ominous sequelae. Nonetheless, the history should be pursued as carefully as possible with both parents and teachers. The participation of parents is especially important; their involvement in supplying facts helps them to understand the child better. They often ask questions of the examiner; they come to comprehend the import of his queries; the process prepares them to accept realistically the status of the child and what can and should be done to help him.

The diagnostic value of the history is attenuated somewhat when the patient is adult. Parents and teachers are not often available, and involving them may not be advisable. The memory of the older patient may be unreliable for facts about childhood, and he can offer only hearsay about events of his gestation and birth. Yet the history of the older patient should be pursued with thoroughness over the entire life history to date, not only the times surrounding gestation, birth, and child development. Traumas, febrile episodes, poisonings, and prolonged anesthesias may occur at any age; minimal brain dysfunction may be incurred at any age.

The questioning of patient and/or parent should trace the extent to which the patient conforms with, excels in, or deviates from expectations in physical, cognitive, social, and emotional behaviors. The guide is the same list of the usual concerns of most parents about their child, used by trained playroom and schoolroom observers (see Chapter 7). The interviewing technique essentially is to allow the spontaneous identification of concerns by the parents, patient, or referring person, and then to explore them more minutely, before moving on to establish or eliminate all the other behavioral possibilities. From a child patient, direct inquiries may produce few meaningful responses. The interviewer should be equipped to use play and storytelling techniques to evoke material to supplement the direct query. The examiner also directly observes the patient in the waiting and consulting rooms, and the parents and their interaction with the child, again noting the physical, cognitive, social, and emotional. The examiner's observations may confirm or question the concerns of patient and parents. They may also identify for exploration symptoms not mentioned by them.

The observations of other professionals who have been associated with the patient are sought when available, and incorporated into the evaluation of strengths and weaknesses. These might include reports from teachers, pediatricians, learning-disability specialists, nutritionists, neurologists, opthalmologists, neuropsychologists, optometrists.

The complete identification of symptoms through the history-taking procedure thus first requires the coordination of observations, concerns, and findings from many sources. Obviously, further symptoms may then be discovered, or verified if suspected, by referral for examinations of a special nature not previously conducted, but the end of the history is the "presenting picture."

Generally it is advisable with all MBD patients to plan the history inquiry over two or more meetings, an arrangement that helps the patient reduce his initial anxiety, stimulates recall, and enables the examiner to confirm or question first observations.

Etiology of the Symptoms

After the symptoms have been identified, their origins must be investigated. Information about when each appeared and under what circumstances may be important to establish their probable etiology. This inquiry, again, covers both the data provided spontaneously by the patient, parents, and other professionals and those brought out by the examiner's questions. The investigation should explore all the etiological possibilities in MBD (discussed in Chapter 2).

Genetic factors. Do the parents or grandparents or relatives have dysfunctions similar or related to those of the patient?

Maturational lag. Does the history of the patient indicate that skills other than the symptom-related one were also acquired slowly? With difficulty? At a time later than usual? Is the patient now of an age when further development in the symptomatic behavior is possible? Unlikely?

Mixed dominance. Has cerebral dominance been established? Are the symptoms possibly associated with a conflict of cerebral dominance? Does the presence of spatial or verbal symptoms coincide with the patient's hemispheric dominance pattern as currently hypothesized?

Neurophysiological factors. Of major concern here is the identification of events that may have caused brain damage, of however slight a degree. These include perinatal events, traumas, febrile episodes, and toxemias. The possible role of neurotransmitters, recently receiving much attention, is still insufficiently documented to permit the interviewer to explore it realistically.

Nutritional factors. The interviewer explores dietary habits with the patient, and with the parents where indicated, to examine the likelihood that nutritional deficiencies or pathologies in eating may be affecting the symptom picture.

Familial, cultural, social, or economic factors. Such influences, when they determine symptoms that parallel or duplicate those associated with MBD, may be operating subtly as well as obviously. A child reading below age and I.Q. level may be responding to subtle or gross family pressures that discourage the acquisition of lexic skill. Or the child may be deterred from progress by a disinterested or financially limited school system. On the other hand, pressures may be extreme in some family and cultural settings and cause some children to give up, others to exist in states of nervous tension that resemble hyperkinesis as they strive to live up to expectations.

Emotional factors. It is well established that symptoms associated with MBD—activity and attention disorders, learning disabilities, sensory-motor dysfunctions, language disabilities—appear frequently among children with identifiable emotional disorders. There are, however, few if any MBD patients who do not manifest some emotional disturbance. The diagnostician seeks here to evaluate the probable extent or degree of emotional factors: Are they primary in the etiology of the symptoms? Or are they secondary responses to the dysfunctions, resulting from anxiety, depression, low self-esteem, frustration, impulsiveness?

Investigation of the patient-parent interaction is important here. Some opportunity to observe this interaction is provided in the waiting room and the consulting room.

Undoing the Symptoms—Treatment Planning

As the case history inquiry identifies symptoms and determines their probable causes, indications for treatment programs begin to take shape in the mind of the examiner. Treatment planning is guided by a principle of parsimony that targets a specific dysfunction with the intervention most likely to be effective for its correction. A minor dyslexia may require only a remedial reading program. A more severe dyslexia with emotional concomitants may suggest psychotherapy in addition to remedial instruction. Parental pressure or anxiety may dictate family therapy. Marked hyperkinesis may call for selective combinations of environmental manipulation, medication, behavioral modification, individual psychotherapy, and family therapy. A late adolescent or young adult who is severely learning disabled may benefit most from vocational training geared to his intact functions.

Interviewing Aids to the Case History Method

This section presents combinations of specific questions that I have found useful in making a case history evaluation of a person suspected of an equivocal neurological disorder. The questions are directed to the possibility of both neurological and emotional disorders, since so often these factors are intertwined. The interviewer will want to keep in mind also those basic queries about motor, sensory, cognitive, social, and emotional factors that were discussed in Chapter 7. Most of those basic queries and the questions that follow may be directed to the patient, to the parents, or to the teacher. Also included are inner-directed queries that I have found illuminating—questions that the examiner asks himself about the patient and about the meaning of the data he is collecting.

Events of Neurological Significance

Since a neurophysiological cause is a prime suspect in MBD, the inquiry must identify any insult or any injury of significance. Six major areas of neurological import usually are pursued:

1. *The pregnancy and birth process.* Any information the patient may have about his prenatal and birth events is sought. Did his parents speak of them? Was his mother bed-confined because of bleeding during pregnancy? Was his birth difficult? Protracted? Was he premature? Did he require incubation? Did

his mother have rubella? Was she ill in any other way? Was she emotionally disturbed? The victim of an accident? Was there Rh incompatibility? False labor? How long was labor? Was he post-term, a large baby, and subject to more than usual pressure? Were instruments used? Were any medications given? Is there any knowledge of his condition immediately following birth? Was he phlegmatic? Any difficulties in breathing, suckling, or swallowing? Convulsions? Deformation of the head? Was Caesarian section performed? The subject of birth is usually most ambiguous, buried in unavailable records, unrecorded information, layers of forgetfulness, and the attenuation and distortion of memory. Nonetheless, it should be pursued. If the patient is a child, the parents should be interviewed, and the pediatrician asked for information.

2. *Developmental history.* Psychotherapists have usually been trained to make inquiries about the emergence of developmental landmarks, feeding habits, toilet habits, posture control, ability to sit, stand, walk, speak, dress. To these should be added specific inquiries about any sensory or motor problems, and any early learning difficulties. Chapter 7 suggests a number of related queries.

3. *High fevers.* The cause, symptoms, duration, treatment, and sequelae of febrile episodes should be investigated. Reaction to innoculations of various kinds should be investigated, since a severe reaction can be equivalent to a serious disease episode. Was the patient ever convulsive or delirious during any febrile experience?

4. *Injuries to the head.* Was any injury accompanied by unconsciousness? Vomiting? Bleeding from the ears? If unconscious, how long? Was the patient hospitalized? How long? Was the patient examined by a physician? Were any special procedures undertaken? EEG? Skull X-rays? CAT scan? Neurological examination? Can reports of these be obtained? Among patients with a psychiatric history, a record of electroconvulsive therapy may be etiologically important to residual memory and cognitive defects, among other problems.

5. *Anesthesias.* Has the patient undergone surgery? How many times? For what? Duration and type of anesthesia in each case? Sequelae, if any? Cardiovascular surgery, on the increase as techniques are refined, continues to result in a significant incidence of postoperative neurological complications; hemiplegia, agnosias, blackouts, and giddiness have been reported.

6. *Poisoning.* Has the patient ever suffered toxemia from foods? Chemicals or gases other than anesthesias? Drugs? Paints? Sprays? Overdoses? Concern is growing about possible adverse effects of medications used in infancy and childhood.

Symptoms Suggestive of Neurological Disorder

The patient's motor behavior can be observed from the greeting in the waiting room, during the walk to the consulting room, and throughout the interview. Gait, posture, rate and character of movement are meaningful. Visible skin is scrutinized for scars, which can be investigated in the inquiry. These sometimes lead to accounts of faints, falls, assaults, or injuries of etiological consequence that would otherwise be overlooked.

Care is given to evaluating speech and thought processes. Any speech disturbance, such as slurring, slowness of reaction, articulation difficulties, perseveration, or grammatical failures should be noted. Too often there is a tendency to ascribe motor difficulties to neurological causes only and thought disturbances to psychogenic ones only. Vague answers, unresponsiveness to requests for elaboration, and seeming lack of insight may signal denial in the psychogenic sense, but they also may reflect a dysphasia. Illogical statements may reflect schizophrenic inappropriateness or looseness of associations, but they may also result from organic impairment.

The major sensory and motor functions, not usually directly observable in the office, developmental progressions, and integrative capacities are explored:

1. Does the patient have any knowledge about his motor development? When he began standing, walking, running, balancing?

2. Does he consider himself clumsier than most people? Drop things? Bump into things? Stumble or fall often?

3. Was he ever hyperactive, or sluggish, slow moving, inactive?

4. Does he recall difficulties in learning? To read? To write? Do arithmetic? The examiner should not be deterred from these queries because the patient is a college graduate or a Ph.D.; learning disability may nonetheless be present. A hearing difficulty may impair acquisition of language. Both language comprehension and expression may be affected, so as to suggest an aphasia or a thought disorder.

Uncovering significant particular experiences can be expedited by observing the manner in which the patient responds to certain questions. The manner in which the patient affirms or denies the experiences asked about in the following questions provides important clinical information, influencing the diagnostician's estimation of the probability that the symptom is indeed present. I have been impressed by the unequivocally affirmative response of some patients and the convincing clarity of their description when asked to illustrate the experience being queried. The responses of some are hesitatingly in the negative, as if something vaguely familiar has been touched upon, but not quite brought into sharp cognitive focus. The responses of others are hesitatingly affirmative, indicating that the patient may not have understood, or may be suggestible. In every case, the request for examples and descriptions guards against false discovery of what is not present.

Many of the following queries are directed toward identifying symptoms of epilepsy, since equivocal epilepsy sometimes accompanies MBD.

5. Has the patient experienced blurred vision or double vision, even when his eyes have been corrected, if necessary? Do moving lights make him tense, uneasy (flickering TV, passing automobile lights at night)?

6. Has he experienced phosphenes—hallucinations of light flashing by the side of the eyes in the dark, or seeming to explode?

7. Has he experienced dizziness not caused by drugs, heat, hunger, fever, hyperventilation, or asphyxia? Has he fainted under such circumstances? Has he had to hold on to keep from falling because the environment suddenly tilted?

8. Has he heard ringing sounds, high-pitched sounds, or an unintelligible rapid voice? The presence of laterality in such experiences should be determined.

9. Does he experience tingling sensations in the fingertips or toes? These are sometimes experienced as electric-like buzzings, as if the person has received a shock. They may be described as itching, with need to scratch the member. Do these members become numb without cause? These sensations must be differentiated from the commonplace feeling after a limb has "gone to sleep" and is recovering. If these sensations have been experienced, inquiry should be made concerning laterality: both sides or one?

10. Does he become angry without apparent cause?

11. Has he experienced blackouts? These are episodes in which while talking with or listening to someone, he is suddenly unable to hear even when his name is called, or he hears the other person but is unable to respond. These states must be differentiated from preoccupation, from which the person can be aroused to respond to a call.

12. Has he experienced altered states of consciousness? These may be reported as feelings of depersonalization. Or the person, fully awake, suddenly begins to dream; he is aware that he is both awake and dreaming. Often the experience is frightening; the patient may fear that he is insane or that he is the victim of mysterious and dangerous forces. These states should be differentiated from daydreaming, which can be ended at will or in response to a summons.

13. Has he experienced an aura-like state in which he has felt strange? Or feared that some nameless, shapeless, unfocused danger may befall him? In such states the patient may be fearful of leaving the home or may require companionship for security. Obviously, these states must be differentiated from both phobias and free-floating anxiety states, a differential diagnosis that is not always easy.

14. Any possible automatic behavior is investigated. Has the patient been doing things he was unaware he was doing? Or started out with one destination in mind and found himself at another, without memory that he had decided to alter his course? Or without memory of how he got to the place where he suddenly finds himself?

15. Favored medications are investigated. Sometimes a clue to a psychomotor epilepsy is found when a patient reports a fondness for some of the older anticonvulsive drugs such as the barbiturates. The amphetamines also have an anticonvulsant effect. Patients may recount that such drugs gave them a sense of calmness and security, of evenness and composure that they lack without them.

16. Disturbances of body image are explored. Has the patient had the impression of alterations in the size of hands, feet, or head?

17. Has he experienced impairment of movement, gesturing, walking?

18. Has he experienced distortions in the apparent shape, size, or distance of objects?

19. Have there been disturbances of speech, reading, calculation, musical skill?

20. Has he experienced difficulty with memory? If so, is it general? Of events? Of material just read? Does it involve words? Inability to find the needed word to say or write may suggest anomia.

21. Has there been any sudden alteration of audition? Increased sensitivity to sound? Music seeming to change into noise? Has there been any fluctuation in the comprehension of speech?

22. Is there increased sensitivity to taste? To smell? Does a favorite odor become unpleasant, then pleasing again?

23. Has the patient experienced any disturbance of spatial orientation? Taking wrong turns? Putting his arm into the wrong sleeve?

24. Has he experienced any impairment of reading? Recognizing numbers, letters, musical notations? Has the visual field become constricted or limited in any way?

25. Has the patient experienced writing difficulties in forming letters, words, or numbers?

26. Has there been any loss of efficiency in writing and reading? Is writing less fluid? Reading less rapid?

27. Has there been difficulty in arithmetical processes? Does the patient recognize numbers when written and spoken? Can he do mental calculations appropriate to age, intelligence, and education?

Examining for Laterality and Cerebral Dominance

Laterality of hand, eye, ear, and foot functions provides insight into a person's presumed cerebral dominance. This data may allow some significant hypotheses concerning etiology; localized cerebral dysfunction, conflict of dominance, or maturational lag may be suggested (see Chapter 2). Most people are right-handed, and so, as with speech, their "handedness" is controlled by the left hemisphere of the brain. However, considerable partial left-handedness and ambidexterity exists in people, and some evidence indicates that in left-handed and partially left-handed people the right hemisphere assumes more control over speech functions than is usual.

"Handedness" may have diagnostic and localizing significance. If a right-handed person demonstrates a right hand weaker than his left in the absence of muscular disease, a left-cerebral-hemisphere difficulty may be suspected. Where the left hand is significantly weaker than is expected in a right-handed person, a right-hemisphere involvement may be suggested. The patient, therefore, is examined carefully as to "handedness." Obviously, the use of the hand in writing helps establish "handedness." When the patient also is asked to go through the motions of driving a nail, opening a door, shaking hands, throwing a ball, or using a fork, differences may be found.

Cerebral dominance also is also explored by having the patient go through the motions of kneeling, kicking an imaginary ball, and stepping on an imaginary bug, to establish which limb is used.

A first step in determining eye dominance is to establish relative visual acuity of the two eyes. Does the patient have a good eye and a bad eye? If the patient needs glasses, they should be worn during this part of the examination. Two conditions of viewing preference are checked: close and far. For the former the patient is asked to put a hole in a 3 × 5 card to one eye, close the other eye, and peer at an object on the table before him. For far-viewing dominance the patient is instructed to stand at one wall or corner of a room while the examiner stands opposite, as far apart as the room permits. The patient is asked to extend one arm, pointing the index finger of that arm at the examiner and sighting along it with one eye closed. The dominance of the eyes also may be explored by having the patient look through a paper tube as if it were a telescope.

Luria (8) suggests a useful eye-dominance test. The patient, with both eyes open, lines up a pencil held vertically in his hand with a vertical line on the opposite wall. While maintaining this alignment, the patient's right eye is covered (or is closed); then the left eye is covered while the right eye remains open. If the pencil appears to move to the right when the right eye is covered, and not to move when the left eye is covered, the right eye is dominant. The opposite result, movement of pencil to the left when the left eye is covered, demonstrates dominance of the left eye.

Determination of ear dominance requires dichotic listening instrumentation and is usually not possible for the interviewer.

"Handedness," "sideness," and cerebral dominance are not always clear-cut. Lateral preference may vary from hand to eye to foot in the same person, or within the organ tested. A person may be ambidextrous, or show a mixed dominance for the eye or the foot, or for two or all of the organs tested. This kind of finding confounds the determination of any lateralized dysfunction, so that the interviewer should be wary in interpreting the observations made.

The foregoing queries obviously do not include all brain-behavior relationships. They do explore the major sensory modalities, paroxysmal phenomena, motor abnormalities, language problems, learning difficulties, and cerebral dominance. Also, they often elicit, by association, accounts of significant events or behavior not specifically covered by the queries themselves.

Projective Queries

Another type of query—the projective question—has similar power to evoke associations that sometimes lead to a neurological clue, as well as supply the psychodynamic material to which they are addressed. Thus a patient asked for the worst thing that ever happened in his life may recount loss of a loved person, or the experience may be a serious automobile accident, or a subictal state. Ten such question areas are suggested here.[1] The inventive clinician can readily add to them.

1. The earliest memory of an event or experience in the patient's life. The age at which it occured. The feeling associated with the experience.
2. A dream history: any dream during childhood that is recalled; recurrent dreams; one or two recent dreams.
3. In the patient's judgment, what is his best quality, trait, or characteristic? His worst?
4. The best thing the patient has done in his life? The worst?
5. The best thing that ever happened to him? The worst thing?
6. If the patient could relive his life what would he change? What would he keep the same?
7. The most pleasant thing the patient can imagine or think of? The most unpleasant?
8. Three wishes the patient would express if they could magically come true?
9. A favorite joke.
10. The worst, the most serious, problem the patient has ever experienced.

The Psychodiagnostic Formulation

To belabor this point, perhaps, the evaluation of MBD requires consideration of many etiological possibilities, many types of symptoms. Among these, emotional factors are prominent: the emotional disturbance of many children is manifested primarily in a learning disorder, while many adolescent and adult patients who are reacting to MBD seek psychotherapy. To guide the interviewer in sorting through the emotional signs and symptoms, I have devised (11) a set of queries that are seldom—if ever—addressed to the patient, but rather guide the interviewer through the inquiry and help him formulate in his mind a reasonable statement of psychodynamic cause and effect. Interventions based upon that statement can then be selected. These questions provide the structure for a neuropsychodiagnostic inquiry as well as a purely psychodiagnostic one.

1. *What is the presenting complaint?* The complaint is the manifest reason for the individual to seek treatment, or for the family to be concerned. It is discomfort that motivates a patient to give up time and money and to accept the invasion of his privacy necessary to obtain relief. The therapist asks himself if the

[1] Drs. Molly Harrower and Bernard Landis have been helpful in their suggestions and ideas for developing this type of investigation. I am most appreciative of their thoughts.

complaint is the real trouble, a derivative expression of the real problem, or perhaps a mask for it.

2. *What has precipitated the complaint?* Emotional disturbances often are better understood when one knows details of the circumstances in which the patient first experienced the complaint. Inquiry may elicit facts about the nature of the stimulus which precipitated the disturbance, the facts that aroused discomfort, anxiety, depression, confusion, uncertainty. They can evoke a history of preceding related events. If precipitating events make no psychodynamic sense in relationship to the complaint, an etiology other than the psychogenic may be involved, some other emotional factor may be causal, or strong defensive denial may be obscuring the facts.

3. *Are there antecedents analogous to the present situation?* The search for antecedents to a current situation is for information to support or refute a tentative hypothesis based on the presenting complaint and its precipitating circumstances.

Verification of a past situation psychodynamically similar to the present one but at an earlier stage in development confirms an hypothesis about psychodynamics, reassures the diagnostician about his view of the causes of the patient's disturbance, and heightens confidence in the treatment interventions he may advise. Even when the present situation does not replicate preceding ones, exactly or in part, earlier incidents still may provide information that rounds out understanding of a current emotional disturbance. Failure to find any related past event may indicate that the disturbance is indeed of recent origin—an important fact for treatment, since it usually increases the probability of favorable prognosis.

4. *What do the symptoms mean?* Symptoms generally may be understood to indicate something beyond themselves. Three levels of meaning are considered: (a) a universal meaning as the result of conflict, trauma, or deprivation; (b) a generic meaning, established through clinical experience and psychoanalytic investigation—for example, in depression, the dynamics frequently found to be causal are inward deflection of rage, loss of love, damage to self-esteem, or deception; and (c) the specific individual nuance of the generic symptom meaning—for example, the family and its culture may encourage acting-out.

When the patient's symptoms can be understood on all these levels, confidence in a psychogenic etiology is reinforced. When such understanding is equivocal or lacking, further exploration through continued interviewing or psychological testing may be considered, or causes other than the psychogenic may be explored.

5. *What is the state of the ego and its functions?* Some function of the ego is affected by every emotional disturbance or behavioral disorder (3). Knowledge of the individual ego functions, the usual manifestations when they are disrupted, and the means to evaluate both strength and weakness in each function enable the diagnostician to identify needed changes and advise effective

interventions (1). Eleven ego functions have been identified and described (2): reality testing, sense of reality, judgment, regulation and control of drives, object relations, thought processes, adaptive regression, defensive functioning, stimulus barrier, autonomous functioning, and synthetic functioning.

A weak or disrupted function does not by itself warrant an effort to strengthen that function by a specific intervention that has been found effective in seemingly similar ego-function weaknesses, since a variety of etiological pathologies—neurological, psychological, cultural—may produce a similar ego deficit. For example, either conflict over rage or sexuality, or the fear of lapses in *petit mal,* may promote aversive object relations. A schizoid-like aversiveness in an aphasia victim may express fear of communication difficulties. The ego expression in each case may be similar, but the effective treatment may be different for each. Etiology is a crucial variable in the use of an ego-function scheme as a guide to intervention.

6. *What changes are required to restore homeostasis?* If the etiology is psychic conflict, resolution of the conflict is expected to reduce symptoms. If the cause is psychic trauma, a gradual discharge of threatening affect and the restoration of adaptive competence is expected to be therapeutic. If the root cause is prodromal anxiety in a seizure disorder, control of the seizures is necessary. This question asks the diagnostician to specify the change or changes—emotional, familial, physiological, or neurological—that will relieve the patient of his complaint. Psychodynamically, the formulation combines the concept of homeostasis with Freud's structural view of personality—ego, id, and superego. Freud's structural view hypothesized an imbalance of major components of the personality caused by neurosis. The hypothesis further suggests how balance may be restored: in one person, the ego may be strengthened either by intensifying or decreasing use of a defense, in another person by redirecting an impulse or mitigating it, and in still another by increasing or decreasing the superego.

7. *What treatment interventions are most likely to restore homeostasis?* The choice of therapeutic intervention should not be limited by the training or theoretical bias of the therapist. Treatment should be one selected from among the array of interventions because that one promises more for shifting the balance in an individual suffering from a diagnosed, that is, an observed and comprehended, disequilibrium. One major consideration is whether there should be any intervention at all, an important caveat. In some individuals, any intervention may worsen an already bad situation: for example, the patient's ego strengths or real-life resources may be inadequate for containing the strains that therapy, however supportive, would almost inevitably evoke in order to achieve the therapeutic goal.

8. *What therapeutic allies are available?* Allies to the therapeutic process can be identified within the patient in his environment, and among his relationships. Intra-patient allies are motivations to change, strong ego functions that may be enlisted to bolster weaker ones, and the desire for pleasure and for work. Exter-

nal to the patient as potential allies are people who can and will support or abet his therapeutic progress. Defective judgment in a patient may be offset if he can be persuaded to accept the counsel of a friend with more rational approaches. The supportive availability of friends and family members as safeguards where there is danger of suicide cannot be stressed enough.

9. *What shall be the sequence in the treatment of this person?* Priorities in therapy should be set by the importance of the various goals to be achieved, that is, their effects upon the quality of the patient's life now and in the future. The probabilities of reaching therapeutic goals are considered. One objective may be quickly and easily reached; others may require long training periods or the slow uncovering of dynamics.

When a neurological problem is possible, first priority may be given to a neurological examination, especially if a proliferating lesion is suspected. Medical consultation and anticonvulsant medication may come first when subictal states are creating anxiety. When a change in attitudes toward a child with MBD is needed to relieve parental pressure, family therapy or conferences with the parents may be chosen as the first procedure, to be followed by remedial teaching or behavior modification.

10. *What is the prognosis?* To answer this question, the therapist reviews the answers to all of the foregoing. And there is evidence (9) that a therapist's clear comprehension of the dynamics of a psychogenic disorder increases the probability of a favorable outcome. Expectation of patient improvement by both therapist and patient (7), motivation, capacity for insight, and strength of ego are all to be considered here as enhancing prognosis. In neurological problems, prognosis may depend upon the known effectiveness of anticonvulsant or antihyperkinesis drugs, the length of interval from an injury, or upon physical factors such as the mass of a lesion.

Where MBD is the primary disorder, the age of the patient combines with the degree of severity of the disorder and especially the quality of therapeutic allies, to determine prognosis. In all degrees of severity, early detection and treatment and constructive family support are major ingredients of treatment success.

The History in Relation to Other Diagnostic Methods

The indispensability of the history appears beyond debate. It often explains the etiology, especially when the observed symptoms are suspected to be caused by neurological factors. And to repeat, identification of etiology enables more precise selection of intervention.

The history also may provide developmental information that details the psychosociobiological development of the person, the context in which he grew, the time and circumstances in which the symptoms appeared, and how they progressed or waned. This information has both diagnostic and etiological significance.

This invaluable diagnostic information does not, however, warrant reliance upon the history alone. Our diagnoses are hypothetical at best, despite the narcissistic investment of some professionals in oracular judgments. For the welfare of the patient, corroboration of a diagnosis should always be sought beyond the history.

Moreover, many histories are unproductive of diagnostic clues. The neurological and psychological examinations are therefore indispensable adjuncts to the history in MBD. All are part of the diagnostician's armamentarium.

Chapter 9

The Neurological Examination

As with almost all matters connected with MBD, debate attends the use of the standard neurological examination in the diagnosis of the disorder. This chapter examines that debate. It reviews the indications for neurological tests, describes the usual or standard neurological examination, and reviews some attempts to increase its effectiveness in diagnosing MBD.

Indications for the Neurological Examination

In some patients, the data from direct observation of behavior, the history, academic records, and psychodiagnostic and neuropsychological techniques will point to the need for a neurological exploration to explain the symptoms. Patterns that suggest a possible neurological etiology include these:

1. The history turns up events of possible neurological impact: difficulties or injuries during gestation or birth, traumas, severe febrile episodes, protracted exposure to anesthesias, toxemias, diseases invading the central nervous system.

2. The patient displays subtle seizure phenomena; these may involve any sensory or motor modality, balance, altered states of consciousness, memory lapses, blackouts, or automatic behavior. Some MBD symptoms (a learning disability or attention disorder, e.g.) may be the consequence of *petit mal* attention lapses.

3. Academic-test and psychological-test data reflect a marked difference

among brain functions, one that exceeds the usual expectation for such scatter. These differences may appear on the Wechsler scales, in pronounced organic indication on the *Bender,* in the lateralization tests, in the projective techniques, and, of course, in neuropsychological testing.

4. A disruptive emotional state (anxiety, depersonalization, *déjà vu,* depression, hypochondriasis) develops that cannot be clearly connected psychodynamically to precipitating circumstances, or to any idiosyncratic meaning to the patient.

5. A sudden emotional change is experienced that cannot be ascribed to specific precipitating circumstances. Such change may be accompanied by sleep disturbances, ravenous hunger and/or thirst, metabolic disturbances, or alteration in sexual appetite.

6. The patient reports a gradual alteration in acuity of vision, hearing, touch, motor control, balance, or in skills such as typing, driving, or playing a musical instrument.

Suspicion increases from possibility to probability as the observations from one source are supported by data from another source or method of examination. The diagnostician must then decide what to do next. Should he proceed with a treatment plan and keep the situation under observation? Refer the patient immediately to a neurologist for examination?

An intermediate step is possible, one that exercises the ethical responsibility not to make judgments beyond one's training, while it safeguards the well-being of the patient and avoids alarming him unnecessarily. This step requires the diagnostician to develop a professional liaison with a neurologist. The cooperating neurologist must be willing to evaluate data communicated to him by the diagnostician from the history, clinical observation, and psychological tests, to estimate the probability that neurological and adjunctive examinations are justifiable. Necessarily, he must be one who gives full weight to cognitive and behavioral manifestations: He must be personally known to be careful and persistent in exploring symptoms of a patient's possible anxiety or depression, language difficulties, limited intelligence, perhaps psychotic behavior.

Where such a professional relationship is enjoyed, telephone conferences with the neurologist can guide the diagnostician. Only when neurological exploration appears justified will the diagnostician have to inform the patient that some of his symptoms may have a neurological base and, if this proves true, that the success of therapy depends upon appropriate medical treatment. If the neurologist reasonably suspects from the data given to him via telephone that an expanding lesion is present, and the patient's life is at stake, the diagnostician must attempt vigorously to persuade the patient to cooperate with the neurological exploration. How far he goes in making the danger to life explicit will depend upon the probabilities delineated for him by the neurologist.

The neurological consultation by telephone should be part of the practicing equipment of the diagnostician in MBD. The diagnostician's willingness to face his own resistive reaction, often unconscious, to the very idea of a neurological lesion is an important aspect of his professional equipment. We cannot minimize the potentialities for pain, loss of function, and death that are possible with a brain lesion, nor can we hide from them. Nor should we overlook the vast reassurance and relief that a patient can enjoy when mysterious symptoms are elucidated. The facts must be sought, this being a matter in which truth cannot be overvalued.

The Standard Neurological Examination

A physical examination of functions of the nervous system, an array of tests with special instruments and radioisotopes, and certain tests requiring minor or major surgical intrusion comprise the usual neurological armamentarium.

The Physical Examination

Although differences in the scope of examination exist among neurologists, my experience is that with most consultants the standard examination focuses upon subcortical central nervous system functions. Cognitive, affective, and behavioral functions are usually not investigated; "hard" neurological signs are given credence but "soft" signs receive scant attention.

According to Voeller (36), four major areas are evaluated:

1. Level of consciousness.
2. Cranial-nerve functions. The integrity of olfaction, vision, gustation, and audition, and the muscle systems involved with these.
3. Gross motor functions. Hand preference, gait, posture, muscle, tone, strength and mass, deep and superficial reflexes.
4. Sensory functions. Generally those tested are the haptic sensations of touch, pain, vibration, and double simultaneous stimulation.

To these DeLeo (7) adds general estimates of some cerebral functions: intellectual, memory, affective, social-behavior.

Essentially, the standard neurological examination is addressed to identifying brain lesions resulting from trauma, stroke, tumor, or other disease. Since the lesion in MBD, if one is present, is subtle, the standard examination produces many negative findings among children suspected of MBD on the weight of other evidence.

Special-Instrument Tests

Special-instrument procedures increase the validity of deductions about the existence, type, and location of any lesion, although, like all test procedures, they have margins of error, more or less wide.

The Electroencephalogram (EEG)

The frequency and voltages of oscillating potentials arising from activity in brain tissue is recorded and measured by the EEG. The test has been widely used for about 50 years, but the validity of its diagnosis of lesion and location is still debated. Positive findings of pathology are generally accepted, but normal findings evoke less confidence, because so many have been obtained in cases of brain pathology later established, by autopsy and epileptic seizures, for example.

EEG recordings are affected by factors other than pathology. These include age, task demands, sensory excitement, levels of consciousness, coughing, blinking, sneezing, metabolic disturbances, and thought disorders. In part, the impaired confidence in validity may arise from the failure to incorporate these factors in the examination, as well as from certain technical problems. Efforts to surmount these difficulties have improved EEG validity.

Norms have been established within limits for the rate, regularity, amplitude, and configuration of recorded tracings. These norms are based upon age, resting state (i.e., metabolic equilibrium), and the absence of known or suspected brain pathology. The persistence of the validity problem is highlighted, however, by findings that a "normal" adult population produces abnormal departures from these norms in 5 to 15 percent of the group. Norms have also been established for children. These are marked by predictable changes in pattern from birth to adolescence, with more gradual changes thereafter.

Good EEG procedures now provide contrasts with the usual waking-resting state, used as a base line. Separate readings will also be taken while the subject is sedated, or stimulated by flashing lights, or performing cognitive tasks such as reading, or when induced to hyperventilate. Single recordings are now frequently compared with others obtained on different days and at different hours.

For decades, the reading and interpretation of EEG recordings was a laborious, time-consuming task, requiring calipers and rulers to measure the characteristics of the obtained tracings, counting each variable frequency by hand, so to speak. Computer technology is replacing this method of analysis and improving the interpretations that result. Computer methods for banding together a number of recordings into a consolidated reading have also contributed to accuracy of diagnosis. Since, despite the available computer and banding methods, visual scanning by the individual electroencephalographer is still widely used, the double-blind interpretation remains a useful check on accuracy.

A fundamental detail of EEG practice affecting validity is the number and placement of the electrodes that pick up the brain's electrical activity. Initially, electrodes were placed on the surface of the scalp. Then needle electrodes were developed, to be placed under the scalp. More rarely, depth electrodes are inserted into direct contact with brain tissue. Now nasopharyngeal leads may be inserted through the nostrils, and advanced into the nasopharynx, relative also to the inferior medial surface of the temporal lobes. The effort in placing electrodes is to record as much as possible of the brain's electrical activity. At present a maximum of about one-third of the brain is available to electro-encephalography. But only a centimeter, approximately, of the outer and ventral medial surface is available to electrodes of any type. Despite their small size, all electrodes are enormous in contrast to the microscopic brain cells, so that each electrode picks up the activity of numerous cells rather than a single one.

CAT Scan (Computerized Axial Tomography)

A relatively new procedure, computerized axial tomography, collects numerous X-ray pictures taken by an instrument that rotates around the long axis of any body part. In our area of concern, the CAT is a scan of the head. Numerous pictures collected from successive sections are collated along the axis by computer into a single composite picture for each section. This allows X-ray studies across and all along the brain, a technique that has proved unusually productive of diagnostic data. Comparison of the agreement between neuropsychological test findings and CAT scans, EEG findings, and standard neurological examinations has found best agreement with the CAT scan (34).

An even more recent development (positron emission transverse tomography—PETT) is reaching beyond structure to the measurement of physiological activity in the brain—edema resulting from injury, blood-brain-barrier permeability, drug actions.

The brain scan is a related but simpler procedure. A small amount of radioactive material is injected, exposing the patient to less radiation than a chest X-ray. Exposures are made in various planes, but not cross-sectionally, as is possible with the CAT scan.

Tests Requiring Minor Surgery

Lumbar puncture. A hollow needle is passed between lumbar vertebrae into the spinal cord. A sample of spinal fluid is extracted and examined histologically for evidences of blood or tumor cells.

Wada test. Amytal is injected selectively into the carotid arteries, anesthetizing each cerebral hemisphere in turn, to determine which hemisphere is the site of any lesion present.

Pneumoencephalogram. Spinal fluid is withdrawn and replaced by air. The air enters the ventricles of the brain and the spaces surrounding the brain, more sharply outlining their size and shape for X-ray pictures.

Angiography. Radiopaque material injected into the blood stream circulates through the brain's blood vessels, enabling X-ray examination of the brain's vascular network.

Brain surgery and biopsy. Surgery allows direct examination of the brain's gross anatomy. Biopsy is the histopathological study of small sections of brain tissue removed from suspected sites.

Value of the Neurological Examination

The value of the standard neurological examination in the diagnosis of MBD is not universally accepted (18). Increasingly the evidence, however "inconsistent and circumstantial," indicates that the neurological procedure is more productive when extended beyond its classical assessments to include equivocal signs, finer signs, and age-specific evaluations of sensory, motor, integrational, and cognitive levels, and when special procedures are added in obtaining EEG recordings (1, 15, 19).

Voeller (36), a pediatric neurologist, suggests that the limitations of the classical neurological examination arise from its relatively limited objective: to find lesions if they are there. In MBD, lesions when present are usually formed early in the life of the patient; they are often subtle and diffuse. Lesions at any time of life vary in character. Some are expanding, others are receding, still others are static; some are gross, some fine to the point of being molecular. Many produce effects far beyond their site, through the process of diaschsis, in which the effects of an acute lesion are transmitted to a remote area by connecting fiber tracts.

The present standard neurological examination is not equipped to rule out the submicroscopic or molecular lesions that are generally believed to be the cause of "soft" signs, according to Gross (11). And Reitan (24) has demonstrated that "hard" signs are not necessarily to be found even in clear-cut neuropathy: 35 percent of patients with diffuse brain damage resulting from cerebrovascular disease produced normal EEGs; contrast studies failed to identify a lesion in 50 percent; all showed only minimal positive signs on standard neurological examination. These findings correlate positively with those of Benton and Joynt (2), who state that behavioral changes after cerebrovascular accidents may be inconspicuous, and discernible only in changes in reaction time, decision-making time, or in short-term memory, and only when compared with the performances of normal peers or with the patient's own pre-pathology level, if that is obtainable. Few learning-disabled children display "hard" neurological signs, and even when present, such "hard" abnormalities do not usually explain much about the learning disability.

The examination, Voeller further notes, is not reliable, in the sense of replicability. Observed findings in a patient vary from one time of day to another, from one day to the next, from one neurologist to another. Additionally, age and I.Q. norms for the neurological examination are vague or lacking, so that the neurological evaluations of patients of different age and I.Q. levels are correspondingly obscure.

In similar fashion, the value of the EEG is questioned (28). Many children in whom MBD is suspected produce normal EEG tracings yet function abnormally in learning tasks or on psychological examination. Hughes (13) reports from a survey of EEG in dyslexia that no studies have been able to correlate types and degrees of abnormality of EEG tracings with prognoses, either poor or better. Nor does any data indicate that dyslexic children with positive EEG spike patterns improve in reading skill when treated with anticonvulsants. A nationwide survey (18) of diagnostic procedures found the EEG "widely and erroneously regarded as the *sine qua non* for the identification of Minimal Brain Dysfunction." The survey was unable to identify any EEG abnormality with MBD or diffuse brain damage.

Yet the neurological examination and its associated procedures cannot be overlooked when brain dysfunction is suspected. Through its evaluation of subcortical levels of behavior, the neurological examination tests for the presence of brain conditions or progressive diseases that may demand immediate therapy. It may detect nonprogressive diseases such as seizure disorders that require continuous medication. Further, the neurological examination may contribute to confidence that the behavioral, perceptual, motor, and cognitive dysfunctions observed are not due to such conditions as parietal-lobe tumors which tend to cause behaviors nearly identical.

A major deterrent to the effectiveness of any diagnostic procedure for MBD is the difficulty in defining the disorder; as we have seen, it is a syndrome of syndromes. The enormous variety of symptoms and causes make cohesive study groups virtually impossible to organize.

Increasing the Value of the Neurological Examination

A key to improving the contribution of the neurological examination here appears to rest in expanding its scope with variations and additions, as discussed below. These are exemplified by Voeller's (36) conclusion that its diagnostic efficiency can be increased not only by efforts to improve replicability and quantifiability but chiefly by scrutiny of a wider range of behavior, language-processing difficulties, subtle parietal-lobe dysfunctions, academic performance, and psychological-emotional reactions. These, she feels certain, are likely to shed more light on learning disabilities than do sensorimotor and reflex dysfunction alone.

Since minimal brain dysfunction is by its nature an "equivocal" neurological disorder, not an obvious one, it can be reasoned that a search for equivocal or "soft" neurological signs would add to the value of neurological examination. This suggestion is but one of the prominent and persistent suggestions for such improvement. Others are to link the neurological with the neuropsychological investigation and to use specialized EEG procedures.

"Soft" Neurological Signs

"Soft" signs are those that "suggest" or arouse suspicion of neurological pathology but are associated only with the slightest discernable dysfunction, if any. They are likely to appear inconsistently or infrequently in a patient, without correlation to other symptoms. So ambiguous are they in their manifestations that Ingram (14) argues that they deter the neurologist from pursuing a proper diagnosis that could be readily identified if vigorously sought. Soft signs should not be categorized as real signs, he seems to argue, lest they distract the neurologist from his pursuit of real neurological disorders, real diagnosis. But he illustrates his argument by citing some seemingly innocuous signs that may have profound neurological import: (1) difficulty in properly placing the hands, lips, or tongue on request may be symptoms of a congenital dyspraxia; (2) a mild speech dysfunction may prove to be due to suprabulbar palsy; (3) left-handedness and clumsiness may be the only manifest symptoms of a minimal hemiplegia.

The argument is not a convincing one against the value of identifying soft signs. Indeed, it reasons forcibly that they may at times point to serious conditions and should not be overlooked. Uncertain signs are ubiquitous in neurology, and signal conditions varying in seriousness. Difficulties in spatial organization, arising from a sensory dysfunction, impair skills in dressing and eating, in judgments of time. Interpersonal relationships may become pathological because of a dysphasia developing in early life. The repeated occurrence of such signs among the emotionally disturbed does not necessarily mean that the signs are psychopathological rather than neurological in origin. They may instead confirm the generally accepted hypothesis that subtle neurological dysfunctions cause emotional disturbance, just as do gross ones.

The convincing argument for extending the neurological examinations in MBD to search for soft signs is that MBD usually is, we have seen, an equivocal disorder, presenting equivocal symptoms. To uncover an equivocal, ambiguous disorder, the presence of hard clear-cut signs can scarcely be the criterion.

Among the many soft signs identified in numerous studies (2, 4, 8, 9, 12, 15, 16, 19, 20, 23, 25, 26, 30) are the following indicators:

Motor impersistence.
Astereognosis (poor haptic perception of objects or forms).
Agraphesthesia (impaired perception of symbols written on the skin, usually of the fingers, with a stylus).
Extinction of bilateral simultaneous stimulation.

Bilateral hyper- or hypo-reflexia of marked degree.

Coordination dysfunctions.

Dysfunctions of balance, usually more marked when visual cues are absent.

Dysfunctions of gait.

Movement disorders in skipping, hopping, standing on one foot.

Speech dyspraxia.

Activity levels either above or below normal.

Difficulties in auditory-visual integration.

Choreiform movements (irregular spasms of limbs or facial muscles).

Slight anisocoria (inequality of diameter of pupils).

Esotropia (convergent strabismus).

Hearing deficits.

Mild visual-field and retinal disorders.

Hypotonia or hypertonia of muscle status.

Positive Romberg sign (greater difficulty standing on one foot with eyes closed than with eyes open).

Difficulties in tandem walking.

Difficulties in bringing a limb from one position to its opposite: from flexion to extension, from pronation to supination.

Past-point disorders in touching finger to nose, heel to toe.

Poor imitation of rapid alternating movements exhibited by the examiner: opposing fingers to the thumb of each hand; hitting one hand alternately with the palmar and dorsal side of the other.

Synkinesis (moving one hand unintentionally while moving the other purposively).

Difficulty identifying right/left body parts.

Tics; grimaces.

Apraxia of face or tongue.

Peculiarities of posture or resting position that indicate persistence of a dominant avoiding reaction.

Clumsiness, tremor, and ataxia may be tested in children as early as three years of age by having the child place marbles in a cylinder whose diameter is only slightly larger than the marbles; smoothness of movement and fair rapidity is usual by three years (18). Other useful tests are repeatedly touching the fingers to the thumb in sequence; alternating movements of the hands; having the child write to dictation so that he may be observed directly for slowness and confusion (15).

A number of soft signs have been assembled into a standard examination by the National Institute of Mental Health. PANESS (Physical and Neurological Examination for Soft Signs) was developed by a drug-evaluation unit in NIMH to test its ability to reflect drug effects. One study (4) found that it did not discriminate hyperactive from normal subjects. As we have seen repeatedly, establishment of cohesive MBD groups that adhere rigorously to diagnostic criteria appears virtually impossible because of the diverse subsyndromes. This experimental difficulty for research does not controvert the use of soft signs to improve the diagnosis of an individual patient. The work of Peters *et al.* (23) shows clearly that the diverse, variable symptoms of MBD require a wide array of different tests if an individual pattern is to be separated out from that diversity. In their study, they applied 80 "soft-sign" neurological tests to 82 boys, aged 8 to 11, with learning disabilities and/or behavioral problems, and to 45 age-matched control subjects. Forty-four of the tests proved to be significantly discriminating. Meaningful to the clinician responsible for a patient is their eminently reasonable rationale that this extensive investigation is justified because no one neurological test can be expected to correlate significantly with a specific cognitive defect. Instead, they hypothesized that where cognitive defects existed, some sign or signs of motor deviation could be detected. Their rationale is supported by Benton's (1) finding in the literature that the most frequently observed neurological sign in dyslexia is some type of motor disturbance. Among these the most prominent is clumsiness. Less frequently reported are dyspraxia, hyperkinesis, motor impersistence, and choreiform movements.

Specialized EEG Techniques

Some recent efforts to improve the general validity of the EEG were discussed earlier in this chapter. The value of these efforts in MBD has received some attention.

The elusiveness of "hard" data in EEG patterns in dyslexia is remarked in the survey of the literature by Benton (1), who reports that the findings are equivocal, with both dyslexia and controls showing similar patterns. His observation that the Visual Evoked Response (VER) may possibly be associated with poor reading highlights the effort to extend the EEG examination beyond its classical techniques, as is being done with the neurological examination. Satterfield (27), for example, reports that the VER is of lower amplitude and is longer lasting in MBD subjects than in controls. Zambelli *et al.* (37) found that impairment of electrophysiological and behavioral selective attention as measured by auditory-evoked responses is correlated with behavioral indices.

An interesting EEG innovation (35) suggests that continuous EEG recordings made while a child is performing a task may show that disruption of learning is correlated with transient EEG abnormalities.

Sklar *et al.* (31, 32) recorded EEG data for both dyslexics and controls under five different conditions that used special spectral binding techniques. The groups were reliably differentiated by two conditions of recording: resting with eyes closed and reading a text. The most prominent difference occurred in the parieto-occipital area during rest periods. Here the dyslexic children recorded more energy in both the 3-7 Hz and 16-32 Hz bands, while the normals recorded more energy in the 9–14 Hz band. During reading activity, the observations of the 16–32 Hz band were reversed, with the normal children showing more activity.

Another difference was observed in the "coherence of activity" between results from variously located scalp leads. In dyslexics, coherence was higher among leads within the same hemisphere. In normals, coherence was higher between similar regions in the two hemispheres. These data suggest hypotheses about cerebral localization of functions and lateral hemispheric dominance.

That EEG differences exist between dyslexics and normals but that more subtle techniques are needed to identify them, the conclusion of the Sklar studies, finds support among other workers. Oettinger's (22) clinical experience is that the EEG *if done carefully* will show abnormality among 50 to 80 percent of MBD children. He takes hour-long recordings, and separate recordings while the child is awake, asleep, subject to photic stimulation, and hyperventilating. If normal findings are obtained, he repeats the procedures on another day at a different hour.

A new technique, BEAM (brain-electrical-activity mapping), appears capable of differentiating the EEG data (both usual and evoked potential) of children with learning disabilities from those of normals. It is a data-consolidation method, presenting findings more concisely than before.

Selection, rather than consolidation, of pattern by computer has led to valuable developmental norms in EEG. Using evoked potentials, researchers have found that normal children of different ethnic and cultural groups all record the same EEG pattern or profile at the same age, while children with learning disabilities within these groups record significant deviations (29).

And Conners (5) notes that a clearer differentiation of dyslexics from normals is likely with an "active challenge" to the brain (evoked potential) during the EEG recordings, especially if the content of the challenge is verbal or semantic.

Even with equivocal and inconsistent findings, the data persistently suggest the value of the neurological and EEG examination in the diagnosis of MBD conditions. To be emphasized are extensive investigations rather than limited ones, credit to "soft" signs rather than insistence upon "hard" signs, and specialized techniques. Myklebust (21) reports an unusually extensive exploration of criteria for the identification, diagnosis, and subsequent treatment of children with learning disabilities. A very large population of 2,704 underachieving children were given opthalmological, neurological, EEG, educational, and psychological examinations. The educational and psychological procedures revealed cognitive deficits, especially in converting auditory data into visual equivalents. Opthalmological findings were negative. The neurological and EEG examinations, however, produced significant rates of abnormal findings, although without definitive patterns. Myklebust concludes that neurological information is essential in the diagnosis of learning disabilities.

Incorporating Neuropsychological Procedures

Among Voeller's (36) suggestions for improving the validity of the standard neurological examination in MBD is the inclusion of many procedures from established neuropsychological test batteries, as discussed in detail in the next chapter. Voeller's suggestion recognizes that cerebral rather than cerebellar dysfunctions are likely causes of MBD; she would therefore explore cerebral dominance, language processing, spatial orientation, and graphomotor and visual-spatial functions, among others.

The mental-status examination as an adjunct to the physical neurological examination is advanced by Strub and Black (33). Their view of the mental-status examination essentially is a survey of the patient's neuropsychological status, although the procedures described are unstandardized and unquantified. They present in detail encompassing procedures to evaluate many cortical functions: language, memory, constructional ability, spatial comprehension, abstract thinking, information, arithmetic, ideomotor and ideational praxia, visual gnosia, right-left and geographical orientation, social behavior, mood, levels of consciousness, and appearance.

Gaddes (10) emphasizes the value of localizing some lesion in learning disabilities, a difficult task facilitated by demonstrating congruence between neurological and neuropsychological test findings. Such corroborated localization is particularly helpful in planning for remediation, he states. Posterior brain dysfunctions may impair visual perception, understanding of speech, tactile form recognition, directional sense, body image, finger localization, long-term memory and pictorial interpretations. These in turn may affect reading, spelling, and writing from copy or dictation.

Frontal-lobe dysfunction may affect oral expressive speech, serial ordering, short-term memory, motor coordination, subtle visual processes, and the ability to make rapid mental shifts.

Left-temporal-lobe disorders may impair auditory perception, understanding of speech, verbal associations and story recall, while right-temporal-lobe dysfunctions may impair spatial perception, pictorial comprehension, and musical skills.

Parietal-lobe disorders may result in deficits in tactile form recognition, finger localization, directional sense, and body image.

Gaddes reports that left-parietal disorders have a high positive correlation with dyslexia, while right-parietal disorders have a similar correlation with visuo-spatial defects. His experience is that the combined neurological and neuropsychological diagnosis affirms brain damage as the cause of the learning disability, thus persuading parents and teachers that the child's deficits are not due to neurosis or parental or cultural influences. Such a combined diagnosis best directs the remediation effort, by predicting the likely future outcome, indicating the residual strengths for development and the areas of dysfunction upon which remedial efforts should be concentrated. Presumably Gaddes' presentation of brain-behavior relationships is based upon correlations between neurological and neuropsychological test findings in cases of demonstrable brain damage. His approach is supported by Klatskin *et al.* (16) who found *WISC* and *Bender* results positively correlated with those of neurological examination in 43 of 50 patients *without* known central-nervous-system damage.

A less definite position is reached by Benton (1) in his extensive and valuable survey on the relationships between dyslexia and neurological disorder. He observes that the evidence as of 1975 favoring either focal or general dysfunction is not firm and that extant studies do not establish a neurological basis for dyslexia. He favors the view that a neurological base is suggested but not identified. He believes research has not been as productive as it might be were dyslexia more precisely defined by types. Were such definitions available, he feels confident that an association would be seen between them and the factors he pursued in the literature (finger agnosia, right-left disorientation, intersensory deficits, sequencing disorders, and generalized language disabilities).

Of interest is the publication, also in 1975, of the finding by Mattis *et al.* (17) of three independent neuropsychological syndromes associated with dyslexia that are not found in brain-damaged children who can read normally (discussed in the next chapter).

Neurological Evaluation During the First Year of Life

The possibility of identifying minor neurological dysfunctions early in life is receiving some attention (3). This may contribute to early identification of infants at risk for hyperkinesis and future cognitive dysfunctions as development progresses, and make possible desirable early remedial interventions. Minor physical anomalies of the head, face, hands, and feet in neonates were found to have a significant, albeit low, relationship with so-called "infant temperament" (irritable, fussy behavior) in 123 of 933 infants screened for these anomalies. The authors postulate that these signs may be possible predictors of hyperkinesis. A longitudinal assessment is ongoing.

Early signs of neurological dysfunction during the first year of life which may develop into later pathological syndromes are detailed by Dargassies (6A). These early signs may be global or minor, motor, sensory, or affective. The importance of baseline age-norms is stressed, and Dargassies presents both normal and abnormal signs for newborns and infants three months to four-to-six months, seven-to-nine months, and 10 to 12 months.

Chapter 10

Psychological Testing Methods

THE PSYCHOLOGICAL TESTING METHODS used in the diagnosis of MBD are chosen to evaluate the complex variables affected by the disorder, in the cognitive, emotional, and neurological areas. The three major types of psychological testing used correspond; they are (1) psychoeducational, (2) psychodiagnostic, and (3) neuropsychological. A fourth type, intelligence testing, is essential to the exploration of every area and is discussed in a separate section to reduce repetition. As will become evident, the types borrow from and give to each other. They are not identifiable strictly by stated purpose, but rather by individual emphasis. Each incorporates instruments and approaches sometimes considered to be under the rubric of one of the other testing types. Some neuropsychological investigators, for example, use the *Human Figure Drawing* procedure borrowed from psychodiagnostic tests. Psychoeducational testing explores cognitive functioning in relation to patterns of lateral cerebral dominance, an approach originating in neuropsychological testing. Also observable is the borrowing of neurological procedures by psychological testers (51) and, conversely, neuropsychological tests by neurologists (90). These cross-overs in practice have developed because cognitive, emotional, and neurological processes are essentially inseparable, and because the major testing methods are similarly so, bound together by principles common to all human measurements. And, of course, victims of MBD are human beings in whom the processes we seek to assess are parts of an integrated whole where every part relates to every other part.

Statistical analyses are fundamental to interpretation of all good psychological-testing procedures, but the test diagnostician should find equally important the clinical data potentially available to him in the psychological-testing process. The ultimate value of test diagnosis depends upon the clinical skill and sensitivity of the diagnostician. An obscure relationship between items, or some innocuous-sounding response may arouse an "aha!" recognition in the experienced clinician who is open to all possibilities. The clinician notes in the subject those matters of personal style, of reactions to difficulty, of preference for working with one task and avoiding another, or for approaching the test elements in an order different from the usual. This chapter argues no magic for psychological tests *per se,* holding that they are primarily extensions of the clinician. Matarazzo (57) sagely advises that one should hesitate to diagnose on the basis of test scores when a person's life history contradicts the obtained results. His observation is that the life history is more reliable for indicating intelligence level than the intelligence-test score.

Some General Guides to Psychological Testing in MBD

Psychological testing makes major contributions to the diagnosis of MBD. Achievement tests of reading, spelling, and arithmetic evaluate learning status according to age and grade norms. They identify both capabilities and dysfunctions. They can highlight specific types of disabilities in dysfunctional areas, and they can direct remedial efforts more specifically than would be possible without them. Mauser's (59) annotated catalogue of instruments for assessing the learning disabled is a valuable reference. It is helpful in communication with the learning-disabled person, parents, remediation specialists, and regular teachers, because it outlines the many separate and definite items that can be assessed and remedied by work and treatment.

Neuropsychological tests are capable of elucidating a wider array of brain-behavior aspects than are the achievement tests; more specifically assessing sensory, motor, intrasensory, language, and other higher-level cognitive processes.

Psychodiagnostic tests illuminate the emotional impact of MBD and learning disabilities, particularly identifying defensive reactions and ego resources for coping.

The wide range of psychological tests available have, therefore, these possible contributions to make:

1. Specification and assessment of disabilities and dysfunctions to which remedial efforts are to be directed.
2. Identification and assessment of strengths and assets, to be used in circumventing dysfunctions, in developing alternate modes of reception and expression, and in bolstering ego strengths.

3. Providing baseline reference for evaluating subsequent change through maturation, remediation, and other therapies.

The last important consideration is receiving increasing research attention. Dykmann *et al.* (27) in a longitudinal study contrasted test data produced by learning-disabled (LD) children with those of normal achievers. The children were first tested when aged 8 to 11, then retested when they reached 14. Originally, the controls had been superior to the LD children only in *WISC* Verbal I.Q.; at 14 the controls were superior in Full Scale I.Q.. One-third of the learning-disabled children decreased 10 points on the Verbal I.Q. while one-half of the controls increased 10 points, a movement in opposite directions over time that meant a widening gulf between the groups. The LD children were especially dysfunctional in conceptual, sequencing, and symbolic abilities, and they were several years behind in reading, spelling, and arithmetic. Not specified is whether these findings reflect the natural course of MBD left untreated, or whether there had been a treatment program, which appears unlikely. The study suggests an hypothesis that this writer has entertained while observing declines in test-performance levels in children over several years, particularly in I.Q. levels. Presuming that a disability will limit the mental age in the function under consideration (arithmetic, for example), that disability may not become apparent until chronological age reaches and passes the thus fixed mental age. Baseline and longitudinal test data are clearly valuable in maintaining an overview of progress or lack of it over the years.

Not only are tests valued for their ability to focus remediation efforts, but also they have been used as retraining methods in the very areas they test. Pontius (66), for example, suggests that the *Trail-Making Test, Part B,* and the *Wisconsin Card-Sorting Test* have remedial possibilities as practice drills where a child has difficulty shifting from one type of task to another.

What constitutes an adequate diagnostic-test battery for the evaluation of MBD? Is any single test capable of identifying and differentiating most MBD cases? Or is a wide-ranging, time-costly procedure necessary? The available evidence sometimes appears contradictory and uncertain, but the numerous varieties of brain-behavior disruptions are likely to result in fewer false-negative findings as test instruments parallel more closely and specifically the wide array of sensory, motor, integrative, sequencing, and cognitive functions that can be minimally impaired.

An example of confusion from an over-simplified approach to diagnostic testing is provided by Hartlage's analysis of the ability of three tests to differentially diagnose dyslexic, MBD, and emotionally disturbed children (35). He reports that the traditional *Wechsler Intelligence Scale for Children (WISC)* analysis did not differentiate among the groups. A special classification system, incorporating *WISC* spatial, sequential, and conceptual discrepancies did differentiate the dyslexic and MBD group, but not the emotionally disturbed group. The *Bender Visual Motor Gestalt Test* identified organic impairment in 17 of 25 MBD children, correctly ruled out organicity in 19 of the 25 emotionally disturbed group, and incorrectly diagnosed organicity in 19 of 31 dyslexic children. The reading part of the *Wide Range Achievement Test (WRAT)* identified 23 of 31 dyslexics, 20 of 25 MBD cases, and 18 of the 25 emotionally disturbed children. The failure of traditional *WISC* scoring in this study contrasts with the diagnostic power of the instrument attributed to it by Clements and Peters (17), who stressed the pattern of subtest scores that a child receives rather than the Full Scale, Verbal, and Performance I.Q.s. And, as Hartlage discovered, a special scoring approach produced differential diagnoses where the traditional approach failed. The successful diagnostician is one able to use a one-two-punch, with both standard and innovative aspects.

Methods for inferring brain damage from psychological tests developed by Reitan (72) have been applied to the diagnosis of MBD by Selz and Reitan (81). These inferential methods are:

1. *Level of performance.* Statistical measures of variability are established for single tests for groups along a continuum, from groups with known cerebral damage to those without it. This enables the performance levels of individuals or groups to be compared with a normative standard. The diagnostician must, however, keep in mind that performance levels on psychological tests are affected by variables other than brain damage. These include genetics, cultural deprivation, educational disabilities, severe emotional conditions, and the normal aging process.

2. *Comparison of results from the two sides of the body.* This intra-individual comparative method based upon right-left differences is free of many problems inherent in other inferential methods. It is basic to the classical physical neurological examination, which compares the right and left side. The extent of difference between the two sides in a given performance is established, for example, in finger-tapping speed or strength of grip. Several different tests of lateralized performance are made at different times during the examination period, to minimize the influence of transient fluctuation of attention and effort. Again, all the possible factors must be kept in mind. Impairment of strength or of finger-tapping speed could be caused by muscle strain, a joint injury, or injury to the peripheral nerve, rather than central damage. Therefore tests of right and left sensory functioning and complex performance tasks are added to the investigation.

Some of the tests will not show differential results if nearly equal damage has occurred to both cerebral hemispheres. Reitan finds the method promising, however, because of the pronounced differences observed between right and left performances in many subjects, including mental retardates, in whom no other neurological evidence suggested damage to only one of the cerebral hemispheres.

The major advantage of the method is its relative freedom from the effects of conscious resistance, pretended impairment, or emotional difficulties. Conceivably, however, a classical hysteria involving one side of the body in its psychodynamics might produce false-positive results.

3. *Pathognomic signs.* A well-known use of specific signs considered indicative of pathology is Piotrowski's (64) list of Rorschach signs indicating brain damage. For example, he labels one sign Impotence and another Perplexity, and associates their presence with brain damage. Such signs of specific deficiencies are believed to be correlated with brain damage more frequently than with any other type of impairing condition. However, acceptance of their validity in the diagnosis of brain damage is not without problems. Being the results of subjective observation by the examiner, they are not easily replicated by other examiners. They produce rather high numbers of false negatives; that is, many patients with clearly established cerebral deficits fail to produce the signs. They are of value in alerting the examiner to the possibility of cerebral damage and as supplements to other measures which yield more quantitative results.

4. *Patterns of test performance.* Measurements obtained from different tests that tend to corroborate each other and also to extend the investigation into more complex aspects of the deficient function make up meaningful patterns. These groupings of measurements involving one function are compared with grouped measures of other functions for the same person.

Selz and Reitan (81) elaborated a complex of 37 rules for applying these inferential measurements to the classification of nearly 60 children 9–14 years old as normal, learning disabled, or brain damaged; they report 73 percent accuracy. Their rules system is reminiscent of the taxonomic key method developed by Russell *et al.* (78).

The reflections of skilled workers derived from their use of psychological tests in the diagnosis of MBD constitute a valuable professional heritage.

Voeller (90) offers those features which she finds make for a good examination battery:

1. Normative data should be available for each of the tests used.

2. The chosen battery should cover a wide range of brain functions (cognitive, motor, sensory, language, spatial) and academic levels. No single standard battery is applicable to all diagnostic situations. The age of the patient, the nature of the presenting complaint, and the examiner's training, experience, and preference all influence the composition of each battery used.

3. The battery (and the examiner, we may add) should be flexibly adaptable to individual clinical situations, capable of exploring in depth beyond the first signs of deficit or capability.

4. Fatigue of the patient is to be avoided. Many test batteries are so time-consuming that a low score may be an artifact of the protracted testing situation rather than a true measure of the patient.

5. The patient should be observed as an individual, not as a mere producer of statistics. His style, self-concept, and coping ability are significant clinical data.

Levinger and Ochroch (51) also emphasize this latter point. They argue against test-by-test descriptions of a subject, and urge the diagnostician to strive to integrate test findings into a complex pattern of assets and deficits, feelings and thoughts. They comment, ruefully and wisely, that a deficit is not the person.

This writer's experience has been that the social aspects of a diagnostic-testing situation almost always provide significant data with which the statistical test data must be compared, for corroboration or for questioning. Spontaneous use of vocabulary or metaphor may exceed the level of test results, and indicate the size of the deficits that have been measured. Additionally, the social-clinical situation allows observation of aspects of the person not assessed by any test: (1) the handling of the physical self in space; (2) the handling of the social self in relationship to the examiner; (3) the handling of the emotional self in coping with stress and difficulty. These observations are at least as important as the numbers that the tests generate. To ignore them is to risk a mechanical diagnosis that obscures the patient's capacity for growth and change.

Intelligence Testing

Psychological testing of all kinds—psychoeducational, psychodiagnostic, neuropsychological—leans heavily on intelligence testing, particularly of the battery type. The Wechsler scales (the original *Wechsler-Bellevue—WB,* the *Wechsler Intelligence Scale for Children,* original and revised—*WISC* and *WISC-R,* the *Wechsler Adult Intelligence Scale—WAIS,* and now the revised *WAIS—WAIS-R*), long established and widely used, are potent instruments in the diagnosis of MBD. Their power resides in the diversity of cognitive and brain-behavior functions tested by eleven to twelve subtests, and the clues to emotional status to be found in the subject's responses. There are similarities in the way the testing specialties use the Wechsler scales, and to avoid repetition, the Wechsler scales are discussed here, before the major testing types, all of which use them.

Reliance upon a single score, and overall intelligence quotient, has long been abandoned, especially in the diagnosis of MBD. Instead the diagnostician looks for *patterns* of responses, for the cognitive abilities represented by the differences in scores on the subtests (i.e., their scatter) and in *factor* scores. Also sought are clues to cognitive processing contained in the subjects' responses.

The diagnostician can make telling use of the many different subtests of the Wechsler scales. These include receptive and expressive language, naming or word finding, arithmetic ability, short- and long-term attention and memory, spatial visualization, constructional praxis, concept formation, graphomotor ability, thought processes, and sequencing.

Most of the functions are tested on a continuum of relative difficulty established by item analysis. Statistical scoring and scaling procedures allow one function to be compared quantitatively with all others. Knowledge of the stimulus modality and the nature of response required, together with the intervening integration involved, enables the diagnostician to derive clinical interpretations from the scores. The six subtests of the Verbal Scale all use an auditory stimulus and require an oral-verbal expressive response. The five subtests of the Performance Scale present instructions in the auditory modality, while the material involved in each subtest is a visual stimulus. The responses required are varied: graphomotor, constructional, sequencing. Briefly, the demands of each of the subtests are as follows:

Information requires recall of names, dates, and geographical, literary, anatomical, and other information. The storage and retrieval of old data is tested.

Comprehension requires judgment, reasoning, abstract and propositional thinking, and awareness of social amenity.

Similarities requires concept formation, and associative and abstract thinking.

Digit Span measures recent memory and capacity to attend and concentrate.

Vocabulary evaluates comprehension and expression of word meanings.

Comprehension, Similarities, and *Vocabulary* supply valuable data on the state of the subject's language skills, as will be developed later.

Digit Symbol evaluates symbol processing and accuracy and speed in matching. A manual motor response is required that can be evaluated for quality of control and placement. The mental functions of learning, attention, memory, and sequencing are involved.

Picture Completion tests recognition of essential details in a parts-to-whole relationship, and judgment. The response required here is an oral-verbal expressive one, unlike the other Performance subtests. Although it is part of the Performance Scale, the *Picture Completion* subtest requires naming and word finding and so may reveal anomic difficulties.

Block Design, a constructional task, involves spatial relations and figure-ground separation, and requires a motor response.

Picture Arrangement tests logical thematic perception and construction, and requires a motor response, with perception and awareness of both logical progress and social relations involved.

Object Assembly, also a constructional task, requires spatial-relations ability and a motor response. Some of the *Object Assembly* subtests involve representations of the human body and may reveal aspects of the body image.

Witkin *et al.* (93) have separated three major areas (factors) in the Wechsler Scales: (1) verbal *(Information, Comprehension,* and *Vocabulary);* (2) attention *(Arithmetic, Digit Span,* and *Digit Symbol);* and (3) perceptual-analytic *(Picture Completion, Block Design,* and *Object Assembly).* These by and large correspond with the three major factors, apart from the "g" factor, originally discussed by Wechsler (92). These were: (1) verbal comprehension *(Vocabulary, Information, Picture Arrangement, Block Design,* and *Object Assembly);* (2) nonverbal or performance *(Picture Completion, Picture Arrangement, Block Design,* and *Object Assembly);*

and (3) memory *(Digit Span, Digit Symbol,* and according to the age of the subject, *Arithmetic* and *Information).*

Wechsler reports a personal communication from F.B. Davis on the scale-score differences between pairs of *WAIS* subtests, differences significant at the 15 percent level. The average difference is three scale-score units, the range is from two to four scale-score units. Differences exceeding three scale points suggest a pathological process. Averaging the scale scores for the subtests constituting each of Witkin's factors allows the examiner to compare the factors.

This method is somewhat limited in sophistication. It does not utilize the overall I.Q. level of the patient being examined, an important point in evaluating levels of subtest and factor scale scores. A three scale-point difference between the verbal and perceptual-analytic factors has a pathological significance that is different with different Full Scale I.Q. scores. The significance is greater when the I.Q. is 100 or lower than it is when the Full Scale I.Q. is 140, for example.

The factor-average scale score may conceal an extreme deviation in a specific function. For example, a patient's average scale score for all factors may be 12. Thus, no difference is reflected. But the contribution of each subtest to each average factor score may tell another story. For example, in the perceptual-analytic factor, *Picture Completion* and *Block Design* may both be 14, while *Object Assembly* is eight. Within the factor, therefore, one subtest function is six scale scores below the others, twice the average for all differences reported by Davis, and strongly suggestive of pathology. This possibility emphasizes the diagnostic importance of examining the scale scores of subtests *within* each factor, as well as the average scale scores for the three factors.

Clinical insights can be obtained from considering the different modalities and processes required by each subtest and the manner in which the patient deals with each task. *Block Design* and *Object Assembly,* both constructional tasks, involve a visual stimulus and a motor response. In *Object Assembly,* however, the subject must form a mental concept of the whole from the parts, without the visual representation of the whole for a guide, as given in *Block Design,* where a drawing of the whole is provided. In some patients, the relative ambiguity of the *Object Assembly* items may reveal a deficit in ideation not identified by the somewhat more structured *Block Design.* Another patient, one who has difficulty separating or interpreting figure-ground relationships, may do considerably better on *Object Assembly,* with less figure-ground interference and less conflict between stimulus card and puzzle parts, than on *Block Design,* where he must conform his construction with an external visual model. This situation may emerge dramatically, with *Block Design* very poor in contrast to a high-level *Object Assembly.* Or in *Object Assembly,* the Hand, visually the most ambiguous item, may be done quickly, with speed credits, while the other three items are constructed more slowly, albeit accurately. A related phenomenon in the reproduction of figures in the *Bender Visual Motor Gestalt Test* is reported by Koppitz (50). Some brain-damaged children, finding the sight of the stimulus card confusing, prefer to look at the design, put it out of sight, and then draw it from memory.

The power of Wechsler scales to assess a variety of language functions needs emphasis, since dyslexia, dysphasia, and dysgraphia are frequently encountered. Dyslexia (except for the reading of arithmetic problems on the *WISC*) and dysgraphia are not tested by the Wechsler scales, as they are by many of the psychoeducational tests. But dysphasia disorders are discernible in the Wechsler-scale scores if the diagnostician is alert to this capability.

The *Similarities* and *Comprehension* subtests both require verbal expressive ability, but differ markedly in their demands on this function. Most *Similarities* items can be satisfactorily answered with a single-word response (furniture, directions, food, metals). Most *Comprehension* items, in contrast, require an extended response with propositional thinking, the interrelating of two or more ideas into a conclusion. Dysphasic disorders become apparent in differences between these subtests. A low-level *Comprehension* score may contrast with a high-level *Similarities* score to suggest a verbal-expressive defect of propositional thinking. The reverse, high *Comprehension* with low *Similarities,* may indicate a deficit of verbal concept formation. When both are low, in contrast to indices of high-level endowment, a major aphasic disorder is suspected. This usually is paralleled by low *Vocabulary,* so that all the subtests of the verbal factor produce an average scale score supporting the presumption of dysfunction. *Picture Completion* may reveal difficulty in word-finding ability that suggests an anomia. This difficulty can be present with or without dysfunctions in propositional expression or abstract conceptualization. Verbal abstraction (*à la* Goldstein) is tested by some items of *Comprehension* as well as by *Similarities.* Indeed, those items on *Comprehension* that ask for meanings of metaphors appear to tap a higher level of abstraction than do the single-element associations required in *Similarities.* One patient who accurately and succinctly defined the similarities of north-west and table-chair, fumbled painfully for the meaning of "shallow brooks are noisy," responding "A little knowledge is a dangerous thing. A lot of bombasm (*sic*), bombastic, dillentantism (*sic*), a flash in the pan."

The scores should be viewed against the quality of the responses. Marked difficulty in understanding spoken instructions may suggest a receptive language disorder. The patient may offer a rhyming or associative response, or may appear not to have heard the word correctly. A patient gave the meaning of *obstruct* as "to build, to wreck," suggesting that the sound of *obstruct* evoked association of both *construct* and *destruct* without comprehension of the separate meanings of the three rhyming words. Expressive language difficulties are apparent in this response to a *Comprehension* item asking how to find one's way out of a forest in the daytime: "Look in the direction of the sun in the area and how I'm set in the area, and the position of the sun and find my way out." On *Picture Completion,* word-finding difficulties may be suggested by the patient's pointing to the missing part instead of naming it, describing the missing part or its use, or indicating the part's function with gestures.

These subtest variations and comparisons create the diagnostic value of the Wechsler scales in MBD. Before proceeding to suggestions for modifying the usual administration procedures to enhance the opportunities for clinical observation, it would be well to look at the history of the scales in neuropsychological testing. Their neuropsychodiagnostic power had for a time been obscured somewhat by the search for single-test indicators of brain damage. Also the *Hold-Don't Hold* category in the Wechsler Scales is not responsive to the wide variety of dysfunctions possible when different areas of the brain are damaged. Wechsler had himself reported that some subtests of the early *Wechsler-Bellevue Scale* were more sensitive than others to deterioration and brain damage, while some brain-behavior functions measured by the scale remain intact (92). The *Hold-Don't Hold* (or *Deterioration Scale*) has been found to be largely ineffective for diagnosis (4).

Another impediment to exploiting the fullest diagnostic value of the Wechsler scales has been the tendency to diagnose brain damage only when Performance scale scores are significantly lower than Verbal scale scores, as though brain damage would produce spatial and motor impairments only. The impact of left-hemisphere damage upon verbal functions, a well-documented phenomenon, was ignored in this limited view. However, even neuropsychological research crediting hemispheric differences and relating deficits in Verbal I.Q. and Performance I.Q. respectively to left-hemisphere and right-hemisphere damage was challenged. In his monumental fifth edition of Wechsler's *Measurement and Appraisal of Adult Intelligence,* Matarazzo (57) reports eight studies (1958 to 1971) that support the cerebral-dominance hypothesis: patients with left-hemisphere damage do less well on Verbal subtests than on Performance subtests; patients with right-hemisphere lesions do the reverse, while patients with bilateral damage perform more like right-hemisphere-damaged patients, doing better on Verbal than Performance subtests. These conclusions have been challenged by Smith (85, 86); his own study of large numbers of patients with lateralized lesions, and the studies of others he cites, did not confirm the sensitivity to differentiate between hemispheres claimed for the Verbal and the Performance I.Q.s.

The nature of the individual subtests of both the Verbal and the Performance scales, examined above, bears upon the confusion. The Verbal scale is not purely verbal nor is the Performance scale purely motor. Aggregate Verbal and Performance I.Q. scores sometimes obscure marked dysfunctions that show up only in scores on individual subtests. Precise diagnosis is better served when each subtest score is examined individually in the context of aggregate scores, instead of relying solely upon comparisons of the Verbal I.Q. with Performance I.Q. (22).

Another error in use of the Wechsler scores has been a tendency to diagnose schizophrenia when a patient succeeds with more difficult items of a subtest after failing easier ones, on the assumption that erratic means psychotic. This tendency involves the corollary assumption that the brain-damaged person, in contrast to the schizophrenic, reaches the upper limit of capability on a subtest and thereafter fails consistently. These assumptions rest upon a questionable further assumption of a high positive correlation between the gradient of difficulty established for a subtest by item analysis and the brain's capacity to succeed with problems of increasing difficulty. But failure at lower levels and success at higher does not necessarily mean schizophrenia. Specific impairments of the brain may affect the matter. The "more difficult" problem may contain words or concepts, or require processes, that remain intact within a patient's brain or for which he was able to establish compensatory routes. The cerebral representation of the elements of the "inherently easier" problem may be impaired, destroyed, or blocked by the specific damage he has suffered.

A fourth deterrent has been the failure to use the Wechsler scales in a clinical-statistical manner with due credit to the individual brain-behavior qualities required of the patient by each subtest along with the scale score it produces. Matarazzo's survey (57) reported only research on the sensitivity of the Verbal-Performance I.Q.'s in neuropsychodiagnosis. No data was available to illuminate the import of intra-individual subtest scatter, which is, as detailed above, where the clues appear. Luria (53) overlooked the clinical potency of the Wechsler scales when he regarded them as psychometric instruments rather than as a clinical method as well. Had he used them with his superb clinical acumen, they might have risen in his esteem; certainly he could have made valued contributions to their use as clinical diagnostic instruments.

As long ago as 1954, Klebanoff *et al.* (47) perceived that the overall scores of the Wechsler were relatively insensitive to brain damage, while the subtests had greater diagnostic power. Later data from Reitan (70) and from Reed *et al.* (68) suggested that Wechsler-scale variables consistently showed more difference between brain-damaged and normal groups than did other measures of concept formation, alertness, and motor functions. The explanation is the capacity of the subtests to assess many of the varied effects of different brain lesions. The Wechsler scales can serve as a mini-neuropsychological battery, providing clues for more extensive investigation. The diagnostician, however, must be wary when making decisions about an individual patient that he does not apply the result of research studies with groups to his single subject as the major diagnostic criterion.

Modifications of usual administration procedures I have found useful to enhance the clinical value of the Wechsler scales in diagnosis begin with identifying the point in each subtest where a marked increase in complexity is presented or a shift in approach is required. On *Block Design,* the number of blocks is increased from four to nine with item 7, presenting both a more detailed test environment and a more complicated visual field. A further complexity is added in the requirement to shift from a 2 × 2 square to a 3 × 3 square construction. The inherent difficulty of the design itself is also to be considered. Item 7 of *Block Design* appears to be far less difficult than item 8, so that the marked difficulty with the other requirements may not be observed until the design difficulty is increased. *Digit Span* presents a linear increase in difficulty imposed by the increasing number of digits the subject must remember; then recall in reverse order is required and the patient's capacity for attention and recall may become heavily taxed.

For *Picture Arrangement* and *Object Assembly,* as well as *Block Design,* the increase in number of units alone, whether pictures or parts, may be enough added difficulty to overtax a brain-injured person's capacity. Of course, this factor cannot be separated from the inherent difficulty of the item itself. But the brain-injured person is prone to "fall apart" under pressure; increased test difficulty of any kind may constitute that pressure, and provide a valuable clinical clue.

Two procedures often are productive of clues to brain damage: the application of stress and testing the limits. They may be inserted without altering the standard scoring methods if introduced after the usual administration and scoring, as an additional step in investigation.

Stress can be used to check a suspected deficit in attention by readministering the *Digit Symbol* subtest, requesting the patient to try to go faster on the second trial than he did on the first. Ability to increase speed without significant loss of accuracy of location and form would suggest that the poorer first effort was due not to organic but rather to emotional or motivational factors. Loss of speed and/or decreased accuracy would suggest the effect of fatigue associated with organic conditions, if muscle weakness, depression, or regressiveness can be ruled out. Stress can be introduced in *Block Design* by readministering the subtest according to the method developed by Satz (79), in which the patient is asked to construct the designs again, block by block, in a plane rotated 90 degrees from the orientation of the design. Reciting the *Digit Span* series backwards adds stress; unusually large differences between the forward and backward series should not be interpreted only as due to anxiety.

Limits may be tested in several ways. Should the patient fail to retain, say, six digits forward on two trials in *Digit Span,* a third set of six digits may be presented. Failure on the third trial confirms the failure as a limit of capability; success does not change the score of failure, but does question that a true limit has been found. Limits may be tested by extending the time allowed on the most difficult item failed by the patient in *Arithmetic, Block Design, Picture Arrangement,* and *Object Assembly.* The patient who has reached the allowable limits on *Information, Comprehension, Similarities, Arithmetic, Picture Completion, Block Design, Picture Arrangement* or *Object Assembly* may be told that there is another solution or arrangement for the last item or two he has taken and failed, and may be asked to attempt a solution different from the first he had offered. Or the patient is told that his construction of a *Block Design* or *Object Assembly* item contains an error. Can he find and correct it? This procedure helps distinguish between a true failure and carelessness.

An explanation may be requested for solutions or responses that appear unusual or bizarre. For *Arithmetic,* one may ask, "How did you get that answer?'' The patient may be asked to rethink his answer without being told it is incorrect. For *Vocabulary, Similarities,* or *Comprehension* answers, one may ask, ''Tell me more about what you mean.'' For *Picture Arrangement,* one may say, ''Tell me the story as you see it.'' With unusual constructions in *Object Assembly,* one may say, ''Tell me about this construction. Explain it to me.''

It may be helpful to test the patient's ability to respond to additional clues beyond those provided by the standardized direction of administration. For example, the examiner may construct part of the solution of an item the patient has failed on *Block Design* and then ask the patient to complete the design. A small portion of the design may be offered first, followed by additional portions if the patient continues to fail after the help provided by the first partial construction. A similar tactic can be used with *Picture Arrangement* and *Object Assembly.* In *Picture Completion,* questions on individual items may be asked that will direct the patient's attention to some element necessary for correct response. If the patient says ''Some legs are missing for the crab'' (item 15), the examiner may ask, after the entire subtest is finished, ''How many legs are missing here?'' while again showing the picture of the crab.

Knowing the extent of the patient's ability to respond to additional clues can be helpful to teachers, especially in remedial efforts, and to work supervisors, in establishing how much of a field or how many clues must be present for the patient to be able to complete a task.

Differentiation between organic brain damage and psychogenic conditions such as schizophrenia has been difficult to establish with the Wechsler scales. Wechsler states that subtests of the Performance Scale tend to be more negatively affected than those of the Verbal Scale in most emotional and mental cases (except for acting-out persons), but that the same is true in brain-damage cases. To resolve this difficulty Birch and Walker (10) sought to distinguish between the ability of brain-damaged and that of schizophrenic children to identify a *Block Design* item they had been unable to construct correctly. Younger brain-damaged adults and children were better able than schizophrenic patients to identify the design they had failed to construct properly. DeWolfe (24, 25) reported that schizophrenics do less well on *Comprehension* (verbal expression) and better on *Digit Span* (attention) than do brain-damaged patients. Watson (91) reports confirmation of these findings in one hospital population but not in another. Another effort at differential diagnosis used the *Similarities* subtest and an error-analysis approach with children. Emotionally disturbed children were found more likely to make an expansive error or to offer a conceptually inadequate response; the responses of brain-damaged children were marked by restrictive errors, such as ''don't know,'' or by no response. This study by Hall and La Driere (34A) is also an example of a clinical approach to test data.

Some success in lateralizing brain damage in a cerebral hemisphere with selected Wechsler subtests has stimulated research with them to locate sites and identify types of cerebral lesions. But the capacity of the Wechsler subtests to localize and identify remains hypothetical at this time. Such precision is not required of them, however, by the diagnostician who is estimating only the possibility of brain damage and the need for specialized consultation where MBD is suspected.

Wechsler's own comments had a somewhat limiting effect upon the use of his scales in neuropsychodiagnosis, tending as they did to assess the scales' values by statistical standards. He did not emphasize their clinical applications in individual patients. He found that the impairments usually connected to brain damage are in visual-motor functions, ability to shift, memory, and synthetic ability. Brain-damaged persons, he concluded, do consistently better on Verbal Scale than on Performance Scale tasks, and brain damage of any etiology produces a typical test syndrome *if the damage is sufficiently extensive* (italics added). The proviso is significant when the search is for *minimal* dysfunctions.

His conclusion that massive brain damage will produce a loss in general intelligence is probably valid. But it did not incorporate the later findings that in adults some lower subtest scores in the Verbal Scale tend to be associated with left-hemisphere damage in a right-handed person, while in a right-handed person some lower subtest scores in the Performance Scale tend to be associated with right-hemisphere damage.

Reitan and Heineman (73) investigated the ability to diagnose brain damage when there is little or no difference between Verbal and Performance Scale scores but one of the sensitive subtests *(Similarities* or *Block Design)* is markedly low. The absence of a difference between Verbal and Performance scales in these situations, Reitan states, suggests a static rather than a proliferating lesion.

The sensitivity of subtests of the Verbal Scale to left-hemisphere damage and of the Performance Scale to right-side damage has stimulated much investigation (49, 62, 63). Parsons and Vega (62) confirmed findings that the *Vocabulary* and *Block Design* subtests have the highest loading respectively in the verbal and perceptual-organizational factors, and that these factors are associated respectively with left-hemisphere and right-hemisphere function. Related results associate *Similarities* subtest deficits with left-hemisphere damage and *Object-Assembly* deficit with right-hemisphere damage. Means significantly lower on *Picture Arrangement* are linked with right-hemisphere lesions by McFie and Thompson (56). McFie (55) reports consistent findings of *Digit Span, Similarities,* and *Arithmetic* difficulties in left-hemisphere disorders, while deficits on *Picture Arrangement, Block Design,* and *Object Assembly* are associated with right-hemisphere damage. These lateralizing signs are, again, specific subtest scores, not aggregate Verbal and Performance I.Q.s.

No similar sensitivity to lateralization was found for the subtests of the *Wechsler Intelligence Scale for Children (WISC)* in a study of subjects with a mean age close to ten years (13). The explanation may be that in the adult, lateralization of function has been completed and then damaged, while in the child it is still developing. Nonetheless, scrutiny of differences between subtest functions of a child with the *WISC* is a good clinical procedure, as is the *WAIS* with adults.

The value of Wechsler scales in neuropsychodiagnosis is illustrated also in the inclusion of nine *WAIS* measures by Russell *et al.* in their approach to diagnosis (78). In addition to the Verbal, Performance, and Full Scale I.Q.s, they incorporate scores of *Digit Symbol, Digit Span, Vocabulary, Similarities, Block Design,* and *Object Assembly* subtests.

Remediation specialists seeking psychoeducational diagnostic clues have related individual subtest scores and patterns of subtest scores to specific learning disabilities. They have also sought to generate suggestions for specific remediation interventions from these scores. Searls (80) reports that poor readers tend to have lower scores on *Information, Arithmetic, Digit Span,* and *Vocabulary* in the Verbal Scale, and *Coding* in the Performance Scale of the *WISC*. The net effect is that the poor readers produce lower Verbal Performance I.Q.s. She analyzes each of the twelve subtests of the *WISC* according to "input" and "output," that is, the sensory and expressive or motor modalities they employ. And, as is characteristic of special-education diagnosticians, she also seeks to identify the particular sensory-motor-cognitive task demanded by each specific subtest. Sequencing ability, she states, for example, is tested by *Digit Span, Picture Arrangement,* and *Coding.* The reader will be aware that the sensory "input" and motor "outgo" are different in each of these three subtests. Other analyses of the functions inherent in *WISC* subtests are presented by Banas and Wills (6) and by Jacobson and Kovalinsky (42). The application of Wechsler-subtest-score diagnoses to remediation is discussed in Chapter 12.

Psychoeducational Testing

This area of psychological testing requires training and skills which many psychologists have not acquired. The academic competence or dysfunction of the patient (usually a child) cannot be properly assessed merely by the administration of some standardized tests. Since the most effective treatment of MBD and its emotional impacts is the earliest possible work on the dysfunction, diagnosis is useful to the extent that it leads promptly to remediation tailored to a patient's specific assets and liabilities and the requirements of specific learning tasks. Thus a sensitive awareness of the elements comprised in learning processes is important in psychoeducational assessment, and the test instruments are useful to the extent that they reveal the components of these processes.

Remedial instruction takes into account both the process by which the child learns and the components of the task he is to be taught. An effort is made to determine how readily a child learns through each sensory modality, and how well he integrates the data received from two or more (e.g., the integration of visual and auditory stimuli necessary to learn to read). The focus of the instruction that will help the minimally impaired child will be less upon subject matter and more upon the processes involved in mastering it.

Johnson (43) has suggested that a learning task be analyzed to determine:

1. Whether it demands a single sense or is intersensory.
2. The sensory modalities involved (vision and audition are most frequently employed in learning, but the haptic modality must also be considered).
3. Whether the task is primarily verbal or nonverbal.
4. The level of the task. (Does it involve primarily perception, memory, reproduction, symbolization?)
5. The expected mode of response. (Is it to be pantomined by pointing, gesturing, or manipulating objects? Or expressed in speech, or writing?)

The purpose of the analysis is to plan how to encourage and develop the child's ability to comprehend and to respond; any prompt success positively reinforces the learning experience.

If the dysfunctional child is to benefit from remedial instruction, the point at which instruction begins is of great importance. Developmental studies as well as theories suggest that normal progression is toward greater differentiation, accompanied by integration. This fact underscores the value of age norms in diagnosis, and indicates that diagnosis should first establish the child's present level, so that he can realistically advance from that stage. Too often, teachers are misled by a child's obvious brightness or discouraged by aversive apathy misinterpreted as mental dullness, and begin their remedial efforts at the wrong level for him.

The experienced examiner knows, for example, that most tests of reading do not allow sufficient actual reading time to permit adequate assessment. A tense child may stumble, hestitate, and grope initially; another child's deficit may not appear until a sustained reading sequence exceeds his short attention span. Again, the arithmetic abilities of a child with a reading dysfunction cannot be properly assessed through arithmetic problems that must be read. And always, an assessment of a child's functioning in any academic area must take account of the child's educational-social-cultural-economic environment. His school or his teacher may be "dysfunctional" rather than the child. His family may set a low value on academic achievement or ambition. His whole culture may devalue academic attainment, either tacitly or directly, in favor of athletic skills, for example. Or economic pressure may orient the child toward skills immediately rewarded with a few dollars, rather than those seemingly nebulous activities, reading and writing.

The skilled and sensitive psychoeducational tester works back and forth between the facts of the test and the facts of the child. The now numerous test instruments are indispensable in the diagnostic process. Steadily increasing, about 325 of them are described by Mauser (59) as a "selected" list of instruments for assessing the learning disabled. He groups them as intelligence tests; preschool readiness tests; motor, sensory, and language tests (a strange grouping); reading readiness tests; diagnostic reading tests; survey tests—general and reading; oral reading tests; diagnostic tests of math abilities; creativity tests; social adjustment—personality scales; vocational tests; and miscellaneous tests.

Many batteries of tests are available. Among these are the *Slingerland Screening Tests for Identifying Children with Specific Language Disabilities,* the *Detroit Test of Learning Aptitudes,* and Valett's *An Inventory of Primary Skills.*

The *Woodcock-Johnson Psycho-Educational Battery* (94) incorporates twelve tests of cognitive abilities (visual matching, spatial relations, blending, memory for sentences, visual-auditory learning, numbers reversed, analysis-synthesis, concept formation, picture vocabulary, quantitative concepts, antonyms-synonyms, and analogies). These are variously grouped to reflect levels in four cognitive factors (verbal ability, reasoning, perceptual speed, and memory), and four scholastic aptitudes (reading, mathematics, written language, and knowledge). To illustrate: verbal ability is assessed by tests of (1) picture vocabulary, (2) antonyms-synonyms, (3) analysis-synthesis; mathematics aptitude is assayed by tests of (1) visual matching, (2) antonyms-synonyms, (3) analysis-synthesis, and (4) concept formation. The battery also contains ten tests of scholastic achievement, grouped into reading, mathematics, and written-language levels. Additionally, the battery measures five interest levels, grouped with two areas: scholastic and nonscholastic (physical, social).

A widely used and respected battery is the *Illinois Test of Psycholinguistic Ability (ITPA)* for children from two years and four months to ten years and three months of age (54). It evaluates: (1) channels of communication; (2) psycholinguistic processes, which involve the interaction between receptive and expressive functions; (3) levels of organization, the level of representation or utilization of symbols, and the automatic, although organized and integrated, level. At the representational level are six subtests. Two are for the receptive process of decoding: (1) auditory decoding, with a single response (yes, no, or nod) requested to questions of increasing vocabulary difficulty; (2) visual decoding with pictures shown for three seconds, and the child asked to find a similar concept amongst a field of pictures. For evaluating the organizing process, there is (1) an auditory-vocal association test which asks for sentence completion and (2) a visual-motor association test in which the child is shown pictures and asked which of four others goes along with the stimulus picture. For the expressive process of encoding, there is (1) a verbal-vocal encoding test in which the child is asked to "tell me about this—" and (2) a manual-motor encoding test in which the child is told to "show me what we do with a _____." For investigating the automatic level of organization, four tests of closure are presented: (1) grammatic closure, requiring the completion of incomplete statements; (2) auditory closure; (3) sound blending; (4) visual closure, in which the child is asked to identify the incomplete visual presentation in a set. Finally, there are two tests for sequential memory, one using audition and the other visual stimuli.

An aid to translating diagnostic findings from the *ITPA* into organized remedial programs is available (45). These programs are organized around the specific dysfunctions uncovered: auditory reception, auditory association, verbal expression, grammatic and auditory closure, auditory sequential memory, visual reception, visual association, manual motor expression, visual closure, and visual sequential memory.

A test battery designed for early detection of potential for learning disabilities is aptly titled *SEARCH* (82). The battery is based upon both clinical experience and factual analysis of data derived from an interdisciplinary individual examination of 447 kindergarten children to whom the preliminary test battery was administered. Vulnerability to learning disability is identified by score levels based upon stanine-level analysis. These levels can be used to assign priorities for educational interventions, proffered in a corollary program called *TEACH* (33) that coordinates its teaching plans point by point with the diagnostic findings of *SEARCH*.

SEARCH tests for 10 factors:

1. Matching (ability to discriminate between and match asymmetric figures variously placed in a right, left, horizontal, and vertical orientation).
2. Recall (immediate recall of the orientation of asymmetric figures).
3. Design (copying of designs of increasing difficulty, a process that requires visual discrimination, praxis, and fine motor control).
4. Rote sequencing (measures recall of commonly heard verbal rote sequences).
5. Auditory discrimination (requires identification of similarities or differences between syllables or words that are either identical or differ by only one phoneme).
6. Articulation (measures ability to reproduce sounds of commonly used words).
7. Initials (tests ability at intermodal dictation, a complex task requiring auditory, visual, praxic, and motor associations).
8. Directionality (assesses spatial orientation).
9. Finger schema (measures ability to perceive and locate tactile stimuli).
10. Pencil grip (assesses maturation of thumb and finger opposition).

To illustrate the principles of covering as many learning processes as possible and of developing and expanding the diagnostic exploration of the individual, the test battery used by Dr. Doris Gray, a psychoeducational diagnostician and remediation specialist, is instructive. Not all tests nor all parts of any tests are administered to any one child; tests and parts of tests are used as needed to assure coverage and selectively to explore deficits as they are discerned. This battery includes: *Peabody Picture Vocabulary Test; Peabody In-*

dividual Achievement Test; Illinois Test of Psycholinguistic Abilities; Benton Visual Retention Test; Boehm Test of Basic Concepts; Detroit Test of Learning Aptitude; SEARCH; Wepman Test of Auditory Discrimination; Slingerland Screening Tests for Identifying Children with Specific Language Disabilities (Forms A, B, C, D); *Specific Language Disability Test for Grades Six, Seven, and Eight; Goldman-Fristoe-Woodcock Auditory Skills Test Battery; Lindamood Auditory Conceptualization Test;* the *Wechsler* intelligence scales according to the age of the subject; *Bender Visual Motor Gestalt Test.*

Psychodiagnostic Testing

The basic psychodiagnostic test battery, that most widely used, surveys intellectual functioning as well as the individual's psychodynamics and emotional status with projective techniques. Additionally, many psychodiagnosticians survey the patient's responses to projective techniques for clues to neuropsychological functioning as well. It is for this reason that many psychodiagnostic test batteries include a brief test or two with specific neuropsychological focus, although psychodiagnostic potency is also ascribed to them.

So it is that the most widely used psychodiagnostic battery, in addition to the Wechsler scale appropriate to the patient's age, includes the *Rorschach,* the *Thematic Apperception Test, Human Figure Drawing,* and the *Bender Visual Motor Gestalt Test.* The individual psychodiagnostician may add other instruments (e.g., *House-Tree-Person,* the *Hand Test*), or substitute the quantitative analysis of the *Minnesota Multiphasic Personality Inventory* for the more subjectively interpreted projective techniques. Some diagnosticians prefer to use the *Benton Visual Retention Test* instead of the *Bender,* because they consider the scoring and norms to be more quantitative. And, because they are looking for neuropsychological clues, some psychodiagnosticians add brief tests of lateral hemispheric functioning.

As will be seen from some of the studies cited later, there is considerable doubt that the projective techniques can identify brain dysfunction. But there is equal insistence that they have a role with the neurological patient to illuminate his emotional response to his dysfunction. The psychodiagnostic test battery may be introduced at either of two points in the diagnosis of MBD. It may be the first step of the process, that point where parents and/or teachers, concerned for a child's social, cognitive, emotional, and possibly physical difficulties, begin to search for clues to help him. Or it may come later in the process, when other diagnostic efforts already have established that MBD is indeed the cause, but the total impact remains to be comprehended.

When psychodiagnostic testing is sought after MBD is established, its major purpose is to identify and illuminate the emotional consequences of the impairments, and the patient's ego resources for coping with them and for undertaking the indicated remedial programs. In these circumstances the diagnostician is alerted to evidences of damage to self-esteem, depression, aversiveness, the quality of impulse control, rationalization, denial, masochism, and megalomania, as well as the nature of family interaction. His subject becomes the impact of MBD, of the awareness of dysfunction and limits, and the pathological defenses that awareness has provoked.

Where psychodiagnostic testing comes first in the process, the diagnostician is alerted both to the emotional state of the patient and to clues to possible cognitive dysfunction. These in turn may indicate the advisability of in-depth exploration through neurological and neuropsychological examination. He must ask himself whether a psychodynamic or neurological etiology, or both, should be inferred from any evidence of emotional disruption or conflict the testing uncovers. To this task of differential diagnosis, a complex one like that with intelligence tests, this discussion of the psychodiagnostic battery is directed.

Projective techniques—the *Rorschach, Thematic Apperception Test (TAT), Human Figure Drawings (HFD)*—are not now usually included in the batteries used by neuropsychologists. Originally the neuropsychologist Halstead used a group multiple-choice *Rorschach* in an effort to detect perceptual deficits. Reitan has also published in years past on the neuropsychological use of the *Rorschach*. And early in the popularity of the *Rorschach* systems of *Rorschach* organic brain-damage signs were developed. Paralleling this was the proliferation of rating scales for evaluating the possible presence of organic signs in the *Human Figure Drawings* technique. Despite this early surge, neither of these techniques has survived strongly in modern neuropsychological test batteries, although a few continue to include the *HFD*. The reason for this change from the early days may be the time demands of testing. Neuropsychological batteries have lengthened with the development of specific tests validated with neurological populations and with the increasing concern for lateralization and localization, to the exclusion of questions of emotional impact.

However, many phenomena appearing in the *HFD* and in *Rorschach* responses may be due to neurological rather than psychological causes. While differentiation of organicity from psychogenesis by projective tests alone is not possible, the psychodiagnostician can, with data from these tests combined with those from the *WAIS* and other tests for lateralization, detect clues on the neurological side.

The *HFD* and the *Rorschach* each involve specific processes: the *HFD* test requires graphomotor representation of a mental concept of the human body; the *Rorschach*, a visual-perceptual stimulus, requires intermediate processes of recognition, integration, and naming, and an oral-verbal expressive response. Dysfunctions in any of these processes may appear during the administration of these tests.

Distortions in *HFD* drawings comparable to those appearing on the *Bender* or the *Greek Cross* (a lateralization test) may appear: poor handling of the pencil and controlling of the drawn line may be observed; bilateral asymmetry may be marked. Pronounced difficulty on the *Rorschach* in arriving at a perception satisfactory to the patient may be indicative of Piotrowski's Impotence sign, in which the subject, aware that his response is unsatisfactory, is unable to correct it. Robot-like human figure drawings may reflect a neurological disturbance in body image or rigidity of thinking and feeling. Over-detailed drawings may suggest the uncertainty of an organically impaired individual or the meticulous control of the obsessive. Fragmentation of the body may arise from neurological dysfunction or from the ego disruption of schizophrenia. Rendering the body outline in short, separate, overlapping strokes may express schizophrenic feeling of vulnerability and fear of individuation through separation, or the organically impaired patient's motor inability to sustain a line. The graphomotor, visual, constructional requirements of the *HFD* technique may be the factors underlying their ability to predict the emergence of MBD symptoms in first-grade school children, as reported by Eaves *et al.* (27A).

Burgemeister (14), in an excellent review two decades ago of systems of *Rorschach* organic signs—those of Piotrowski (64), Hughes (39), Ross and Ross (75), Dorken and Kral (26), and Baker (5)—found that their etiological import could go in any of several directions. Her own research and clinical experience identified the following *Rorschach* indices to be of greatest value in suggesting organicity:

1. Repetition of responses, if occurring in a person of upper-level intelligence.
2. Perplexity.
3. Impotence.
4. Automatic phrasing.
5. Perseveration of content, even when asked to vary the response content. (Note: this is a limit-testing technique.)
6. "Pickiness"—emphasis upon small details.
7. Indications of feeling a threat to the integrity of the self in the content of responses.
8. Impairment of organizational ability.
9. Personalization of responses, suggesting impairment in abstract thinking.
10. Prominence given to color in a response with passive content.
11. Indications of a catastrophic reaction of anxiety, usually in the inability to muster a response.

Burgemeister emphasizes that the *Rorschach*'s value in neuropsychodiagnosis depends upon integrating its data with those from other tests.

Awareness of the possibility of multiple etiologies prompts the diagnostician to review carefully all the data from the *WAIS*, lateralization tests, the history, and interviewing.

The uncertain differential diagnostic meaning in *Rorschach* findings became apparent in the mixtures of organic and neurotic features that prevailed in the epileptics studied by Delay *et al.* (23). The *experience types* obtained showed them to be either *constricted,* with relatively good social adjustment, or *extratensive,* with poor social adjustment. Thus, the etiology was not differentiated by the *Rorschach;* it could have been organic disease, the individual's response to his disorder, or to some purely psychogenic factor.

Baker (5) believes that the neurodiagnostic use of the *Rorschach* has focused upon cognitive aspects of the patient's approach to the blots rather than its major value, which is identifying the impaired patient's emotional reaction to change in ability to cope, resulting from brain dysfunction. She suggested some of the major differential diagnostic difficulties with the *Rorschach:*

1. Hysterical symptoms arising from emotional response to brain dysfunction are similar to those observed in psychosomatically and somatically ill persons.
2. The patient with both a functional psychosis and mild brain damage may defy differential diagnosis.
3. The most difficult differential diagnostic problem is probably presented by the patient of low intelligence, poor education, and immature, hysterical personality.

Despite the difficulties, the psychodiagnostician must consider both the cognitive and the emotional in assessing brain dysfunction. The necessity for caution and skepticism concerning any single explanation or etiology is stressed by the recurring clinical and research observation that many of the same symptoms are found among brain-dysfunctional, physically ill, and emotionally disturbed individuals.

The responses of neurologically dysfunctional persons to projective techniques reflect both the nature of the processes involved in the task imposed, and the patient's emotional response to changes in coping ability. Birch and Diller (12) hypothesized that anatomical brain dysfunction produces either subtractive (lost sensory capability) or additive (psychological disturbances) alterations in behavior. The degree of psychological disruption does not necessarily correlate with the amount of tissue damaged. To test their hypothesis, Birch and Diller examined five hemiplegic patients who showed Piotrowski's signs of organicity on the *Rorschach* and five who did not. This separation enabled them to identify consequences of "neurophysiological" disturbances (additive): labileness, disorientation, convulsions. In a second experiment, ten hemiplegics were divided into groups of five according to whether they exhibited "additive" or "subtractive" features. A correlation of + .77 was obtained between the number of additive features and Piotrowski's signs. They conclude that so-called organic signs on the *Rorschach* reflect neurophysiological (additive) rather than neuroanatomical (subtractive) disturbance. A low percentage of both *Popular* and *Good-Form* responses was useful in distinguishing between their additive and subtractive groups of patients. Lower *Response Total* and paucity of *Human-Movement* responses were not so helpful; they are also found in depression and therefore may be caused by the individual's reaction to his illness rather than being primarily a result of neurodisintegration. The most discriminating *Rorschach* indicators, Impotence and Perplexity, were shared with other clinical groups. Perseveration appeared in 90 percent of organic patients and 50 percent of nonorganic patients. While scores and signs from the *Rorschach* test can be associated with brain dysfunction, the absence of organic signs may be a false positive, not proof that the individual does not have brain damage. Birch and Diller conclude that the *Rorschach* is more sensitive to the emotional behavioral consequences of brain dysfunction than to the brain dysfunction.

Birch and Belmont (11) turned from traditional *Rorschach* scoring methods to the kinds of cognitive demands the *Rorschach* task imposes:

1. *The visual-verbal task.* The subject is given a complex visual stimulus and responds with an oral-verbal expressive report. Figure-ground shading, shape, and color are organized within the person's ideational capability and content. The end result of a complicated process, the patient's response is scored "Well Defined" or "Poorly Defined."

2. *The perceptual-analytic task.* The patient is asked in the inquiry to identify the components of the stimulus incorporated in his response. This requires the patient to review actively the possible characteristics of the blot, but also may evoke new responses. The review is scored "Well Analyzed" or "Poorly Analyzed."

3. *The verbal-visual task.* This is a testing of perceptual limits. An additional perception is suggested to the patient. His ability to alter his original perception to one in accordance with the verbal suggestion is scored "Accepted" or "Rejected."

The protocols of 18 left-hemiplegic patients in the seventh decade of life were compared with those of 16 orthopedic patients of the same age without brain damage. First scored according to Klopfer's system, the protocols were then rescored for the three tasks described above. The major difference was in the perceptual-analytic task, where the brain-damage group had greater difficulty analyzing their perceptions into components and parts. No significant differences were found in the visual-verbal or verbal-visual tasks. The Klopfer scoring system identified some of the brain-damaged group as less productive, while others in this group were similar to the nondamaged group in response total. Productivity was inversely related to clarity of percept: higher proportions of clear-cut percepts at the visual-verbal level were offered by patients with low productivity than by patients with high productivity. Low productivity was also associated with better performance in the perceptual-analytic and verbal-visual tasks.

Belmont and Birch (7) hypothesize that low-productivity patients may have found a relatively constricted area in which they can function adequately. Goldstein described similar patients who functioned well as long as their environment was constant and clearly defined, enabling them to limit sensory input or their response to it. The higher-productivity group, unable to develop protective limitations or not having done so, continued to react to many stimuli with inadequate responses. Reminiscent of these observations are the findings by Delay *et al.* (23) of bipolar *Rorschach* "experience" types among epileptics: "constricted" types were more frequently associated with better social adjustment than were the "expansive" types.

An extensive analysis of *Rorschach* organic systems and signs is provided by Goldfried *et al.* (32) for the diagnostician who may wish to pursue matters of validity and reliability in detail.

The *Thematic Apperception Test (TAT)* generally is unproductive in differential diagnosis. Sometimes a severe anomia, visual-perceptual difficulty, or oral-verbal expressive disorder is apparent. For Card 1, for example, a patient may be unable to name the violin as such, or may misname it as a guitar or another very different stringed instrument. Often in MBD this card provides clues to a cognitive dysfunction, with themes depicting the difficulty of the boy pictured in mastering the violin and in the depression, damage to his self-esteem, or his parent's disappointment that result. Beyond that, of course, the *TAT* themes provide insights into emotional strengths and weaknesses, an important factor in the diagnosis and planning of treatment of MBD.

When the psychodiagnostic examination is early in the diagnostic process in suspected MBD, heavy reliance is placed upon the Wechsler scales for clues differentiating cerebral dysfunction from emotional disturbance. In support of this effort, lateral dominance of hand, eye, and foot are established (see Chapter 8), and some simple tests of lateral hemispheric functioning and of spatial-constructional praxis are added to the psychodiagnostic battery.

Tests of Lateral Hemispheric Functioning

In these tests the patient is not being compared with others but with himself—one side of his body against the other, a type of function associated with one side of the brain against another. He provides his own norm.

The Heimburger-Reitan Method

An easily administered lateralization test was developed by Heimburger and Reitan (38), who chose four among the 36 tests of aphasia from the original *Halstead-Wepman Aphasia Screening Test,* predicated upon the established dominance of the left hemisphere for language and of the right hemisphere for spatial and constructional functions.

The patient is shown, successively, a line drawing of a square, one of a triangle, and one of a Greek cross. He is instructed to reproduce each of the drawings without lifting pencil from paper. He is asked to name each figure, and then to spell the name of each. The examiner then says an unexpected sentence, "He shouted the warning," which the patient is asked to repeat, then to explain, and lastly to write down. None of these simple tasks has been practiced by most patients. Language skills of naming, spelling, and explaining are tested after constructional praxis is assessed. These simple tests, requiring little time, provide some material for hypotheses concerning language or spatial dysfunctions derived from the patient's performance on the Wechsler scales. The tests have been made part of the neuropsychological "key" method developed by Russell *et al.* (78), who offer a five-point-rating scoring scale for the drawings of the Greek cross. Clinicians who are just beginning to use the method will find their scale helpful.

Motor Tests

Quickly administered simple motor tests for assessing the extent to which lateralization is intact are the *Purdue Pegboard,* finger-tapping speed, and strength of grip, measured by the dynamometer, with three trials averaged for each hand. Instrumentation for testing finger-tapping speed can be constructed at relatively small cost, using electronic circuitry to avoid testing strength rather than speed. The electrical circuit is completed by the finger, activating a counter. Three trials of ten seconds each are administered and averaged for each hand. Dysfunction in the left hemisphere, for example, may affect verbal skills and also the speed and strength of the contralateral hand.

The simple efficiency of these methods is that each patient provides his own norm. Dysfunction is hypothesized if the dominant hand is slower than the other hand, or if the nondominant hand is significantly slower than the dominant hand. The nondominant hand, in my experience, usually averages ten fewer finger-tapping contacts than the dominant hand during a ten-second period in an undamaged individual, but research is needed to establish norms and grades of significant difference.

The *Purdue Pegboard* (19, 67, 89) performs a similar function. Starting with the dominant hand, each hand is tested separately. Then both are tested simultaneously. The three tests are repeated and the results for each averaged, giving scores for the dominant hand, nondominant hand, and both hands. Administration takes only about ten minutes; norms are available (19).

Tests of Spatial-Constructional Praxis

The *Bender Visual-Motor Gestalt Test* is a complex visual-motor task, although the subject is instructed to copy relatively simple designs. Analyzed by Koppitz (50), it concerns at least four processes: (1) perception of the stimulus; (2) comprehension of what is seen; (3) translation of the perception into a planned motor act; and (4) the motor act. The functions tested, therefore, are both receptive and expressive, and Koppitz reports that most often impairments when present involved both processes.

Long-established signs of organic dysfunction on the *Bender* are: rotations, when the designs are drawn in an axis different from the one in which they are presented; distortions in reproduction; collisions when designs are run together; disproportion between components of the design; use of circles, loops, lines, angles, or straight lines for dots; use of angles or straight lines for curves; and perseverations. Koppitz has evolved a clinically rich developmental approach to these *Bender* signs. She notes that each of the distortions made by dysfunctional persons on the *Bender* will occur in the productions of all children at some point in development, making age norms essential since an age-appropriate distortion does not signal dysfunction. Should it persist beyond the age when additional capability is expected, it then has diagnostic import. Lower I.Q. has been found to be associated with increased rotation, and this factor must be considered in evaluation.

Scoring systems to objectify interpretation are available: Pascal and Suttell (63), Koppitz (50), Hutt and Briskin (41), and Hain (34). Pascal and Suttell differentiate two types of rotation: type I, the usual rotation of 45 degrees or more; type II, special instances of rotation on designs 4, 5, 6, and 7, and rotation of more than 45 degrees on design A and part of design 3. Freed (30) reports that nonpsychotic neurological patients produced significantly more type II rotations than did psychotic or neurotic patients.

Many diagnosticians have added a memory component to the *Bender,* by asking the patient, after the usual administration, to draw as many of the designs as he can recall. The procedure is difficult to evaluate, however, because of the connection of memory to intelligence, the varying complexity of the designs, and the decreasing time intervals from the exposure of the first design to the last. These difficulties may be eliminated by introducing the memory component *before* the usual administration. Designs A, 3, and 4 are exposed, each for a five-second interval. Each is then removed, and the patient is asked to reproduce it from memory. The usual administration procedure then follows, using all of the designs. Comparison can be made of each of the three designs reproduced from both memory and direct copy.

Stress can be increased by using Canter's *Background Interference Procedure (BIP)* (16). The *Bender* is administered first in the usual way, with each design drawn separately on a sheet of blank paper. Other tests (e.g. *WAIS, Rorschach*) are then administered, to erase memory of the designs. The patient is then asked to draw the designs again, on paper that now contains a background of randomly placed intersecting curved lines.

Koppitz (50) has identified signs of brain damage in the *Bender* drawings of adults. If brain dysfunction disrupts the complex receptive-expressive visual-motor function that, she hypothesizes, is assessed by the *Bender,* regression in that function is displayed in these signs:

1. Excessive time.
2. Tracing designs with the finger.
3. Placing finger on part of the design being drawn.
4. Preferring to draw from memory because sight of the card is confusing.
5. Rotating both card and paper to draw, then returning the paper to the presenting position after finishing the drawing.
6. Uncertainty about the number of dots and circles, despite checking them several times.
7. Hasty drawings erased and corrected with much effort.
8. Expressions of dissatisfaction and efforts to correct the drawing.

Some of these signs are similar to Piotrowski's (64) *Rorschach* clues to brain damage. Both tests present visual-perceptive tasks, the *Bender* requires a graphomotor response, the *Rorschach* an oral-verbal expressive one. Increased time, tracing, and finger anchoring have been clinically observed in persons with impaired visual-perceptive processes.

The ability of the *Bender* and the Canter *BIP* to diagnose brain damage has received only equivocal research support. *Bender* drawings of brain-damaged patients were significantly differentiated from those of psychiatric patients by scoring of their reproductions, but not by time scores, in a study by Rosencrans and Schaffer (74). Brain-damaged patients scored lower than did non-brain-damaged patients when the *Koppitz Developmental System* was used (61). The *Hutt-Briskin* system was reported to be effective only in identifying brain damage in patients of Borderline of Dull Normal intelligence (43). And it has been observed that the *Bender* identifies brain damage only in the most obvious cases. Tymchuk (87) reports the *Bender* to be more effective in separating groups of brain-damaged persons from the non-brain-damaged than in identifying individuals.

Canter suggests that his *BIP* method distinguishes brain damage from schizophrenia because it presents mild arousal conditions (15). Kenny (44) reports that the *BIP* discriminated brain-damaged children from both emotionally disturbed and control groups better than did the *Bender.* Adams *et al.* (1), however, find the *BIP* much less sensitive to brain damage in children than in adults. Adams (3) found the *BIP*'s contribution to the diagnosis of brain damage in mentally retarded children uncertain, and also that it failed to differentiate hyperkinetic boys from controls. In another study, Adams (2) found little difference between the *Bender* and the *BIP* drawings of heterogenously brain-damaged adults and those of non-brain-damaged adult psychiatric patients.

Smith (83) reminds us that the *Bender* was designed originally to explore emotional disturbances, not brain damage, and he advises the use of the *Benton Visual Retention Test* (9) instead. The *Benton* scoring system is illustrated and easy to follow; normative standards evaluate children and adults for "number correct" and "error" scores according to age, sex, and intelligence levels. There are three equivalent forms of the test. A memory test is incorporated in the design for its administration; the patient is first asked to reproduce designs from memory five, ten and/or 15 seconds after each exposure, then the direct-copy task is given. The designs incorporate right and left peripheral figures sensitive to homonymous hemianopsia and to unilateral spatial inattention. The two administrations of the test, recall and direct copy, together take about ten minutes.

Neuropsychological Testing

The many symptom clusters or subsyndromes observed in MBD and the variety of brain-behavior relationships that can be affected must be matched by a wide-ranging neuropsychological test battery to search them out. Intelligence, psychoeducation, and psychodiagnostic testing all provide clues. But the brain-behavior disruptions suggested by these often require further, more minute exploration, within the purvue of the neuropsychologist (28, 37, 52). The tests he will use will vary with the individual psychologist's background, training, experience, and immediate interests. There is no standard neuropsychological test battery. Extensively used at present, however, are the *Halstead-Reitan* tests and the *Luria* battery; the approaches of the two differ.

Neuropsychological Approaches

Luria's approach emphasizes the acumen of the neuropsychologist, the developed capacity within the clinician to move surely and swiftly from observation to evaluation to judgment. Standardized tests are deployed not in a pre-prescribed order but rather selected on the spot in response to the unfolding situation in the patient observed by the clinician, who may invent tests to meet an unusual situation. Here, the psychologist himself is the primary test instrument, reacting with diagnostic judgment to how the patient performs, not to what he scores. Scoring and standardization of Luria's battery is currently being researched in America by Golden *et al.* (31A) based in part upon Christensen's (16A) adaptation of Luria's battery.

The Halstead-Reitan model, in contrast, places the test instrument and the test battery in the forefront, emphasizing the scores that emerge. Each test is statistically validated. Tests are incorporated according to their ability to assess specific brain functions; the battery assesses as wide a range as possible of these functions. New tests are devised to meet perceived needs, but the battery is applied in standardized, prescribed fashion to all patients. While clinical style is defined by such standardization, clinical acumen, of course, remains in the neuropsychologist, to use as he may.

A recent development from the Halstead-Reitan approach is the "key" method of neuropsychodiagnosis, in which reliance upon test scores is most pronounced. The method is derived from systems used by biologists in classification of specimens by orders, genera, and species. Scores, like specimen characteristics, are checked against statements in the key listing. If the score or characteristic matches the first statement, the pursuit of the key follows the directions given by the statement. If there is no match, the next statement is consulted, and so on.

Neuropsychological Test Batteries

Halstead developed 27 tests in his monumental and pioneering effort at diagnostic insight. These he eventually reduced to ten, and from these he obtained the *Impairment Index* according to which the patient was or was not diagnosed as brain-damaged.

Reitan, who worked with Halstead, extended and refined the battery to include a wider range of functions than did the original *Halstead* battery. His battery, *Halstead-Reitan,* assesses simple motor functions, sensorimotor functions, and psychomotor problem-solving processes. These are at a relatively simple level of brain-behavior relationship, but their power is enhanced by comparison of the two sides of the body in each function. Higher-level functions assessed by the battery are: symbolic and communicational aspects of language, visual-spatial relations, abstraction and concept formation, and general intelligence.

Among the tests making up the *Halstead-Reitan* battery from which the *Impairment Index* is derived are these:

Auditory Imperception Test. This test seeks to determine if the subject can perceive simultaneous bilateral sensory stimulations. Each ear is tested separately to make sure that it is functioning; then a series is offered in which stimulation to one side is interspersed with bilateral simultaneous stimulation.

Seashore Rhythm Test. This is a subtest of the *Seashore Test of Musical Talent,* adapted for this battery. The subject is asked to differentiate between thirty pairs of rhythmic beats, some of which are similar, some different. Reitan uses it for older children and adults, but finds it somewhat difficult for younger children and does not use it for the five-to-eight-year age group.

Speech-Sounds Test. Sixty nonsense words with variants of the "ee-ee" sound are heard, spoken in multiple-choice form, using a tape recorder. Intensity of sound is adjusted to the subject's preference. The subject selects the syllable which he believes has been spoken from the four alternatives presented for each stimulus.

Fingertip Number-Writing Test. Numbers which the subject cannot see are written on the fingertips of each hand and the subject is asked to name each so written. The numbers and sequence of writing are standardized. Four trials are given for each finger of each hand. X's and zeros are used for children between five and eight because number recognition is usually too difficult for them.

Tactile Form-Perception Test. The subject is asked to identify pennies, nickels, and dimes through touch alone. Each hand is tested separately. Simultaneous bilateral stimulation is also introduced, by requiring the subject to identify coins placed in both hands at the same time. Coin recognition is not used with children under eight. Another version uses plastic figures, a cross, square, triangle, and circle, as stimuli, to be matched by the subject against pictures of the stimulus figures.

Tactile Finger-Recognition Test. This procedure tests ability to identify the fingers on each hand, as a result of their stimulation, according to a system for reporting the finger touched worked out beforehand with the patient. Some prefer to report by the finger's number, others prefer to use other terms. To ensure that the patient is able to report reliably, some patients are allowed to keep their eyes open for practice. Forty trials in all are given, four for each finger on each hand.

Critical Flicker-Frequency Test. An electronic instrument housed in a sound-proof container presents intermittent light at variable frequencies. The subject adjusts a knob to increase the rate of flashing of the light to a point where the light appears to be steady. The intermittency frequency at this point is recorded in terms of cycles per second.

Time-Sense Test. To check both visual and memory components, the subject presses a key, releasing a sweep hand to rotate on a clock face. The subject is asked to allow the hand to rotate ten times, then stop it as close to the starting point as possible. During 20 trials, the subject observes the rotation. The clock face is then turned away and he attempts to duplicate the performance without visual control. After ten trials based upon memory sense, ten visually controlled trials and ten memory trials are interspersed.

Hand-Hand Test. Each hand is touched separately to establish that the subject is able to identify that hand, then bilateral simultaneous stimulation is interspersed with unilateral stimulation, and the subject is asked to identify whether the right hand, left hand, or both hands have been touched.

Trail-Making Test. In the first of two sections, 25 small circles numbered from 1 to 25 are distributed upon a sheet of white paper and in scattered order. The subject draws a line from 1 to 25 in numerical sequence as quickly as he can. The second section also presents 25 circles; some are numbered from 1 to 13, others are lettered A to L. The subject draws a connecting line, progressively alternating between numbers and letters, as fast as he can. Ability to shift is involved. The score is the time taken to complete each part.

Halstead Category Test. A milk-glass screen upon which the stimuli are projected tests a patient's ability to perceive categories among the stimuli. Beneath the screen is an answer panel with four numbered levers. Two hundred and eight stimulus figures are available for projection. The subject is instructed to depress one of the levers each time a picture appears on the screen. This will cause either a bell or a buzzer to sound, corresponding with the "right" or "wrong" answer. The subject is instructed before the test begins that the stimuli are divided into seven groups and that each group is bound by a single principle which appears throughout the entire group. Thus on the first item in any group his response is pure guess work, but as he progresses, the feedback of right or wrong (bell or buzzer) indicates to him the accuracy of his responses. This allows the patient to test one possible principle after another until he develops an hypothesis; this is thereafter reinforced positively by the consistent ringing of the bell. The beginning and end of each group is announced to the subject.

Reitan also uses finger-tapping-speed and strength-of-grip tests, and has developed a version of his battery for children.

Russell *et al.* (78) use scores from 41 tests or subtests in their key structure. These include some of the *Halstead-Reitan* tests, an aphasia examination, and the *WAIS*. Rating scales have been developed to improve quantification in some tests, such as the Greek cross of the aphasia examination. Scores are obtained for the visual fields and the sensorimotor functions of each side of the body.

Rourke (77) has selected his extensive neuropsychological battery for children to cover the many elements he has found essential for full exploration of suspected MBD: sensoriperceptual abilities (tactile, visual, auditory, and intersensory), motor skills (force and accuracy), psychomotor abilities (manipulatory, steadiness, graphomotor), language abilities (receptive, expressive, associative), higher-order concept-formation and problem-solving abilities, memory, sequencing, and attentional abilities. He uses these tests: *Halstead Neuropsychological Battery for Children; Reitan-Indiana Neuropsychological Test for Children; Klove-Matthews Motor Steadiness Battery; Reitan-Klove Lateral Dominance Examination; Reitan-Klove Tactile Form Recognition Test; Trail-Making Test for Children; Test of Auditory Ability; Wechsler Intelligence Scale for Children; Wide-Range Achievement Test; Peabody Picture Vocabulary Test.* Rourke justifies the three and one-half to eight hours required for administering this battery by its broad intent, which is to contribute to habilation, rehabilitation, and remedial procedures as well as to evaluate the possible presence, type, location, chronicity, age of onset, and prognosis of brain damage.

In one study using the battery, Rourke and Finlayson (76) divided learning-disabled children, matched for I.Q., into three groups: those uniformly deficient in reading, spelling and arithmetic (Group 1); those relatively good in arithmetic as compared with their ability in reading and spelling (Group 2); and those relatively deficient in arithmetic but with average to above-average levels in reading and spelling (Group 3). Groups 1 and 2 proved superior to Group 3 on measures of visual-spatial and visual-perceptual abilities. Group 3, as might be predicted, were superior to Groups 1 and 2 in tests of verbal and auditory-perceptual abilities.

Rourke advocates both adequate norms for all tests used (something not always available) and the heterogeneous testing of a function supplemented by other more homogeneous measures. He cites the *Coding* subtest *(WISC)* as an example of a heterogeneous test involving speed and accuracy of eye-hand coordination, visual and symbolic memory, and attention. While this subtest is a "factor analyst's nightmare," the subsequent application of more homogeneous measures of each of the component functions improves the possibility of specifying the deficit or deficits making for poor performance on the *Coding* subtest. Such enhancement of precision in diagnosis is provided by Smith's *Symbol Digit Modalities Test* (84); here symbol processing is tested through both written and oral modes, and by requiring the patient to respond by pointing after the usual oral response to the *Digit-Span* subtest.

Smith (83) at the Neuropsychological Laboratory at the University of Michigan uses an extensive yet time-economical test battery that takes about three hours to administer. His principles of test selection are to use specific tests of specific functions, to test the same function via various modalities where possible, and to use some tests tapping more than one function. In addition to his *Symbol Digit Modalities Tests* and the two-modality testing of *Digit Span* in the Wechsler scales, he uses all the other subtests of the *WISC* or *WAIS;* the Verbal, Performance, and Full Scale I.Q.s; the *Hooper Visual Organization Test; Raven's Progressive Matrices;* the *Benton Visual Retention Test* (from memory and direct copy); the *Purdue Pegboard* (each hand separately and both hands simultaneously); *Right/Left Body Parts Identification; Peabody Picture Vocabulary; Double Simultaneous Stimulation* (face and hand); *Color Naming, Color Matching, Verbal Recognition, Reading Recognition; Singing; Reading Comprehension of Simple Commands; Oral Comprehension of Simple Commands; Memory for Unrelated Sentences; Writing;* and *Human Figure Drawing.*

Neuropsychological Testing in MBD

Much effort has been devoted by neuropsychologists to the differential diagnosis of MBD, brain-damaged, and non-neurologically-impaired subjects. Reitan (69) compared these groups according to: (1) levels of performance, (2) patterns of relationship, (3) specific disabilities, and (4) right-left motor and sensory differences. He found the right-left differences to be the most discriminating. The MBD children are worse than normals, not as bad as the brain-damaged. Reitan and Boll (71) similarly found MBD children scoring between brain-damaged and normal controls on an extensive neuropsychological test battery.

Benton (8) believes the evidence justifies the assumption that brain damage or dysfunction in MBD is not actually minimal, but major in extent. He cites observations that it takes more extensive damage in children to produce aphasia than it does to produce the same degree of language dysfunction in adults, and that children with established, demonstrable cerebral disease may manifest MBD symptoms either with or without classical neurological symptoms and with or without "gross mental deficiency."

The questions underlying these neuropsychological debates are whether or not the MBD child is indeed brain-damaged to some degree, and whether or not neuropsychological tests of brain damage may be validly used to identify and assess the MBD syndrome. Klatskin *et al.* (46) report agreement in 43 of 50 cases between neurological examinations turning up minor signs only and findings from the *WISC* and *Bender.* Crinella (20) was able to discriminate between normal controls, cases of verified brain damage, and cases of suspected brain damage in a testing procedure that encompasses 90 variables. While he found so much variation between the brain-damaged and MBD subjects that he questions the use of brain-damage tests to identify MBD, he also found the MBD group to be functioning better than the brain-damaged, less well than the controls.

No value is ascribed to psychological tests for diagnosing central-nervous-system dysfunction by Conners (18). He cites the observations of Hartlage (36) and others that most tests imply a unitary concept of brain damage, are normalized on small populations, have poorly matched controls, lack specificity in scoring, do not account properly for age and acuteness of injury. The major fault, Hartlage finds, is in grouping the heterogeneously brain-injured into a single sample, when no single behavioral pattern may be expected in them. In an effort to delineate patterns of scores representing homogeneous groups, Conners factor-analyzed all the test scores of 267 children, 6 to 12 years of age, referred for treatment for behavioral and/or learning disorders on the *WISC, Bender—Koppitz* scoring, *Porteus Maze, Wide-Range Achievement, Frostig Test of Visual Perception,* and *Draw-A-Man.* These were then divided into separate patterns of factor scores or "cluster types":

1. Good impulse control, low I.Q., poor learners.
2. Inattentive, low achievers, poor learners.
3. Very poor impulse control, poor learners, moderately attentive.
4. Bright, high achievers, good impulse control, slightly inattentive.
5. Attentive, good learners, generally above average in most areas of functioning.
6. Very good learners, poor impulse control.

Conners concludes that psychological tests may be more useful in describing functions than in diagnosing central-nervous-system dysfunctions, in refining categorization of patients, suggesting etiological hypotheses, and identifying subgroups who may have "unique responses to therapies."

Such "clustering" with concomitant implications for treatment was accomplished by Mattis *et al.* (58) in the thoroughgoing study of dyslexic children presented in detail earlier (Chapter 4). Their results deserve summary here. They identified three patterns of neuropsychological-test data in dyslexic children without brain damage that were distinguishable from the patterns found in brain-damaged dyslexics and brain-damaged readers. One cluster of dyslexics was characterized by anomia and disorders of comprehension, imitative speech, and speech-sound discrimination of "e" rhyming letters. A second group showed primarily articulatory and graphomotor dyscoordination but had normal acousto-sensory and receptive language function. The third group presented visuo-perceptual disorders with Verbal I.Q.s higher than Performance I.Q.s.

Neuropsychological evidence is offered by Pirozzolo (65) that dyslexia comprises at least two independent disorders, each the result of a different form of neurological dysfunction, visual-spatial and auditory-linguistic.

Many studies report ability to differentiate children with MBD, hyperkinesis, learning disabilities, and dyslexia from normal controls on the basis of a single test or two (21, 27, 29, 46, 60). But such gross discrimination alone is inadequate for fulfilling the major purpose of diagnosis: directing treatment. Only the comprehensive neuropsychological battery has that potential in the service of a treatment-oriented clinician. An illustration of the point is the history of a battery of tests for the early detection of learning disabilities *before* otherwise normal children suffer the emotional damage of school failure. Such a battery, the *Predictive Index,* was developed by de Hirsch *et al.* (22A) and consisted of *Pencil Use,* the *Bender,* the *Wepman Auditory Discrimination Test, Number of Words Used in a Story, Horst Reversals Test, Gates Word-Matching Subtests, Word Recognition I* and *II,* and *Word Recognition.* Subsequently, Eaves *et al.* (27A) added the *Draw-A-Person Test* and *Name Printing,* calling the expanded battery the *Modified Predictive Index (MPI).* The battery identified 44 percent of school failures as having MBD and another 44 percent as at high risk for such failures. Additionally, the composition of the battery directed specific teaching efforts.

The typical neuropsychological battery today is so inclusive, and produces so much data along so many variables that the clinician's ability to handle the mass becomes increasingly difficult. Knights (48) is attempting to cope with that problem by the computer storage of individual T-score profiles on 17 tests and 106 test variables. The scores of a newly-tested child are compared with those of every other child previously tested (more than 1,500 at the time of the report), and the print-out includes the coefficients of correlation with the stored scores, case numbers, and names and principal symptoms of the five best-matching problems. These aids should prove increasingly valuable in diagnosis. Meanwhile, the task of translating test data into diagnosis and diagnosis into treatment remains that of the clinician.

III

TREATMENT

Chapter 11

Treatment: An Overview

THE BEST TREATMENT of a person found to have minimal brain dysfunction is a program addressed as precisely as possible to the combination of limitations he suffers. In addition to work on them, the most promising program for him is likely to include measures for restoring or preventing disruption of his social and family relations, ameliorating or preventing emotional disturbance, and planning and preparing vocational competence in due time. Several principles guide this orientation to treatment for the MBD patient:

1. The specific impairments of the individual direct an individual treatment plan, a point that cannot be overstressed. MBD patients cannot be successfully treated as a homogeneous group.
2. A combination of different treatment efforts is usually needed. Possibilities include remedial education, speech training, perceptual and motor training, environmental manipulation, counseling and/or psychotherapy of parents, counseling and/or psychotherapy of the patient, group therapy, family therapy, nutritional guidance, social work, medication, correction of visual and auditory problems, and behavior modification (3, 5, 11, 17).
3. Strengths, identified as zealously as deficits when the patient is examined, are developed as compensation for deficits.
4. Periodic review of progress is essential to modify treatment and, for a child, to exploit developmental changes.
5. The multimodal nature of an MBD treatment plan requires that one professional on the treatment team act as its coordinator and overseer, a necessity detailed below.

The recently adopted national Public Law 142, by mandating treatment for the learning-disabled child, has highlighted the inadequacy of the diagnostic information usually available to educators charged with providing one type of treatment in MBD. They now increasingly complain that they also have inadequate guides to classroom interventions. This lack derives from many causes, chief among them some bias toward one of the many possible eitiologies in each case of MBD, a bias often toward inappropriate treatment efforts. For example, drugs are inappropriate for a child whose hyperactivity on careful exploration is found to be a symptom of anxiety (2). After years of failure, an accretion of effects may obscure the real cause in another child, perhaps even poor instruction, or resignation, depression, or low self-esteem (6). In many children, the impairments go beyond specific deficits and emotional reactions. The child can affect parents with his outbursts of anger, guilt, or despair. The impairment can stigmatize the child, and predicate adverse attitudes of teachers and others to him (14). The many possibilities caution the diagnostician to avoid labeling any individual by a predetermined set of criteria—social, educational, psychological, neurological, genetic, or whatever. Like any other patient in the best of worlds, the MBD victim must be seen as an individual with personal needs specific to him rather than, say, as a social problem (16), or a candidate for a certain medication.

One model of multimodal intervention strategy has been evolved by Feighner and Feighner (5) for the treatment of hyperkinesis. It outlines, first, a far-reaching diagnostic assessment, then choices among medications, behavior modification, curriculum counseling, followed by training for the patient's teachers and use of videotaping to illuminate for parents their interaction with their child, and finally, continuing coordination of therapeutic efforts with child, parents, and school.

The treatment programs of 100 disadvantaged children with learning disabilities by the Learning Disability Clinic at Sinai Hospital in Baltimore reflect the range and variation that grow from careful, multidisciplinary diagnosis of a heterogeneous group. Their educational recommendations included: placement in a learning-disability class or a special-education class or school; a change of class within the regular school; continuing at present grade level beyond the usual promotion time; tutoring by the staff of the clinic, the class teacher, or a teacher's aide; consultation with the regular class teacher by the diagnostic and remedial teacher. Medication was recommended for 36 children. Social recommendations for 67 children included family counseling. In six cases, medical or psychiatric care was advised for other members of the family whose problems were affecting the child. Protective changes in living arrangements were made in seven cases. Referrals to other social agencies were advised in 12 instances. Individual counseling was arranged for 32 children; 5 received group counseling. Speech therapy was recommended for 13 children, eye examination for 19; one child received a hearing aid.

A large sample of 5,212 school children were examined by Lambert *et al.* (9)

for evidence of hyperactivity. Of these, 1.2 percent were identified as meeting criteria for the disorder. Medication was or had been the treatment for 86 percent of this group, at the time of the study, in the recent past, or in the more remote past. When medication was the primary therapy prescribed at the time and stress in school appeared, other therapy modalities were prescribed congruently. These included: counseling for parent of child (50 percent); special education (41 percent); consultation at school (39 percent); diet therapy (32 percent); motor therapy (9 percent). With a similar approach, Oettinger (13) regards drugs as the keystone of MBD therapy, but acknowledges that full treatment also offers remediation, counseling, physiotherapy, and environmental control.

Schackenberg (15) avoids identifying one therapy as primary, and describes how the treatment of an MBD child may combine tranquilizers; psychotherapy, either individual, family or group; special education; perceptual-motor training; or behavior training.

Even a single aspect of MBD—for example, derivative emotional problems—presents a complex situation that in turn requires more than one kind of treatment. Muir (10) separates three major considerations in diagnosed emotional problems attending MBD: (1) the individual's intrapsychic emotional reactions; (2) his interpersonal or social interactions; and (3) the family's interactions or dynamics. Muir suggests that treatment of these factors, depending upon their combination, will require one or more of the following: joint family conference, a series of conferences with the child, family therapy, individual therapy, home-management counseling, teacher conferences, and education programs with the community and peers.

While the importance of a case coordinator or manager has only recently been proposed in MBD (6A, 12), the role has been explored and debated in the post-hospital treatment of chronic psychotic patients, whose needs are multiple and complex, but whose prognosis is far less favorable than that of the MBD patient (4, 8). With MBD, the pattern seems equally necessary but far more promising.

Ochroch's (12) advocacy of the case manager in MBD treatment goes to the heart of the enormous difficulty faced by families of child and adult MBD victims in obtaining thorough diagnosis, and then in finding appropriate treatment, sometimes not available locally, in coordinating the many kinds of data and their sources, in dealing with the spread effects into family and society, in getting cooperation from education and government authorities, and in monitoring and evaluating the patient's progress. Many patients and their families are overwhelmed by the enormity of this task, about which they have little or no information. The family, Ochroch justly argues, needs one central person with all the needed information about the child who can comprehend the implications of the information for child and family. And, we may add, the adult MBD patient no less than the child needs the help of a central coordinating professional.

It is true that professional education does not now include training in the skills and responsibilities or tasks of the case coordinator or manager. Nor are there many practicing professionals willing to serve in the role. The case-coordination function, so obviously needed, is still largely a concept. It is a service need, like so many others, not currently being filled, but one which professional training institutions and government agencies must be pressed to meet. Hope for this future development prompts its discussion here. And it is in the hope that many parents and patients, becoming better able to confront the reality of their situation, will demand this service that the knowledges, tasks, and skills of the case coordinator are outlined here in the form of a job description. This overview of the treatment of the MBD patient presents an idealized program. While it is realistic on the basis of the needs of these patients, all too often it is still unavailable in the real world of professional services.

The case coordinator in MBD knows: (1) the many possible etiologies for any symptom; (2) where to pursue further the diagnosis of the various etiological possibilities; (3) the local treatment resources and how to obtain them.

The case coordinator in MBD has at least these tasks:

1. He takes a history, if not done before, and gathers all earlier records, to assure completeness.

2. He coordinates the various diagnostic findings and recommendations, and pursues their clarification wherever fragmentary or contradictory.

3. He evolves a treatment plan, setting priorities according to the diagnostic data and its import.

4. He makes the necessary referrals according to the treatment plan.

5. He works closely with parents and family to secure their contribution to diagnosis and treatment, to help them understand the complexities and ambiguities of the patient's situation and his realistic prognosis, to assure their understanding of the child's assets as well as his limitations. He acquaints them with possible limitations in available treatment services as well as with the attitudes of other professionals with whom they may have to deal, and helps them to understand the impact of their MBD child upon family interactions—all with the intent of making the family part of the therapeutic team.

6. He serves as communication center for treatment personnel, child, and parents. Here the coordinator promptly circulates important data and developments in the case, to forestall the discouragement of both remedial teachers and parents when no feedback is provided. To prevent such isolation the coordinator may convene periodic conferences of the team, with the parents involved as warranted. Especially important is an initial conference at the beginning when diagnostic data from the various sources are coordinated, a treatment plan evolved, and responsibilities assigned, where the family is essential.

7. He acts as advocate or ombudsman when needed services are withheld

or nonexistent; for example, he helps parents to negotiate for necessary school services and government services mandated by law.

8. He regularly monitors information from the various treatment sources, being especially alert to the negative side effects of drugs prescribed, maintaining easy access to the case physician.

9. He is continuously available by telephone or in person to intervene in crisis and emergent situations.

10. He regularly assesses developments, changes, and need for modification of plans, writing reports in understandable, jargon-free language, available to the parents.

The case coordinator thus establishes and sustains an alliance with several professionals, with the child, and with parents, explaining to the child and parents all that is involved in the cooperative effort, supporting both through the vicissitudes of the course of treatment. Providing a stable center during periods of eruptive, reactive behavior, and counteracting the defensive denial and aversive isolation that are likely to develop in the patient, the coordinator not only starts the process but also holds it together.

The coordinator may be any member of the team drawn into the working therapeutic alliance, but must value the communication process and be willing to allot the time required. The time requirements are not overly demanding: the initial planning conference may require about two hours; later work is variable in length. During a crisis he may be needed frequently, by telephone or in person. Ordinarily, he may schedule only occasional telephone calls and one-hour conferences. With young patients personal consultations may be necessary only at the beginning and end of the school year.

Finally, a concept of parsimony guides the decisions of coordinator and all other members of the treatment team. The treatment process for patient and family is a long and costly one at best; optimism and motivation, and confidence in the professional will all drain away if a random, shotgun "we'll hit it with something" approach is adopted. Each step is selected for its probable appropriateness and effectiveness and explained to patient and family.

The effort in treatment always is to reduce as much as possible the discrepancy between potential and achievement (6). Seldom if ever is the discrepancy eliminated in MBD. Sometimes a specific deficit is not responsive to intervention. Then negative psychological consequences for patient, family, and community often intensify, and these become the focus for treatment. Or practical treatment may be less than total. The "ideal" goals must be modified by realities. But these possibilities should not deflect or dilute the effort with each patient to help him realize the use of all his endowment in both the unimpaired functions and the treatable ones.

From the reports of specific treatment methods surveyed in the following chapters, the impression is strong that no consistent theory has yet emerged about how interventions work. But even stronger is the fact that many MBD children respond to the input of remedial efforts. Growth in any child is a function of "input times development," and more of all these are needed by the MBD child. He also needs unusually careful selection of the inputs.

Remedial workers in MBD differ in orientation and emphasis, but most are alike for the most part in their dedicated response to the special needs of special children. A characteristic of the successful professional working with MBD patients is innovativeness and willingness to develop the necessary extensive armamentarium of "skills, techniques, and materials" (7). Unlimited by bias toward any one approach, the effective worker in MBD is able to develop individualized programs from among the available options as indicated in each case (1).

Chapter 12

Remediation Through Special Education

A CHILD SPENDS about 1,400 hours of the 8,760 hours in each year in school (13). When that child labors with learning disabilities that do not improve, he is subject to the accretion of thousands of hours of failure, humiliation, and severely damaged self-esteem. Well conceptualized psychoeducational remediation is the major element in the complex treatment programs these children need.

Based on careful diagnosis, habilitation and rehabilitative programs can be guided by assessment, both prior and ongoing, of his assets and liabilities, and give him his most direct help.

Several general principles emerge from a scanning of special-education literature. First is the value of early beginning, with normal progression toward greater differentiation, accompanied by integration. As discussed earlier, careful diagnosis should first establish the child's level of capability, so that instruction can advance from that stage, lest a teacher, misled by one child's obvious general brightness, begin remedial efforts at too advanced a level, or discouraged by another child's aversive apathy misinterpreted as mental dullness, begin it too low.

The length, or size, of units of instruction is best adjusted to the attention span of the individual child. Repetitive drill usually is avoided, so as not to provoke perseverative behavior, although patient repetition of information is helpful with hyperkinetic children (43).

Remedial instruction can be focused hypothetically upon a specific brain function—for example, perception, categorization, peripheral motor manip-

145

ulations. Encouraging manual manipulation of parts may abet a child's ability to focus on the task at hand, as in learning numbers by using a number wheel.

The acquisition of facility in one learning strategy has been found to be transferable to other learning situations (36), so that unexpected gains may result from a remedial program. But these are in their very nature unpredictable, and not counted upon.

Reinforcement of any gain is an important element in remediation. Reinforcement reduces uncertainty and confusion. It helps the student identify the structure in a task or the learning process that increases "cognitive economy" by reducing the task of information processing (17).

The many teaching aids professionals have developed, either to bypass deficits or to mitigate them, are ingenious; they bespeak both the devotion and the creativity of workers in this field. Teaching directionality, for example, can be facilitated by placing bracelets of different colors on the right and left wrists of the child, and the same colors on the corresponding wrists of the teacher as they face each other. And certain diagnostic tests can be converted into learning tasks; Pontius (39) suggests the training possibilities in such diagnostic tests as the *Wisconsin Card Sorting* and *Trail-Making B,* where the goal is to improve the child's ability to shift.

Children with intractible dyscalculia can be taught to use hand calculators, those with agraphia to type, or to use a tape recorder, to present their reports and test responses orally instead of writing them; dyslexics may assimilate much information auditorily from tape-recorded material that as printed matter would be beyond their reach. Dyslexics can also improve their reading ability through intersensory reinforcement by listening to tape recordings of the same material they are trying to read. This strategy has been used successfully with learning-disabled adults who were not correctly diagnosed or fully helped when they were children. It uses intact channels of communications as compensatory methods; the adult is taught to dictate instead of writing or to use a pocket calculator instead of floundering with mental arithmetic (14). Circumvention of a dysfunction has its opponents, who consider the use of calculators superficial and of limited effectiveness in the remediation of dyscalculia. Weinstein (49) uses instead intellectual exercises that require analytic thought, with immediate feedback to the student on the accuracy of his strategies. Occasionally she presents tasks that can be solved spatially rather than numerically.

For hyperkinetic children especially, the quality of the classroom environment is stressed by workers who subscribe to the stimulus-overload hypothesis. Littleton and Davis (30) advocate control of sound and light, in addition to a small class size (see Chapter 13).

For all dysfunctions, cooperative interaction of professionals is imperative; psychologist and teacher must work together to identify promising areas for intervention and practical applications of diagnostic findings (40). Where discriminating diagnosis and placement is not the practice, children with different disabilities requiring different teaching methods are likely to be placed together in one class where all receive the same instruction, willy-nilly (16A).

Major Approaches to Remediation

In some respects the state of theory in the field is chaotic. Remediation is influenced by divergent theories of where, how, and when interventions should be directed. Each camp reports successes. Some argue for cost economy to meet the enormous social problem posed by the extent of MBD in the school population. Others maintain that the precise tailoring to the complexity of learning disabilities which they advocate is inescapable.

A valuable effort to bring some theoretical order to the field is presented by Kirk (27). He finds that remedial efforts generally follow one of the three orientations described below.

Skill Training

Skill-training interventions focus more upon the task to be taught, less upon the child and what is going on in him. The teacher does not make inferences about underlying processes, but instead relies on behavior and environment. First, determinations of what the child can and cannot do in a specific task are made. The behaviors needed to do the task are identified. Goals are set, and the teacher organizes a systematic remedial program with reinforcement. The procedure, Kirk observes, is simply a more refined and complete version of the methods used by all good teachers.

Abrams (1), a strong advocate of "psychoeducation," gives primacy to the teacher's or "learning therapist's" work with specific deficits as the agent for change in the MBD child.

The skill-training orientation is essentially a behavioral approach, emphasizing incremental learning steps. Operant conditioning, discussed later in Chapter 15 on behavioral modification, is used increasingly in remedial instruction (37). The process starts with a step already within the child's repertoire of mastered skills. Graded steps are introduced successively, producing gradual alteration of the child's set. Reinforcement at each step is intended to make the next step possible.

Treatment of a perceptual and concept-formation disorder is described by Levi (28). Through persistent peripheral prodding, primarily auditory, an 11-year-old boy was taught over a year of special training to understand the notion of category, to acquire a set of categories, and to scan categories in order to select from them. Significant improvement in this capacity was accompanied by improvement in school grades.

Initial introduction of concrete rather than abstract material within a structured program, with changes introduced slowly and carefully, is recommended with hyperkinetic children by Schrager *et al.* (43).

Some remedial instructors prefer to work first on the improvement of attention as such with behavioral methods, rather than with any content, since ability to pay attention is prerequisite to all learning. Cantwell (10) recommends that the learner verbalize self-directed commands before responding to a task. He finds errors can be reduced by training in better scanning and search procedures and in delaying response. For hyperkinetic children Littleton and Davis (30) recommend structured classroom procedures, with activities carefully sequenced and maintained over time with little change. With sequences set in levels of progressive difficulty, success at one level is assured before the next more difficult one is undertaken. The teacher intervenes at any point to clarify, and each child is encouraged to practice in order to reach competence.

Many good teachers rely upon the diagnostic information provided by test instruments to guide their incremental training. The *Illinois Test of Psycholinguistic Ability (ITPA),* developed by McCarthy and Kirk (33), is widely used. It identifies deficit areas and serves thereby as a guide to remedial instruction, without providing specific instructional tasks. A similar nonprescriptive use of the *Wechsler Intelligence Scale for Children (WISC)* is described by Searls (44), to identify specific dysfunction affecting reading. Poor readers, Searls reports, tend to score lower on *Information, Arithmetic, Digit Span, Vocabulary* (sometimes), and *Coding.*

The acquisition of ''strategies'' that can be applied to improve mastery and decrease the time required for learning is used in another approach (36).

A so-called ''competency'' method is offered by Faas (15), who seeks to remediate selectively by choosing instructions from among 370 identified ''competencies.''

Process Training

Process training is based largely upon an analysis and correction of processes operating in the child, not upon the nature of the task to be mastered. It assumes that success depends upon mastery of certain underlying processes. Reading, for example, requires adequate functioning of several processes, visual discrimination and sound blending important among them. While the remedial instruction takes into account analysis of the components of the task, the major effort is to determine how well this child learns through each of his sensory modalities and how well he integrates the data from two or more sensory modalities (6). Werner and Kaplan (49A) have influenced this trend with their hypothesis that the child moves from global perceptions and reactions to an increasingly differential and hierarchal organization. Consequences of this process include separation of the self from objects and other people and less domination by the stimulus field around him. The parallels with the psychoanalytic concept of progression from primary- to secondary-process thinking are striking.

Understandably, neuropsychologists, neurologists, and opthalmologists are among the major advocates of process training. Bogen (9) reasons that process remediation should account for the differential lateral dominance for verbal and nonverbal methods of thinking. Reitan (41) urges training for the dysfunctional cerebral hemisphere where such localization can be established. But the effectiveness of remedial instruction in general is questioned by Luria (31, 32). His studies suggest that intact systems should be encouraged to take over the tasks of impaired systems, to circumvent the deficit, so to speak. He demonstrates ingenious substitution of visual for auditory abilities, and vice versa, to develop competence when one sensory modality has been impaired.

Dysfunctional auditory word discrimination has been demonstrated in MBD children by Parr (38). Adams (2) has shown that cerebral dysfunction in learning-disabled children resulted in poorer tactual than visual form recognition, while discriminatory ability was improved when bisensory methods were applied.

A concept of latency in responsiveness has been developed by Belmont (5) into a perceptual-motor training principle. The concept holds that the impaired portion of the brain responds more slowly to excitation than does the rest of the brain. Where a dysfunction is unilateral, stimulation may be applied to the impaired side before it is applied to the intact side. Or the stimulation to the impaired side may be intensified, while that to the intact side is kept lower.

Indirect contributions to the correction of learning disabilities are attributed to what may be called process-training procedures that in themselves do not contribute directly to the acquisition of cognitive skills. Sensorimotor skills and conceptual ability are said by Bierbauer (7) to be developed respectively through games and play and through the use of everyday objects to illustrate categories.

Imparting direction to uncontrolled movement in hyperkinetic children, another example, is reported enhanced by music therapy (19). Two forms of the therapy are described: the *receptive* is listening to music; the *active* is movement to the music. Success is reported in improving concentration, time and space orientation, visual- and audio-motor coordination, ability to direct movements, and ability to make decisions and choices in life tasks, as well as in active attitudes towards the self and the environment. Music therapy also sometimes made possible the discontinuation of drug therapy in this group.

A related dance-therapy method is reported by Schmais and Orleans (42) to convert the motor symptoms of MBD into positive experience. They believe that to concentrate solely upon educational subjects (task training) is to suffer from ''tunnel vision.'' Their concern is with the *process* of performance, not with achievement. Their exercises emphasize body awareness: balance, eye-hand-foot coordination, rhythmicity, expressivity, flow of physical effort, and use of body weight as a force. Awareness of space and interaction are also sought.

A complex and detailed method for correcting sensorimotor deficits in MBD children through the use of physical therapy to alter abnormal muscle tone and movement is described by Norton (35). This detailed assessment tests for soft neurological signs such as aberrant sequential sensorimotor behavior, those reactions normal earlier that persist beyond the developmental level for the age of the child. Smoothness of movement, flexibility, and balance are assessed as the child is asked to assume a variety of positions. Observations are recorded and guide the therapist in training the child in specific movements that are purported to result in more organized behavior, suggestive of improved central-nervous-system integration.

Process-Task Training

The third orientation gives equal weight to analyses of the child and the task (27), integrating the two analyses into the remediation effort. Improved visual discrimination, for example, will be sought by using letters and words, rather than nonlanguage material. ''Prescriptive'' techniques are associated with this method. Some description of this approach is found in the catalogue of Academic Therapy Publications (11). It coordinates some 18 diagnostic-teaching instruments with 13 language skills and processes, eight motor skills and processes, and ten similar aspects of arithmetic. Skill and mental process appear inseparable in their presentation.

A promising use of the *Wechsler Intelligence Scale for Children* as a diagnostic guide to remediation is offered by Jacobson and Kovalinsky (24). They identify an educational implication of each subtest of the *WISC-R,* and from that generate recommendations for remediation at specific grade levels. Poor *Digit Span,* for example, they relate to inattention, poor memory for words, articulation disorders, poor basic reading skill, and possibly impaired audition. After hearing is checked and corrected, if necessary, they prescribe games and tasks geared to four grade levels: 1 to 2.5; 2.5 to 3; 4 to 6; 7 to 9. At the simplest level, the student is asked to listen, to name a sound he has heard in the room or outside it. At the most complex and difficult level, sentences of increasing length are presented for recall. In similar fashion, the educational implication of each subtest is presented, with teaching tasks for specific grade levels. Sources for teaching material are provided. A psychologist may argue more with the processes analyzed for the subtests than with the tasks prescribed for remediation. The authors' analysis of *Comprehension,* for example, is that comprehension is judging solutions in practical situations, but they overlook its demand for expressive speech, where a dysfunction may indicate some degree of aphasia.

A more integrated approach to skill-process remediation is the *TEACH* method developed by Hagin, Silver, and others (22). The method is guided by the diagnostic leads from a corollary device, *SEARCH,* designed by Silver and Hagin (45). This method, discussed in Chapter 10, identifies the priorities for intervention, which are then related to items supplied by the *TEACH* structure. The structure consists of 55 teaching tasks, of which 45 are single modal, 10 intermodal. The 55 tasks are organized into five clusters; these merit description here, to illustrate the possibilities for integration of skill and process teaching.

The *Visual Cluster* teaches discrimination, recall, sequencing, and figure-ground processes necessary in distinguishing the features of forms, letters, and words, starting with simple forms and progressing to more difficult symmetric shapes. Children whose *SEARCH* profiles indicate difficulties with *Matching* and *Recall* need training in this cluster of tasks.

The *Visual-Motor Cluster* teaches the motor patterns necessary for writing: control of fine movements, monitoring the direction of movements, and targeting movements in copying symmetric and asymmetric forms, then letters. Difficulty with the *Designs* section of *SEARCH* directs training to this cluster.

The *Auditory Cluster* trains the child in progressively finer discrimination and recall of the sounds that make up words, in recognition of rhyming words, and in ordering and blending of sounds within words. Skill is developed in arbitrary sequences (time and codes) and meaningful sequences (songs and stories). Children with low *SEARCH* scores in *Rote Sequencing, Auditory Discrimination, Articulation,* and *Initials* need training in this cluster.

The *Body-Image Cluster* directs training to the mapping of finger schema and to left/right orientation. These body-image concepts need development in children showing *SEARCH* difficulties in *Directionality, Finger Schema,* and *Grip.*

The *Intermodal Cluster* trains in the matching of temporal and spatial location of initial-consonant sounds, consonant blends, and diagraphs, and in associating visual symbols with their auditory equivalents. The child with *SEARCH* difficulties in *Initials* and *Articulation* is taught this cluster.

TEACH provides stimulation in the areas of deficit, to develop the underdeveloped or impaired neuropsychological skills necessary for learning reading, writing, and spelling. It teaches perceptual accuracy, first in single modalities, then in intersensory modalities. Learning tasks lead the student through three levels of complexity: (1) *recognition* of similarities and differences; (2) *copying* procedures that require a motor response, while the teacher continues to provide structure; and (3) *recall* tasks, in which the child with reduced cues from the teacher builds his own structure for responding. The fundamental hypothesis is that learning, a complex process, cannot proceed if a dysfunctional modality is ignored. If the teacher gives immediate feedback when the child makes an error, the frustrations of trial and error are avoided. Aids are presented in the modality required by the task being taught; a stronger modality is not substituted for a weaker one, as in the circumventing strategies. Left to right progression in a horizontal series of symbols is practiced, with consistent use of the child's preferred hand.

There are probably as many theoretical schools of sensory training as there are senses. Some argue for teaching to the intact sense, even though it may not be primary to the task. Others press for strengthening the weaker sense, while still others advocate the use of bisensory training to promote reinforcement of what is being learned. *TEACH,* we have seen, concentrates on the modality inherent in the task being taught.

A different approach to modality training is practiced by Zentall (50). When dysfunctional auditory skills are found to cause problems in learning sounds of letters, in blending sounds into words, and in sounding out words, he argues for the use of visual stimuli in instruction wherever possible. Math, spelling, and reading tasks, for example, can be learned by use of flash cards and tachistoscopic presentation. Zentall does acknowledge, however, that strengthening of the weaker modality is often required, as in presenting sequentially lengthened tape-recorded stories for practice in recall. He also uses bisensory tasks, helping the child to construct visual images to reinforce the auditory.

Intersensory exercises, designed to improve the various areas of auditory perception, have been designed by Behrmann (3). These include learning tasks in discrimination, location, separating figure from ground, translating auditory stimuli into motor tasks, or the auditory stimuli to visual and then to oral expression, blending, sequencing, following directions, memory, interpretation and intonation, rhyming, and comprehension.

A single-sensory approach to audition is reported (18) that distinguishes between sensation and cognition. This discriminatory ability in turn is based upon auditory comprehension. Also to be considered in this schema are the motor aspects of speech; apraxia slows comprehension as well as expression. Training here is directed toward correction of amplitude, concentration in speech upon simple auditory stimuli or constructs, and the graduated stage-step improvement of auditory memory, first using a simple sentence, then using the same sentence embedded in background noise.

The visual modality has received as much attention as the auditory in task-process remediation. A lively controversy between the professions of ophthalmology and optometry has developed around the use of optometric training, such as that provided at the Optometric Center in New York. The debate centers on two questions. Is there a significantly greater association of peripheral eye defects among the learning disabled than among normal readers? Is there any value in the visual training provided by optometrists after diagnosis? Flax (16) describes and challenges the negative answer to both questions advanced in a joint statement of the American Academy of Ophthalmology. He examines the references used by this coalition to support their negative conclusions and finds serious omissions that would counter the weight of their argument. Optometry claims a significant contribution to the improvement of learning disabilities, with selective visual training through muscle exercises, ocular pursuit, special prescriptive glasses, and training in neurologic organization (lateral dominance and balance, for example).

Visual abnormalities—subtle dysfunctions in ocular motor control—were reported in a broad survey of the literature (34) to affect adversely the processing of visual information and thereby contribute to learning disabilities. Optometric training seeks to improve the aiming precision of the eye, its focusing capability, and binocular fusion by the use of corrective lenses and corrective training with instruments that provide feedback, showing the patient when he is using his eyes correctly, and how to make any necessary correction.

With the rationale that the interpretation of stimuli received via one modality is reinforced by simultaneous stimuli from another modality, Behrmann (4) has developed a multisensory approach to visual perception as he did also for auditory perception. His exercises include tracing, blackboard copying, motor responses to visual stimuli, tracking, motor responses to tactile-visual stimuli, integration of auditory-visual stimuli, motor responses to kinesthetic-visual stimuli, discrimination of parts from wholes, visual sequencing, figure-ground discrimination, and gains in vertical visual integration and comprehension.

Remediation of Dyslexia

Dyslexia, of all the many disabilities associated with MBD, is the most troubling to parents and the most burdensome emotionally, socially, and economically to the MBD victim. For that reason a review of the work on its remediation is given a special section here, although it will become evident that earlier discussion applies here as well.

An important volume on the state of dyslexia, its theory, diagnosis, and treatment, edited by Benton and Pearl (6) discusses the four approaches to remediation summarized here for their thought-provoking contributions. Dyslexics, reasons Johnson (26), are similar in some respects, different in others. This variation mandates individually oriented remediation based upon specific diagnosis. There is no single therapeutic approach; therapy is not accidentally effective or ineffective. She chooses three interventions as desirable. (1) The Orton-Gillingham approach simultaneously links a variety of language stimuli—visual, auditory, kinesthetic—and gradually fuses small components into a more complex whole. (2) Fernwald in 1943 reported the first effort in MBD remediation, Johnson says, to provide successful experiences to counteract negative ones, emphasizing kinesthesia. Words are written or printed in large size, one to a card. The child traces each with his finger until he can write it from memory. Tracing is discontinued when the child is successful. Thereafter the child looks at the word, then writes it from memory while saying it. (3). The third group of methods advocated by Johnson are use of color phonics and of modified alphabets, with an emphasis on individual sensory preference. Phonics are reinforced by color coding; a mirror enables the teacher to show the child the proper placement of tongue, lips, and jaw. The method facilitates sequencing. In the special modified alphabet she urges, the standard alphabet is increased so that each grapheme represents a single phoneme, to try to overcome the difficulties of the irregular spelling patterns in English. The work uses the individual's preferred sensory modality if it can be identified.

Guthrie (20) differs sharply with Johnson. He argues for his focus on the dysfunction, as opposed to her reliance on the residual strengths. He is task oriented, basing instruction on the major components of reading, while Johnson, he states is process oriented, focusing on vision and audition. Guthrie's schema includes four components of reading, in which dyslexics are inferior to normal readers and on which remediation should be focused: (1) decoding accuracy, the translation of written or printed language into speech; (2) decoding speed, the rapidity with which decoding is done; (3) semantic segmentation, a process of locating target words in a paragraph, with fine discrimination between spoken words required; and (4) semantic construction, the meaning of words and clauses united in the text and from long-term memory. Remedial reading instruction, he urges, should focus on the deficient cognitive components of reading, instruct the child in all components of reading, provide intensive interaction between teacher and child, and maximize the time given to direct reading instruction.

An equally vigorous approach is that of Zigmond (51). The failure of a child to learn to read, she states flatly, is the failure of the teacher to teach. She sees dyslexics as primarily children who are "hard to teach"; most of them could learn to read if taught properly. She reserves the term "dyslexic" for that small group who do not respond to specifically individualized instruction. She cites Woodcock as identifying at least 45 ways to teach reading. These include variations of alphabet modification, structure flexibility, part-whole meaning, sensory modalities, means of presentation, and environmental characteristics. Her comments find support from Levinson and Nissenbaum (29), who consider the prevalence of learning disabilities to be in fact a teaching disability. The LD child learns when instruction is geared to his needs, and schools in the United States, they believe, reward the "left-brained" child and punish the "right-brained" one.

A point of contention among specialists is whether dyslexia is due primarily to a language disorder or to a visual-perceptual dysfunction. Velluntino (47) reports that the literature most frequently cites deficiencies in visual perception and memory. More recent findings, including his own, dispute the notion that visual deficiencies in verbal processing are "possibly associated with basic language problems." The need to consider both visual perception and central processing in special education is clear.

Choosing a Remediation Approach

Therapists, patients, and families are confronted with a bewildering array of fact and opinion, hypothesis, and theory. The task of selecting a remediation focus is not made easier by the insistent certainty of the advocates for one approach or the other. One insistence is justified—that upon matching individual diagnosis to individual therapy, although this is sometimes opposed as economically unfeasible as public policy.

But how to choose more specifically? How, for example, to select an orientation from among the task, process, or task-process types? Are the circumventing strategies using tape recorders and calculators to be disparaged for attempts at correction by more basic process-directed instruction aimed at the limitation? Shall instruction be single or bisensory? Exploit the intact sense or seek to develop the weak one?

The age of the MBD victim may well be a determining factor in such choice-making. The younger the child is when MBD is identified, the more receptive is his brain to process training, and the more time is available to test the child's response to the process method. With careful monitoring, later decisions can be made either to continue with the process method or to switch to a more task-oriented approach, or even to some circumvention. But no one should rest assured that there is "all the time in the world." A stubborn bias against circumventing strategies, for example, may doom the child to prolonged failure, with concomitant accumulating damage to self-esteem. And generally, the adolescent or young adult benefits most from the quickest remediation or amelioration of the dysfunction, from the quickest mastery of adequate coping strategies. We have available for answering these questions definitely much advocacy but little research. Assuming the local availability of an adequate armamentarium of remedial interventions, the best choice appears to rest upon diagnosis, time in the individual's life span, and his emotional state.

Siting Remedial Instruction

Most remedial instruction in the United States is provided within public school systems, and debate about the location of such instruction within the system is lively.

Where should these highly specialized educational procedures be offered? Will the child's self-esteem be damaged less if he receives special instruction away from a regular class of nondisabled children, and the rest of his program, usually music, art, gym, shop, and home economics, with the regular class, as in "mainstreaming" pattern? Or should he receive all instruction in a separate special-education class? No definitive answers are available at this time. Hagin and Silver (21) consider remedial intervention best centered in "school resource" rooms, to which reading-disabled children go three to five times weekly for 30-minute sessions. This arrangement, they found, best assures communication between school and clinical staffs, so that diagnostic findings for each child can be integrated into learning tasks. Helsinger (23) reasons that the heterogeneity of the MBD group itself clearly indicates that more than one type of program is necessary; those children of "good" physical and emotional control and intelligence do best when special classes are integrated within regular programs, while those with lower intelligence levels and hyperactivity require a special educational setting.

Clements and Peters (12) observe that since MBD is a medical designation requiring a complex treatment team, schools have emphasized the educational aspects to make administratively possible the development of programs for these children. Such programs tend to be of three types, based pragmatically upon severity of symptoms:

1. An *educational group,* again divided into three subtypes: (a) the child remains in a regular class with a slight modification in his program; (b) the child spends most of his time with a regular class but is released for specified periods to a resource room, for individual instruction by teachers trained in special education; or (c) the child attends a special class for the full day with specially trained teachers.

2. A *special group for the training of central processing functions of the brain* concentrates upon deficits in visual and auditory perception, cross-modality integration, motor skills, and coordination.

3. A *special-therapies group,* providing medication, psychotherapy, family counseling, and special consultants for the schools. The hypothesis for such a program is that the major ingredient of a comprehensive, individually prescribed program is a protective learning environment, to be provided until with time and maturation the child can reach a functional level of CNS maturity and integration, "possibly enhanced by specific training."

For many children, this hoped-for level of maturation may never be reached; the special-education needs of older students are now recognized by increasing numbers of colleges and universities. Curry College, for example, regularly accepts 10 percent of its 350-member freshman class from among learning-disabled students. Initially they pay an extra fee for special help during the first year, when they are instructed in the use of techniques for circumventing their disabilities and are given untimed tests.

Some school systems provide little or no remedial instruction or offer only token services that fail to meet the needs of many MBD children. Traditional tutoring as we know it is also inadequate. And so some parents must employ remediation specialists privately for after-school instruction, or find and pay for private remediation after-school centers or private remediation schools that the child attends full-time. These adjunctive services to public school systems are relatively rare; they are largely unmonitored for standards of adequacy.

For the most part they are to be found in large urban centers, occasionally in suburban areas, and rarely, if ever, in rural sections.

Remediation and the Law

The need for adequate remediation services is a national problem, so widespread is the occurrence of MBD, and so many are the victims still of school age. The national scope of the problem is being recognized in laws passed by the Congress that mandate remediation services in every school district to those children who need them. Governmental recognition of the national need is reflected in a 1977 memorandum from the then-existing U.S. Department of Health, Education, and Welfare. The memorandum encourages collaboration between vocational education, special education, and vocational rehabilitation. Recent laws, based upon the "mainstreaming" concept and the increasing number of options available to the learning-disabled person, support this collaboration (48).

Under the Vocational Education Act Amendment of 1976 (P.L. 94-482) 10 percent of the federal funds allocated for vocational education are to be spent on the handicapped, a category that now includes the learning disabled. These services include courses designed to lead to employability; the presentation of the services in a way that permits the handicapped person to benefit from them; teachers, tutors, special devices; and job placement. Training time provided may be extended as necessary, to enable the student to benefit or to acquire a new skill. Twenty percent of federal funds are allocated for the academically or socially disadvantaged, usually defined as those whose reading, writing, and arithmetic skills are two grades below age-grade level.

The Education for All Handicapped Children Act (P.L. 94-142) requires an "individualized education plan" (IEP) for each eligible handicapped child between the ages 3 and 18, a plan designed to meet the child's needs and abilities in classrooms, hospitals, institutions, or at home if homebound. The IEP may include special education that will lead to employability.

The Rehabilitation Act of 1973, Section 504, provides equal educational rights for the handicapped child, and forbids discrimination in student admission by any college or postgraduate program receiving federal funds. The act also emphasizes that the administration of the tests used by colleges and universities must not discriminate against the handicapped by virtue of sensory, manual, or speech skills.

Many specialists in the field are less than sanguine about the beneficial impact of these laws. Johnson (25) is concerned that the definition of handicap is too rigid and that children with mild to moderate degrees of dysfunction will not receive the special training they need. The lack of sufficient numbers of well-trained remedial teachers skilled in reading, writing, language, and arithmetic is deplored by Spano (46). He reminds us of Cruickshank's 1977 observation that the learning-disability situation in our schools is an "educational catastrophe." "Mainstreaming" does not meet the special needs of MBD children, according to Levinson and Nissenbaum (29), because the regular classroom teacher usually has had little or no training in learning disabilities. In practice, the ability of our numerous school systems to respond to the laws is affected by each state's interpretation of the laws, court decisions regarding the laws, pre-existing state and local laws and programs, existing physical facilities and fiscal resources, and the quality of political support for the measures promulgated.

Every learning-disabled child in the United States certainly does not have ready access to the special diagnostic and teaching services that might benefit him. Quality and quantity of services available varies widely as does administrative dedication to providing these services, and, especially, devotion to identifying the child who needs them. The value of "mainstreaming" remains debatable. Many parents are still ignorant of the services they may obtain for a child if they explore and push for them. And the incidence of learning disabilities in some communities is so high that all the special educational facilities and funds they might muster are inadequate for the need.

Chapter 13

Environmental Manipulation

MAKING CHANGES IN the environment is often necessary to improve attention and decrease distractibility often encountered by the hyperactive child.

In Strauss's concept (4), hyperkinesis results from brain damage that affects perception and leads to difficulty in filtering out or ignoring the irrelevant and disturbing. Flooded by unfiltered, unblocked stimuli, the child reacts with a flood of responses. The prescribed intervention for this etiological inference is to modify the child's environment while he is being instructed, to reduce stimulation and protect him from intrusions, thereby facilitating attention and releasing his capacity for learning. The rationale is that the quality of his sensory experience is improved when the MBD child's concentration is focused and sustained upon the stimuli of the task.

Recommended measures include reducing the number of objects in the room, removing clocks that tick or move, disconnecting bells that may ring, removing the telephone, locking doors, placing the child's desk so he faces a screen, a blank wall, or a corner away from other students, carpeting floors, acoustically treating ceiling and walls, placing storage cabinets behind doors, and installing opaque windows (2, 3). Short periods of instruction that alternate in content, and may be interspersed with opportunity for discharge in play or listening to music, are recommended, resulting in a day designed to provide changing activities (1).

The presumption in this approach is that the hyperactive child is in a constant state of endogenous over-arousal or near over-arousal, so that even ordinary exogenous stimuli are excessive for him and add to his compulsion to discharge in motor activity the tension of over-arousal. Since heightened motor activity decreases capacity for attention, learning disabilities are created. Stimulus overload is the diagnosis; stimulus decrease is the treatment.

Again, as with so many aspects of MBD theory and practice, there is opposition to the stimulus-overload hypothesis. Zentall (6) argues that the hyperkinesis itself is an effort to *increase* stimulation: visual, auditory, haptic, kinesthetic, and motor. Hyperkinesis in his view is a response to understimulation or stimulus deprivation; the overly active child is seeking to satisfy a stimulus hunger, to supplement available stimulation in the environment through increased activity. Zentall finds support for his view in medication therapy, where findings suggest that the hyperkinetic child who responds well to amphetamines is in a state of under-arousal, and he observes that the sedative barbituates, contrariwise, tend to increase hyperactivity in such a child. This, of course, suggests a reasonable hypothesis explaining the paradoxical effect in some children of stimulant medications which reduce rather than increase their activity. He believes that behavior-modification techniques are successful because the reinforcement procedures employed increase stimulation.

He also reports in another study (5) that playground activities usually provide this needed stimulation, so that observable differences between normal and hyperactive children are reduced in this type of environment. Additionally, increasing distal visual and auditory stimulation significantly reduced the observable activity of hyperactive children in a quiet sitting-and-waiting situation. Increases in relevant stimuli added to rote-task situations reduced motor activity and improved situation performance. However, when stimuli are added to task situations that involve the child's learning disability, or to those that are not repetitive and boring, increased activity and disruption result.

Zentall concludes that the treatment of hyperkinesis should be directed toward manipulated optimal stimulation, not to stimulus reduction, on the hypothesis that the hyperkinetic child needs more stimulation than does the normal child to maintain the same level of performance. He recommends a treatment regimen that adds selected stimulation to the learning situation while maintaining its essential structure. His overview of available research suggests that increased stimulation is beneficial when added to the "distal" environment, either at the completion of the task or during the task situation if the task is overly familiar or requires rote procedures.

The probability is great that both theories—stimulus reduction and optimal stimulation—are applicable, given the varieties of etiology in hyperkinesis. It is known that stimulant drugs work well with some children, not so with others. The reasons are obscure. Meanwhile, an empirical approach to stimulus manipulation with the individual child is worthwhile.

Chapter 14

Pharmacological and Nutritional Therapies

MEDICAL PROFESSIONALS—chiefly psychiatrists, pediatricians, allergists, and nutrition specialists—manifest an increasing interest in MBD, especially in hyperactivity. They have largely addressed the troubling symptoms—socially disruptive behavior, impulsivity, and abnormal motor behavior, so-called conduct disorders—rather than the cognitive and emotional consequences of MBD (102). In fact, the large diagnostic category, MBD, is often used too loosely in reviewing the medication therapies, when the usual medical effort is to correct one subsyndrome of the syndrome, hyperkinesis. The medications usually are not directed to the numerous other subsyndromes: dyslexia, dysgraphia, dysfunctions of spatial visualization, or constructional ability.

Mitigation of the disruptive and often damaging behaviors in hyperkinesis is hoped for, sought, and welcomed gratefully by troubled parents and children. The medical remedy, through prescriptive drugs and diets, is seen as concrete and direct. Pharmacological and nutritional interventions are also seen as relatively inexpensive, in contrast to psychotherapy and behavioral modification. Many school authorities hope that the reputed quieting effect upon hyperactive children of stimulant drugs will reduce the need for long-term, costly therapeutic and remediation programs. And many people have greater faith in the medical model than in either the educational or psychological ones, while still others find a disorder less stigmatizing socially and emotionally with a medical diagnosis and treatment for it (2).

Pharmacological Therapy

A survey in the Baltimore public schools by Krager and Safer (59) in the early 1970s found that 1.07 percent of the children in its elementary grades were receiving stimulant medication. In two years the number had risen to 1.73 percent, an increase of 62 percent. The increase was found in the children of both the poor and well-to-do, although overall the well-to-do children showed a higher rate of usage, probably due to their easier access to medical care. The authors comment that, based upon general estimates, 3 to 8 percent of all school children are hyperkinetic, so that those in Baltimore who need medications are not all receiving them.

The study epitomizes the increasing use of stimulant medication since Bradley (17) in 1937 first reported on the paradoxical quieting effect of amphetamines in the treatment of behavior disorders in children. Currently, Whalen and Henker (100A) dispute the contention that the use of stimulant drugs is increasing at an "alarming" rate. But the increase is not disputed. After World War II, research into psychotropic medication increased and more varieties became available. Slowly at first, but increasingly of late, their use in the treatment of MBD children, especially the hyperkinetic ones, has increased. A more recent national estimate is that about 2.3 percent, or nearly 700,000 of about 30 million, are suffering from hyperkinesis (51). Some have speculated that the observable increase of hyperkinesis is due to the current retention of these children and adolescents within the school. Earlier they were often allowed, perhaps encouraged, to leave school to work or look for work as soon as legally permitted

The personal plight of these many victims is grave, the probable consequences for them in life are equally grave. Any intervention that can improve this plight is to be welcomed. An attempt to evaluate the possibilities of medication in the treatment of hyperkinesis is not an easy task, so numerous and vigorous are the arguments pro and con.

How the Drugs Are Believed to Work

The drugs used, chiefly stimulant medications, have reduced the restlessness and increased the attention capacity of a sizeable number of children diagnosed hyperactive, although not all of them. This pacifying reaction to stimulants has been termed "paradoxical," and explanations of its mechanism are sought in hypotheses about the neurophysiological state producing hyperkinesis.

An earlier hypothesis postulated that hyperkinetic behavior is the discharge of over-arousal in the cerebral cortex, the over-arousal state being caused by an inherited deficiency of neurotransmitters that prevent the cerebral cortex from inhibiting incoming stimuli and outgoing motor responses in a normal way.

The stimulant drugs, in this hypothesis, are believed to correct this deficiency of neurotransmitters by stimulating their production, thereby increasing the inhibitory capability of the cerebrum.

A more recent hypothesis holds the contrary view that the cerebral cortex of the hyperkinetic child is in a state of under-arousal, that the child's accelerated activity is an effort to promote arousal, somewhat in the way in which a state of hypothermia may cause convulsive shaking that leads to hyperthermia. In this view, the effect of stimulant drugs is not paradoxical but produces its benefits through direct stimulation of a stimulus-hungry brain (18, 106), thereby decreasing the need for external stimulation.

Studies of evoked potentials recorded during task situations suggest support for the later hypothesis (50). Capacity for attention and electrophysiological activity were observed to become "normalized" in response to a stimulant in a drug/placebo experiment (56). But a study of arousal through skin conductance and temperature and of responsivity through reaction time and pupil size contests the hypothesis that the stimulants raised subnormal arousal levels. Higher-than-normal levels of arousal were found in unmedicated MBD children (105), and while the stimulant drugs increased the already high arousal levels, they did not appear to affect the responsivity deficits. Some hyperactive children are hypoaroused, some are normal, some are hyperaroused; thus one research team calls the evidence "confused, confusing, and controversial" (67).

A unique pharmacological approach uses seasickness medications in dyslexia and dyspraxia, on the hypothesis that dyslexia results from a cerebellar-vestibular dysfunction. Frank and Levinson (44) claim, without offering data, improvements in reading, writing, spelling, arithmetic, spatial organization, balance, coordination, speech, and emotional adjustment.

Our understanding of how these drugs work is far from clear. On the one hand, strong evidence indicates that they are more usually effective when there are soft neurological signs and a history of perinatal difficulties (55, 68), while another line of investigation (101) suggests that emotional variables in the parents, including love and anger, account for a sizeable percentage of the variation in response to medication. And, of course, the placebo effect must always be considered. A spate of recent reports tends to increase uncertainty that the action of the drugs is indeed as specific as believed. The stimulants are suggested to produce favorable response in children (a) with attention difficulties but without hyperactivity, (b) with conduct disorder, and (c) with other diagnoses (22A). In an earlier study, Whalen and Henker (100B) failed to find differences in activity levels between hyperactive and non-hyperactive children in global ratings made by teachers and parents, and in electromechanical recording. Zahn et al. (105A) failed to observe differences in autonomic effects between hyperactive and normal children in response to stimulant drugs, and conclude that the beneficial effects reported by both groups (decreased motor activity, increased attention) are not dependent upon increases in arousal. And Rapoport *et al.* (78A) report in a similar vein that stimulant drugs appear to affect normal and hyperactive children and normal adults similarly in producing decreased motor activity, increased vigilance, and improved performance on a learning task.

The Drugs Used

The stimulant drugs most often appearing in the literature, alone or in comparison with other drugs, are methylphenidate (Ritalin) and dextro-amphetamine (Dexedrine). Far less frequently reported are caffeine, magnesium pemoline (Cylert), and Deanol. Methylphenidate appears to be regarded most favorably among drugs in the armamentarium (41, 46, 47, 73, 87, 89). Some studies report little difference between methylphenidate and dextroamphetamine (26, 28, 48), while both were rated superior to caffeine (48). Caffeine alone, in pill form or in whole coffee, is reported favorably in two studies (40, 49). Arnold *et al.* (8) found that methylphenidate and amphetamine were significantly better than placebo or caffeine, but did not differ significantly from each other. Magnesium pemoline (Cylert) was judged a good alternative when compared with dextroamphetamine (27). Levoamphetamine has compared favorably with dextroamphetamine in minimizing aggressive, hostile behavior, but not where high anxiety was associated with the hyperactivity (9). Also reported as effective alternatives to the amphetamines and to methylphenidate are captodiame hydrochloride and thioidozime hydrochloride (25). Chess (23) found that Tofranil (imipramine), an antidepressant, reduced hyperactivity, as did Greenberg *et al.* (47), and that Librium, Valium, and Haldol, all muscle-relaxing tranquilizers, are successful in controlling tics. Anticonvulsants may be considered where the EEG records abnormal brain waves (5).

Side Effects

Many of the principal side effects of stimulant drugs are discussed later in this section in the survey of the controversy surrounding their use. They include irritability, appetite and weight loss, growth stunting, blunting of affect, insomnia, headaches, elevated blood pressure and heart rate, and a potential for abuse. Careful consultation of the *Physicians' Desk Reference*[1] will provide more specific and complete details on a specific drug.

General Medical Approach to the Problem of Hyperkinesis

An overview of the way many physicians approach the diagnosis and treatment of hyperkinesis is useful in formulating an assessment of the stimulants.

[1] Published annually by Medical Economics Company, Oradell, N.J. 07649.

Sandoval *et al.* (83) obtained responses from forty-eight physicians asked to rate the importance of certain indicators in the diagnosis of hyperactivity. These included history of the dysfunction, personal medical history, family history, school history, physical examination, and laboratory findings. Each physician was also asked his preferred diagnostic label for hyperactivity and his therapy recommendations from among drugs, neurological consultation, counseling or psychotherapy for the child and/or parents, consultations with the school, motor-skills training, and special education. To elicit these judgments the cooperating physicians were asked to respond to a standardized set of vignettes describing cases that varied in age, severity of symptoms, and the response of school and parents.

The diagnostic label most used was *Hyperactivity of Unknown Origin.* Usually the diagnosis given was said by the physicians to be based upon behavioral indicators rather than upon data from the physical examination or laboratory findings although these were given in the vignettes. Cerebral stimulants were the medication most frequently prescribed. The treatment recommendations indicated that the respondent physician considered the alternatives and did not follow a single, fixed approach to treatment. Neurological consultations were most frequently advised. Two-thirds recommended school consultations, one-half prescribed psychotherapy. Recommendations for school consultation were high where the school and parents expressed concern. Psychotherapy recommendations for the child were high where his anxiety was high, and high for the parents where they were anxious and desperate for help in coping. The physicians did not regard positive neurological findings as helpful in a practical way, even though such consultations were frequently prescribed; they viewed hyperactivity as a behavioral rather than a neurological disorder. And despite their recommendations of concomitant treatment interventions, they favored the stimulant medications as the treatment of choice.

Evaluating the Role of Stimulants

A lively ongoing debate on the role and effectiveness of the stimulant medications in the treatment of hyperkinesis also examines the basic value of the drugs employed. Do they help a significant number of hyperactive children? Are they applicable to all or most of the children diagnosed as hyperkinetic? Do they do more than quiet the child, that is, do they improve cognitive and social functioning? Do they supplant the need for other types of treatment? Are the actual and potential side effects serious? Vigorous proponents and opponents are countered by many voices of moderation that recommend individualized use of the drugs while guarding against misuse.

ADVOCATES

The numerous proponents of the use of stimulant medications are firmly convinced of the drugs' efficacy. Prominent among these is Wender (99) who reports that about 25 percent of MBD children have a "specific therapeutic" response to amphetamines that is more than merely quieting, that these drugs promote psychological growth through their action in decreasing activity and impulsivity and improving social behavior and cognition. Wender provides a thorough and well documented approach to the management of amphetamine treatment. He reports his clinical experience that many children who do not at first respond satisfactorily to amphetamines often do so when the dosage is increased, and that many children are able to tolerate relatively large doses without evidence of side effects. Participants at an HEW Conference (79) estimated that among those children for whom use of the drug is warranted—those who have not responded to interventions that manipulate education and environment—beneficial results are obtained in one-half to two-thirds of the cases.

Wender also argues (98) that stimulant medication is the treatment of choice for hyperkinesis, that existing "hard" data support the short-term efficacy of the drugs, and that there is no comparable support from "hard" data for family and/or individual counseling and psychotherapy. Further, he sees long-term indications that the difficulties associated with hyperkinesis persist beyond childhood, and often require medication life-long, in a model patterned after that for epilepsy and diabetes. He acknowledges that the behavioral benefits obtained from the drugs do not extend to cognitive functions.

Also a firm supporter of drug efficacy, Solomons (92) maintains that when the medications do not bring improvement it is because the dose is inadequate and should be increased, even to "seemingly alarming" amounts (such as 160 mg of methylphinedate or 75 mg of amphetamine daily). He favors continuation as long as the drug is beneficial, "years if necessary."

The assumption in drug advocacy appears to be that the psychological problems in hyperkinesis are secondary to the social ones that result from behavior with a physiological cause in the nervous system. Barcai and Rabkin (11) see the hyperactive child as unable to learn effectively or to find rewards in intellectual activities. His hyperkinetic behavior leads him to reject the classroom and to be rejected by his peers and teachers, and escalates to truancy and dropping-out. With educational, social, and familial satisfaction blocked as his difficulties increase, the child seeks satisfaction and self-esteem elsewhere (in delinquency, for example) or withdraws aversively. Unlike Wender, these advocates see use of drugs resulting in improved cognitive and learning abilities, attention span, and classroom behavior.

Earlier studies indicated decreases in hyperactivity and irritability accompanied by increased attention span and improved performance on tests of motor coordination (23, 25, 57, 58, 99). Improvement was measured by teachers' ratings of classroom behavior, parents' ratings of home behavior, and performance on various tests of attention, motor behavior, and cognitive functioning.

Forty children treated with dextroamphetamine are reported significantly improved on the *Fels Rating Scale of Classroom Behavior* by Comly (26). In a survey of 197 children treated with either Ritalin or Dexedrine, the author also found significant improvement, with the effectiveness of both drugs approximately equal. He observed side effects similar to those manifested by adult users of these drugs (sleep problems, irritability, jitteryness, appetite suppression), with an increase in the side effects as the child becomes adolescent.

Forty-two children aged 6 to 13 diagnosed as generally learning disabled were rated by Denhoff *et al.* (36) on the *Davids Rating Scale for Hyperkinesis,* then randomly assigned to receive Dexedrine or placebo. Rated again after three weeks, the children were switched from Dexedrine to placebo and from placebo to Dexedrine. Three weeks later the children were again rated by parents and teachers. Significant improvement in ratings by teachers were obtained for the drug treatment groups. However, when the children were redivided into two groups on the basis of the likelihood of whether or not they were hyperkinetic, no significant improvements in behavior were found for the non-hyperkinetic. This trend, suggesting that more manifest the hyperkinesis the better is the judged response to the medication, appears consistently in the studies reported.

Conners (28) reported significant improvements for medicated children, compared with those who got the placebo, in I.Q. equivalents as derived from the Harris-Goodenough system of scoring *Human Figure Drawings.* Sixty-nine children referred for academic or behavioral problems were randomly assigned to Dexedrine, Ritalin, or placebo groups, and produced human figure drawings before and after a three-week treatment period. The two drugs were found equally effective. The improvements in drawing are attributed to the medicated child's increased ability to attend and willingness to follow directions. Another possible explanation is the finding that methylphenidate had a "direct positive effect on visual-perceptual motor deficits" observed in hyperkinesis and learning disabilities. The positive effects are reflected in improved handwriting (63).

In a subsequent study, Conners *et al.* (27) assigned eighty-one children diagnosed as MBD randomly to receive Cylert, Dexedrine, or placebo. Before and after an eight-week treatment period they were given a battery of psychological tests and rated by teachers, parents, and clinicians. Significant improvements with both drugs were again reported.

The effectiveness of methylphenidate in treating hyperkinesis is reported by Satterfield *et al.* (87). Ratings by teachers indicated significantly greater improvement for the medicated children than for the placebo controls. Moreover, those children who responded well to the drugs were found to differ from those who responded relatively poorly in these ways: prior to receiving medication the good responders had "greater resting-mean amplitudes, more slow-wave activity (low frequency power), more movement artifacts...larger evoked cortical responses" and lower skin-conductive level (SCL). Their findings, while supporting efficacy of medication, also suggest that hyperkinetic children differ in responsiveness, indicating that the drugs should not be used indiscriminately, even within this group for whom they promise so much.

Another electroencephalographic study (56) found that methylphenidate corrected the attentional disturbances in hyperkinesis while normalizing electrophysiological indices during sustained task situations.

The continued use of methylphenidate from childhood through adolescence is supported by Mackay *et al.* (73) in their study of 10 MBD patients. Improvements were recorded in the *Raven's Progressive Matrices*, neurological examination, EEG, and an educational-progress report prepared by parents and teachers.

Similar improvements in response to methylphenidate are reported in Burdock's *Children's Behavior Inventory*, but not on the Goodenough *Draw-A-Person* or *Benton's Visual Retention Test* (89). Improvements with the same drugs are described (90) in attention *(Digit Span* and *Coding* of the *WISC)*, visual-motor skills *(Bender Visual-Motor Gestalt Test)*, and behavior in special and classroom situations rated by parents and teachers.

Methylphenidate is reported to decrease extraversive behavior (72), generally to improve objective and subjective measures (64), and to contribute to a more favorable relationship with the child's mother, with the result that she becomes less controlling (54). Elsewhere the drug is reported to make hyperkinetic children more compliant, thus improving relations with their mothers, although the drug-treated children initiated fewer social reactions (13).

Parents and teachers are cautioned by Feighner and Feighner (39) not to expect miracles from the drugs because they do not permanently alter behavior, although they can improve academic work and response to other treatment efforts.

In a study of over 1,000 children on methylphenidate, Fischer and Wilson (41) observed its significant effect in reducing hyperactivity and distractability, thereby allowing for more purposeful behavior. They add that the drug has some undesirable side effects: increased blood pressure, anorexia, and potential abuse of the substance.

The proponents of stimulant medication apparently agree uniformly upon the ability of the drug to inhibit hyperactivity and irritability and increase attention span. Some disagree about whether these benefits extend to improved cognitive abilities. If they do have this effect, the improved cognition appears to derive from increased ability to sustain attention when it might otherwise begin to falter. Just this action was specifically demonstrated in hyperkinetic children with methylphenidate; a group found able to attend only in the early stages of a task, given the drug, was then able to sustain concentration for longer periods (53). In another study (12) the drug increased the time the child spontaneously spent in a given activity, and decreased the number of activities engaged in. Improved attention allows the perception of stimuli that otherwise might escape the child, stimuli needed in the learning process. Thus, dextroamphetamine given to hyperkinetic boys was reported to improve the auditory perception of "rapidly occuring acoustic stimuli and their temporal sequence" (71). Amphetamine is reported also to increase recall of words heard (97).

Some disagreement exists among the advocates about whether the potential for side effects of drugs should be of serious concern, with a few expressing cautions, but most emphasizing a preponderance of benefits.

OPPOSING VIEWS

Other research and reviews of stimulant medications for hyperactive children indicate that despite improvement of attention and of extraversive behaviors, no significant cognitive, social, or emotional improvements result, either brief or lasting. Some studies also report that the improved attention span itself is of limited duration.

The effects of stimulants in improvement of attention were studied in relationship to recall over measured time by Rie and Rie (80). Short-term gains were recorded, but not long-term gains. The authors note that these short-term gains do not presage ultimate scholastic gains.

Repeatedly, increased capacity for attention without effect on cognitive and educational skills is reported. Improved performance on the *Digit Span* and *Coding* subtests of the *WISC* after methylphenidate was not accompanied by improved levels on verbal-content subtests (45). Barkley (14), something of an advocate of stimulant therapy, concludes from an extensive review of research that the drugs appear to improve attention span, on-task behavior, activity level, and disruptive behavior, but still result in little academic change. In eighteen studies using fifty-five objective measures of scholastic achievement and productivity, the drugs appear to result in beneficial changes in less than 17 percent of these measures. Negligible educational gains were found by Aman (6) in a review of research. Adelman and Compas (3) found in a similar review that the amphetamines produce mild to moderate improvement in nonacademic functions, but no change in reasoning, problem solving, or social and emotional functioning.

Of more serious import in evaluating the role of stimulants are those few studies that indicate that hyperactive children do better in some important measures without drugs than with, or when on placebo than when on drugs (20, 43). A significant argument is advanced by Cunningham and Barkley (34). They observe that interventions that focus only on hyperactivity will not improve academic achievement, while interventions geared to improve scholastic functioning will also decrease hyperactivity.

Opponents of medication contend that proponents are too sanguine about possible side effects. Adler (5), an otherwise thoughtful advocate of the drugs, concludes that there is ''...no evidence of growth stunting found due to stimulants other than possibly a 1/2-inch difference (sic) in a child to be 5'10''.''

Side effects were prominent among hyperactive subjects studied over long time periods without social and cognitive improvements in a survey (91) of the work of prominent researchers: Drs. Jan Loney, Judith Rappaport, Robert Sprague, and Gabrielle Weiss. The treated patients were acutely aware of and disliked appetite suppression, insomnia, and stomach cramps. (My observation is that some drug-therapy advocates appear to minimize the latter complaint by calling them "tummy aches.") The researchers believe that height and weight effects seem unrelated to the drugs, and may be due to the hyperactivity itself.

Evidence for potential drug abuse appears equivocal. On one hand, the medicine's unpleasant side effects as well as the general social aversiveness of hyperactive boys may deter them from drug experimentation as adolescents and young adults. However, their impulsivity exposes them to the risk of experimentation.

Undesirable long-range effects of the stimulant medications are the concern of many moderates. Laufer (62) sought information about this issue in a questionnaire sent to 100 patients who had begun treatment between the ages 3 and 18 (mean age at time of inquiry, 19.8). No addictions were reported; only three of 56 respondents had used other "uppers"; four described themselves as excessive drinkers, 92 percent were not.

The most serious concern of the eminent researchers surveyed (91) is that the problems associated with hyperactivity continue into adolescence and adulthood, with little difference found between those who as children received stimulant medication and those who did not. Difficulties with inattention, cognition, and social skills remained. The hyperactive and aggressive child fared worse in adulthood than did the child who was hyperactive but not aggressive. A somewhat reassuring observation is that delinquent behavior in adolescence among the hyperactive is not necessarily a precursor of criminality in adulthood. Barkley (14) concurs that long-term psychosocial adjustment is unaffected by earlier stimulant drug therapy.

The "zombie" effect produced by the drugs in some children causes some professional objection to the drugs. The effect causes anxiety in many children and their parents, but it is frequently glossed over by the administering physician as "quieting," "paradoxical," or even "desirable" since the child's behavior no longer disturbs teachers and peers. Schain (88) flatly states that this zombie effect is not acceptable, that while the child so treated is not presenting behavior problems, he remains a social isolate and is not learning. My experience is that hypoactivity is a real and critical a problem as hyperactivity.

Charges of indiscriminate use of stimulant medication have led to scrutiny by professionals and government agencies (79). In part, the concern was caused by the wide use of "uppers" by both adolescents and adults, the "speed" culture that developed around abuse of these medications, with an increase in frequency of addiction and health impairments. In part also, the concern was aroused by the strong advertising campaigns of drug companies, and by the casual, injudicious manner in which some physicians prescribed the drugs.

Pressure from anxious parents and exasperated teachers also plays a role, so there is some risk that a child may be "chemically abused" in the quest for acceptable behavior. Krippner *et al.* (60) find that medications are often the first device in treating hyperkinesis rather than the last resort; they call for attention to Fish's (42) caution that stimulants are the choice only for selected hyperactive children, and that some may not need any medication.

Some of the etiological assumptions made by stimulant-therapy proponents have been criticized, as has the design employed in their studies to establish efficacy of the drugs. Walker (96), a physician, contends that society is too cavalier about drugging the hyperactive child. He cites treatable physical causes of hyperkinesis seldom explored by physicians in their investigations, such as improper oxygenation, inability to tolerate and assimilate glucose, and inadequate levels of calcium,[2] who instead prescribe methylphenidate and thus mask the child's symptoms. The drug is an hallucinogen, more potent than LSD, and its long-term effects are not known. He advocates that hyperactive children should be carefully examined, not quickly drugged. Elsewhere (95) he, too, cites evidence that children receiving the stimulants do not progress academically any better than hyperactive children who do not get the drugs. He is among those who observe that long-term studies indicate the drugs subdue but do not result in social adjustment any better than that of those who are not medicated.

A similar stance is taken by Rie *et al.* (81) and Sprague and Sleator (94). Both groups question seriously that Ritalin improves learning ability. Rie *et al.* believe the drugs reduce or remove both "the behavioral impediments to learning and the affective investment in learning." They reason that teachers are likely to misread behavioral changes for improvements in academic achievement. They are sharply critical of the studies in which sole reliance is placed upon the drug as treatment and upon uncritical acceptance of parents' and teachers' evaluations.

Also critical of the use of the "subjective" reports of teachers and parents to guide physicians' decisions about medication, Neisworth *et al.* (77) state that physicians rely heavily upon anecdotal rather than clinical data both in electing to medicate and in subsequent monitoring of drugs' effects.

Along with a survey of the literature, Levine *et al.* (65) collected data, largely subjective in nature, from examinations of thirty-seven hyperactive children and from extensive field interviews with school nurses, social workers, psychologists, teachers, and principals in the Chicago area. They, too, found indications that teachers are overly inclined to identify behavior as hyperactivity and to urge visits to physicians, suggesting the desirability of medication. They too are concerned that other etiologies are overlooked and that psychogenic factors operate more frequently than is generally recognized.

Schain (88) stresses a compelling need for research methods and designs capable of assessing the effects of the drugs, independent of the uncertainties from subjective ratings by teachers and parents. Drug research is found

---

[2] To these causes may be added nontoxic blood-serum levels of lead (35).

seriously defective by Nash (76) because of ongoing unsolved difficulties in classifying the disorders being investigated, in measuring behavioral changes, and in identifying the individual characteristics of those who do and do not improve. Douglas (38) observes that virtually all of the better-designed studies are short-term, however, and that the therapeutic effect ends almost at once when the drug is withdrawn. I would add that short-term studies obscure possible long-term side effects.

Perhaps the severest critic of the research done on medication of children is DiMascio (37), who states that only a few of the many drugs available have been assessed with large numbers of patients. The effect of differences in dosage has not been explored in a systematic way; adverse reactions have not been well documented and little data is available on the impacts of these drugs on the maturing process. And, finally, important patient factors have been largely ignored in the studies: diagnostic homogeneity, severity and chronicity of illness, and age, maturational level, and sex of the child.

The fact that the drugs do control and subdue, and are used for that purpose primarily, is the theme developed by Conrad (29) into an interesting social-political hypothesis. The drug therapy of hyperactivity has resulted, he states, in the "medicalization of deviant behavior," one of the most effective means of social control. This control became possible as pharmacological research became more sophisticated and found more subtle correlates with human behavior. The real humanitarian benefits that seemed possible made the use of this research tempting, especially in the school systems, and so the use of the drugs has proliferated. This wide use is accompanied, reasons Conrad, by some seriously negative aspects. Since drugs are the province of medical experts, their views rather than those of society are likely to dominate concepts of what behavior is deviant. Certain behavior begins to be tagged with a medical diagnosis when medical control of that behavior seems useful. This situation, he reasons, will result in the assignment of causality for complex social problems to individuals rather than to society, a process of "blaming the victim." In hyperkinesis, for example, the medical diagnosis may obscure other causes: family, classroom, and/or school conditions. Ultimately this depoliticizes the deviant behavior. In diagnosing hyperactivity in so many children, Conrad suggests, we may be overlooking the need to analyze the school system.

A MIDDLE COURSE

Both proponents and opponents of stimulant-drug therapy are inclined to see some merit on the other side, without relinquishing their firm stands. Advocates acknowledge that the drugs have little impact on cognitive functioning; opponents concur that they reduce disruptive behavior. Oettinger (78) views the drugs as the keystone of the treatment of hyperactivity, but acknowledges that a treatment program must be more comprehensive, and include remediation, counseling, physiotherapy, and environmental control. Benoit (15), also a physician, believes that the drugs should be used only in the most specific way, and only for those children who are hyperactive under all conditions. She is particularly concerned that the child in whom the root cause of hyperactivity is anxiety not be treated with the stimulants. Her orientation is multi-disciplinary for both diagnosis and therapy, and her insistence is that therapy consider the possible needs for special education, guidance for child and for parents, help with emotional and behavioral problems, environmental manipulation, and special placement. Others see stimulant therapy only as a last resort, should all else fail. Like Benoit, Levinson and Nissenbaum (66) emphasize the importance of searching for all possible causes of a specific child's hyperactivity. For example, they remind us that a reasonable possibility occurring regularly is the dramatically increased demand from teachers for more classwork and homework as the term nears its end.

In this middle ground, professionals attempt to maximize the benefits from the medications and minimize the hazards. This group emphasizes extensive diagnosis to determine the necessity for the drugs for the specific child, and their applicability to him, careful monitoring and management of the treatment once begun, and objectification of report data to replace the anecdotal.

Cantwell (22) urges recognition that hyperkinetic children are a heterogeneous group, so that the drugs, even when useful, may be so only in some areas of each child's limitations. Associated with these differences, Cantwell finds differences in response to the medication, the drugs being ineffective for about 25 to 35 percent of hyperactive children. Therefore he urges careful diagnosis before starting medication and recognition of the possible need for other concurrent interventions, especially if there are learning disabilities.

Satterfield, particularly, sought with his colleagues (84, 85, 86, 87) to identify the neurophysiological variables among hyperactive children that make for good or poor response to the medication. Left unanswered is whether the good responders might also respond favorably to other interventions, and what can be done to help the poor responders. In a similar vein, Burnett and Struve (21) observe that MBD children who also show both neurological and EEG abnormalities have a better response to medications than do those with normal neurological findings. A review of the literature by Klicpera (55) indicates that the children who respond well are those identified by diagnosable soft neurological signs, greater motor restlessness, and greater attentional difficulties.

A nonphysiological view of drug response is offered by Loney et al. (69). They found that children whose parents they would define as good "managers" (consistent, warm, firm, predictable, sensitive) respond better to the drugs than do those whose parents are poor managers (rejecting and neglectful).

Most hyperkinetic children have specific learning disabilities in addition to hyperactivity, note Conrad et al. (30), who add that medication alone is sufficient treatment only for those with no learning problems. Abikoff (1) finds that hyperactivity always affects cognitive functioning, that cognitive training is an indispensable supplement to stimulant therapy, that both are needed to manage disruptive classroom behavior.

Another moderating trend calls for a more realistic view of the potential benefits of the stimulant medications, either as providing an early stabilization but not a cure (65), or as properly limited in goal to achieving behavior that will elicit a more favorable response from a teacher to a child (81). This view accepts the drugs' capacity to reduce intensity without improving efficiency in responsive behavior, goal orientation, and social learning (100). But others will not accept such limited goals. Schain (88) believes the goal of stimulant therapy should be to support the child while lengthier, more laborious interventions (remediation, family therapy, individual psychotherapy, behavioral modification) are given time to take hold.

A major plea among moderates is for objectifying data wherever possible. A study of the medical records of 135 boys treated with CNS stimulants by Loney and Ordoña (70) found evidence that *physician factors* influenced, in a confusing way, the diagnosis, the treatment choice, and the evaluation of clinical improvement. Progress notes by different physicians were not entered at consistent times, and judgments of a child's response to the medication were loose and unsystematic, as were the reporting and evaluation of side effects. To counter these tendencies, they recommend a clarification for physicians of the concepts of diagnosis, therapy choice, and progress evaluation.

Objectification of data at every stage of the diagnostic and treatment process is advocated by Neisworth *et al.* (77). They urge that diagnostic reports and impressions be translated into objectively defined school and home behaviors and that objective standards be applied to evaluation of the severity of deviant behaviors—for example, the duration of sustained on-task behavior, the frequency and length of interruptions and lapses. They call for an attempt at situational validation of the diagnosis through the same evaluation of other children of the similar age and development in the same classroom. They would require continued collection and evaluation of objective data about target behaviors after drug therapy has begun.

A recent volume of collected papers (16) presents an overview of the confused evidence emanating for stimulant-drug research and use, and in doing so represents a plea for improved cooperation among the various disciplines in the identification and treatment of hyperactive children.

Lambert *et al.* (61) are optimistic about the trends they see in planning for the hyperactive child on the basis of individual differences. They observe an increasing emphasis upon differential diagnosis, multiple etiologies, and differential therapies. They see a need for more research to identify types of hyperkinetic children according to demographic factors, home environments, developmental progress, school characteristics, school behavior, and medical findings.

Some guidance through the conflicting and confusing evidence was provided by a national conference on the use of the stimulant drugs with behaviorally disturbed children convened by the Department of Health, Education, and Welfare (79). The participants, concerned about indiscriminate use, nonetheless also cited the value of drugs as a recourse for those children who fail to respond to remedial instruction, operant conditioning, family counseling, or environmental control. The drugs properly managed have a role in the treatment of hyperkinesis. It should be no more acceptable to deny a child this benefit when appropriate for him than to make him the unwitting victim of drugs inappropriately administered. For the physician, improved diagnostic and treatment standards clearly are indicated. For the nonphysician clinician working with the hyperactive child, and for parents and teachers, some knowledge of the effectiveness to be expected from the drugs and of the principles that should govern their administration is imperative.

Once again we confront the obvious need for a specific approach to each individual. The value and the danger of stimulant drugs must be considered in the totality of the individual's situation. The support systems available to a given child may be so promising and/or his hyperactive behaviors so minimal that drug therapy would have a very low priority among options for him. Or remediation, behavior modification, or psychotherapy may not be taking hold, making drug therapy a necessary and potentially valuable adjunct. Or a family situation may be so desperate, so threatened with serious disruption by the otherwise uncontrollable hyperkinetic behavior of the child, that high priority must be given to prompt control of that behavior. Which is more desirable: a hyperactive child bereft of either or both parents, or a ''zombie'' whose family is intact? Obviously there is no easy answer. Happily, few situations are so extreme. The decision in each case should derive from a weighing of both the good and bad effects, from an evaluation of the trade-off possibilities. What will be gained? What will be lost? Knowledge of the effect of the hyperactivity upon parental and peer relations, of the need for and probable response to other treatments, and knowledge of the stimulant drugs, how they work, how they should be managed, are all necessary to the decision. The clinician cannot accept or reject them indiscriminately.

Management of Drug Therapy

Specific experience with these drugs must guide the physician, usually a pediatrician or child psychiatrist, who prescribes them for a hyperactive child. A thorough diagnostic exploration should precede drug treatment, one that considers the full range of possible physical, psychological, environmental, familial, and social causes in the child's symptoms, to rule out those for which stimulant medication would be contraindicated. Stimulant medication should not be prescribed as the sole treatment intervention, or even the primary one, in my view, but rather as a potentially useful adjunct. The physician should be knowledgeable about the values and the sources of special education and psychotherapy and counseling for both parents and child, as well as with the possibilities of environmental manipulation.

The physician should prepare both parents and child in a realistic way for the drug regimen. The preparation should include the setting of realizable goals that all of them understand. Any inflated expectations should be curbed with the facts and limits about probable behavioral changes, improvement in attention, learning, and social behavior. All should understand the impossibility of predicting the child's response to the medication before trying it out. The parents should understand that if the child is depressed, withdrawn, or learning disabled, the drugs alone are not sufficient therapy, but that the hyperactivity must be moderated before other treatments can be tried to help those conditions.

The possibility of side effects should be discussed with the parents, with care exercised that any bias of the physician does not dominate the parents' elections. Their right as well as their responsibility is to decide which is more undesirable, the child's behavior or the possible side effects. Parents do need information to guide their choice, including the fact that the side effects sometimes reported are not necessarily probable in each case, and that they dissipate quickly when the medication is discontinued. The risk of evoking a decision stimulated by suggestibility in some parents is outweighed by their responsibility and their right to make the determination for their dependent child in this medical matter. The facts of the prognosis should also be presented to the parents, who should understand, contrary to the general belief that hyperactivity always improves at puberty, that some children remain symptomatic into young adulthood and may require continued medication, and that we have no technique available to predict this possible outcome.

Parents should be made responsible for administering the medication, regardless of the age of the child. The child should be told the reason for this: that measuring how well the medicine works depends on knowing that it is being taken exactly as prescribed. As the child becomes adolescent this requirement is likely to run afoul of the youth's need for autonomy and individuation, and may have to be relaxed. If the physician has established a good working alliance with his teen-age patient, the possibility of carelessness when administration of the drug is made the adolescent's responsibility is reduced.

Drug dosage is an aspect of the treatment regimen where the physician's experience is most important. Effective dosage may not necessarily be correlated with the age or height and weight of the child. Manipulation of the size of dose and timing of administration are crucial in obtaining a maximum response. Some children do best with alternating periods on and off medication. Others do well with weekends as medication-free periods. Still others may do well when the drug is suspended over the summer, although arrangements for resuming if necessary (on vacation trips or at camp, for example) should be made in advance. Generally a titrating approach to dosage level for each child has been found advisable, beginning with a low level, and slowly increasing the dose to the point where either benefits or extreme side effects appear.

Careful study of dosage levels and resulting effects are reported by Sprague (93) for three types of stimulant drugs. He observes that desired behavioral effects tend to increase more rapidly with increased dosage than do undesired side effects, until a point where a reversal recurs in which side effects increase and learning performance and social behavior deteriorate. Larger doses are required to reach peak enhancement of social behavior than of learning performance. Indeed, if maximal social behavior is sought by increase of dosage, cognitive functioning is likely to deteriorate. Sprague hypothesizes that it should be possible to achieve a dosage that balances the desired enhancement of both learning and social behavior without obtaining "deleterious side effects." A more realistic aim would be one for the least possible side effects, since his curves show some side effects from the smallest doses prescribed.

Each child should be considered to have an idiosyncratic response to any drug and be carefully tested for the drug and dosage most suited to him. Withdrawal from medication should also be titrated in order to avoid any rebound or "crashing" response. Feighner and Feighner (39) find that it usually takes four to six weeks to establish the best maintenance dose for a child, with adjustments made at one- to two-week intervals. As to timing, ideally, according to Laufer (62), the effects of a single dose in the morning should last through the homework period without a rebound at pre-bedtime; some children may need an afternoon dose as well. In some cases, the doses required to calm the child are so high that learning is clearly inhibited (94). For them, it may be advisable to schedule instruction periods three to four hours after the drug is administered, when the blood-serum level is decreasing. The desired point is one where the child is in control of his activity and attention, neither incapable of control nor excessively controlled. Obviously, this balance is not always easily attained, but it should remain the physician's goal. The effort to attain it requires dedication of time and interest.

An hyperactive child and his parents should not undertake a stimulant medication regimen unless the physician can assure its continuous monitoring. Monitoring requires seeing the child at frequent intervals until maintenance dosage is reached, and at longer intervals thereafter to check on response and side effects. Proper monitoring includes periods of suspension of the drug during the school year, to test whether or not the drug is still needed. Regular serological and other laboratory tests are essential as safeguards. Periodic objective testing of cognitive functions, attention, and motor skills should be scheduled, along with regular and frequent feedback from parents and teachers, again, with objective rather than anecdotal data desirable. Monitoring is an indispensable feature of a medication regimen in order to adjust dosage to short-term and long-term changes in response. It is mandatory where medication is administered over a period of years.

Cautiously used after thorough diagnostic procedures, with adequate medical control, and with practice of the safeguards pertaining to any long-term intake of any drug, these medications can be a reasonable, at times an invaluable, part of the therapeutic armamentarium. A final comment: the physician must know how and when to end drug therapy as well as when and how to start it.

Stimulant Therapy of the Adolescent and the Adult

Arnold *et al.* (10) report a 22-year-old college student who, after seeing a film on hyperkinesis, sought psychiatric help. The film had convinced him that he was and had long been hyperkinetic, fidgety, mischievous, with attention difficulties in studying. After an unsuccessful trial with methylphenidate, and with placebo studies made, he responded favorably to dextroamphetamine, with improved concentration, less anxiety, but increased depression. The depression is not usually the response of normal adults, but does coincide with that reported in hyperkinetic children.

There is growing recognition of the possibility that a sizeable number of adults diagnosed schizophrenic have histories of MBD and that their disorder may be a variant of MBD rather than classical schizophrenia. Huey *et al.* (52) report the case of a 23-year-old man suffering confusion, ideas of reference, and auditory hallucinations. Multiple hospitalizations and courses of treatment with neuroleptics were not successful. Revelation of a history of MBD led to the prescription of methylphenidate that produced significant improvement within three days. The favorable response had continued throughout four months of outpatient treatment with the drug at the time of the report. This study does not differentiate possible hyperactivity from MBD in the patient, a situation that detracts from the value of many psychiatric studies. Moreover, subclinical epilepsy has been found to result in schizophrenic-like symptoms that respond favorably to anticonvulsant drugs (among them the amphetamines) but are exacerbated by neuroleptic medications (75).

The emotional and behavioral problems associated with MBD and hyperactivity undoubtedly can persist into adolescence and adulthood, and in some cases can intensify into severe psychiatric problems obscuring the MBD etiology. Where the symptoms of hyperkinesis are prominent in these cases, the stimulant medications may be worth a trial, on the same careful basis as is advised with children and also keeping in mind the potential benefits from other treatment modalities as well.

Moderates who emphasize remediation and psychotherapy in the treatment of hyperkinesis also acknowledge the contributing role of medication (74) that may necessarily be continued into adulthood. Safer and Allen (82) found that teenagers get benefits from the medications similar to those for children; their comparative study was of drug effects of treatment initiated at different ages (before 8, at 13 or later, or before 8 and continued into the teens).

Children who responded well to the drugs continued to do so into their teens. Effective dosage levels may not necessarily correlate with age, height, or weight. Hyperactivity and inattentiveness remained problems into adolescence, but aggressivity decreased and there was no evidence of drug abuse in the teen years. In fact, the teenagers were found more resistant to taking medication than were children.

Nutritional Therapies

During the two decades before this writing, hypotheses were advanced, and are still being tested, about the roles of allergens in food and of vitamins in the etiology of hyperkinesis. Because they coincide with the crusading interest in natural food and megavitamin treatment for a host of diseases, including lupus, and often evoke partisan fidelity rather than skeptical scrutiny, these hypotheses and the evidence concerning their operation and effectiveness should be understood by parents of hyperactive children and the professionals responsible for their treatment.

Diet-Control Therapy

Feingold, an allergist, has postulated that some children are extremely allergic to food dyes and preservatives, as well as to salicylates that occur naturally (see Chapter 2). These substances are found in many commercially prepared foods: soft drinks, ice cream and sherbet, dry cereals, candy, delicatessen meats such as bologna, salami, and frankfurters, and mustard and ketchup. Tomatoes, apples, oranges, and cherries are rich in salicylates.

  Since advancing his original allergy hypothesis, Feingold has leaned toward the view that the effect of these food factors is upon the neurotransmitter system. There is increasing evidence that the nature of food ingested influences the rate at which the biochemical precedents of neurotransmitters are absorbed into the brain. Dietary treatment of some neurological and psychiatric disorders is being tested, on the basis that these disorders are caused by an imbalance or deficiency of the transmitters in certain relevant areas of the brain (103, 104). Feingold reports that elimination of these factors from the diet of hyperkinetic children helps about 40 to 50 percent of them. He has not been able to predict how a child will respond. Twenty thousand hyperactive children are now believed to be on the Feingold diet, one that decreases or eliminates the intake of synthetic coloring, flavoring, preservatives, and salicylates (51). Feingold's hypothesis has been extremely difficult to test because of the required double-blind conditions. It is virtually impossible to eliminate most of the suspect items from a child's diet without the child and the parents being aware of it. Moreover, until very recently, no data was made available on the doses of food additives considered necessary to produce hyperkinetic behavior.

The same research difficulties are inherent in the report of Crook (33), an allergist, who studied the effects of diet on 182 hyperactive children. After a thorough medical and psychological examination, the children were tested for food allergies by a sublingual-provocative method. A follow-up questionnaire sent to the parents resulted in 129 full and 35 partial responses. Of these, 128 parents "believed" that the child's hyperactivity was caused by suspect foods. In order of frequency of citation these were sugar, color additives, flavoring, milk, corn, chocolate, eggs, wheat, soy, citrus fruits, and pork.

More objective evidence of individual sensitivity to substances making for hyperactivity is found in a study by Swanson and Kinsbourne cited in a survey of the research on Feingold's hypothesis (51). They found that low doses of suspect food additives produced no negative effects. They administered a high dose, 150 mg, of a blend of nine widely used food dyes, to 20 hyperactive children who for five days before had been on a diet free of the additives. The on-task performance of 17 of the 20 children was adversely affected, while 20 non-hyperactive children were unaffected by an identical dose of the additive.

An example of a contradictory and possibly biased study is the recent review reported by the Nutrition Foundation, which is supported in the main by the food industry. They find no association between hyperactivity in children and their diets in a survey of studies of 190 hyperactive children in seven different centers. Children and parents were unaware of whether they received neutral food or foods containing dyes accepted by the U.S. Food and Drug Administration (FDA). The review's conclusion is criticized because of the low doses used (26 mg instead of the 200 mg that the FDA estimates is the average amount consumed daily by children), and because only dyes, no other additives, were given to the children. The director of the FDA, reacting to this debate, sees the "suggestion" of a link between some foods and some hyperactive behavior, but judges the evidence to be inconclusive (19).

A careful review of the studies of food additives and hyperactivity failed to find support for a claim that 50 to 70 percent of hyperactive children improve on additive-free diets (103).

Megavitamin (Orthomolecular) Therapy

Cott (31, 32) advocates a treatment using large doses of vitamins. His hypothesis, derived from Linus Pauling, is that biochemical disorders whose etiologies are found in allergies, foods, and environmental pollutants impede learning, and that large doses of vitamins and minerals in addition to proper nutrition create the "optimum molecular environment for the brain."

No real research has been published to evaluate this hypothesis in MBD. Vitamins are assigned on an "empirical" basis. They are combined with stimulant medications because the two are "compatible" and because "the vitamins potentiate the actions of most drugs." But Cott also claims that most MBD children treated orthomolecularly improve without the use of drugs. Cott lists the particular vitamins prescribed and the doses, which are determined by the weight of the child, below and above 35 pounds.

The orthomolecular approach as presented might be termed megavariable. Chizeck (24) challenged the conclusions of an American Psychiatric Association task force that the orthomolecular approach to the treatment of schizophrenia is invalid, and defended it as one incorporating "stimulant drugs, tranquilizers, special diets, vitamins, and supportive counseling." A careful review of the role of vitamins in the brain activity of normal and disturbed subjects found no evidence from "properly conducted studies" that megavitamin treatments affected improvement in schizophrenia (103). On the other hand, Adler (4) in a review of the orthomolecular approach finds it a valid biochemical alternative to stimulant drugs and behavioral modification. Because it is so difficult to identify the exact content of the orthomolecular treatment as now presented, I prefer to consider megavitamin therapy as a separate entity. Arnold *et al.* (7), advocates of stimulant-drug therapy, found no support for megavitamins. Prior to the study 31 MBD children were randomly assigned to a trial on megavitamins or placebo. Only two children—both on placebo—responded so well that stimulants were judged unnecessary.

Comment

Both megavitamin therapy and diet control would appear to merit a trial before resorting to stimulant medications, since these drugs are in my view a last resort in the most difficult situations. Caution must be exercised, however, to guard against the possible deleterious effect of high doses of some vitamins, for example, the mineral-chelating potential of large doses of Vitamin C. While therapists cannot speak with certainty about the potential effects of drugs and diets, parents are justified in trying therapeutic experiments with them where the negative odds, checked with physicians, are not too great.

Chapter 15

Behavioral Modification

THE TECHNIQUES OF BEHAVIORAL MODIFICATION have found increasing acceptance in the treatment of hyperkinesis. Even staunch defenders of stimulant medications acknowledge with measured reluctance that behavioral methods are sometimes effective where pharmacology fails, and are often effective when combined with medication (34). They add that while expensive and time consuming, behavioral-modification methods are certainly more desirable than "insight psychotherapy," which they consider unproved in diminishing "behavioral deviance." Confusing the issue even further is the conclusion that neither behavior modification nor medication produces gains that persist over time or from one setting to another (33A). A more moderate opinion is offered by Strupp (33), who observes with favor an increasing rapprochement between behavioral modification and psychodynamic techniques. At present, psychotherapies of all varieties and emphases are being mustered to help the MBD patient unlearn, relearn, and learn. In Fine's case-study review (9A), the treatment chosen for 14 of 21 children with hyperkinesis was behavior modification while the other seven were treated with diet management, family therapy, perceptual-motor training, and psychotherapy.

Hypothetical Propositions

Behavioral modification has a clearly stated hypothetical basis, one that may make it seem especially well-conceptualized amongst the morass of theories,

182

subtheories, and passionate beliefs that surround MBD. All etiologies except problems with the learning process are rejected. Ross (29), for example, rejects the theory that organic, emotional, and cultural factors are causal in learning disabilities, and instead pins the blame on the "unspecialized instruction" in most classrooms. The problem, he avers, is educational, not medical or social; its prevalence implies a social dysfunction, not a personal, individual one. But a reading of some other behavioral literature suggests that apparent clarity or firmness of statement is not synonymous with consensus or with actual freedom from ambiguity.

Strain and Shores (31) focus on the individual's behavior as causal. The child creates his own social environment by the specific quality of his actions: the passive withdrawn child provokes rejection; the physically aggressive child elicits hostility; the positively interacting child is rewarded in kind by peers.

Behavior, states Ross (29), is influenced by its consequences. (Why then, one might ask, does a child whose behavior elicits rejection, continue with that behavior?) He holds that the events that follow immediately upon an act determine whether or not the behavior will be repeated when similar circumstances again occur. Ross here refers to reinforcement, a basic concept that in behavioral-modification theory leads to the inference that normal and abnormal behavior differ only in the nature of the reinforcements each has received in the past (17).

While rejecting consideration of etiological factors as having no place in a treatment plan, Nirk et al. (24) stress concentration upon specific behaviors in the treatment of hyperkinesis. Yet the operation of etiological factors is implied in their view that the behavioral change is sought not as an end goal in itself, but rather as the only way one can feel that "certain psychological structures have changed within the child," i.e., that the child is developing, maturing.

Both clarity and consensus can be found, however, in the behaviorist insistence upon specifying the acts it seeks to modify. These acts are termed the "interfering" behavior. "Social skills" is not a specific limiting, defining term. It can be, and usually is, understood differently by different people. Thus, "social skills" does not identify the behavior to be modified. Closer to the behaviorist goal of specified behavior is this list of specific social factors: smiling and laughing, greeting, joining, inviting, conversing, sharing, cooperating, complimenting others, playing, physical appearance, and grooming (15). As another example the term "aggressivity" is not used to describe a child's behavior. Again, specifics are preferred: hitting, swearing, punching. Parents of children being treated by behavioral methods, confused by the seeming clarity and simplification, may be grateful to learn that a specific aggressive act has been reduced in frequency from 12 to 1 each day. But if that act is fire-setting or eye-gouging, the importance of the quality and gravity of the specific acts becomes obvious.

Another goal of behaviorist specificity is an approach to the treatment of hyperactivity that sorts out for focus of work certain aspects of the behavior:

regulation of activity, sustaining of attention upon relevant tasks, control of impulsivity, and self-verbalization (24).

An insistence upon specificity and definition is a significant contribution to any field of knowledge. It is one to be sought in MBD work, in behavioral as in other treatment approaches. With this ideal, behavioral modifiers have contributed to understanding the acts of victims of MBD by particularizing as much as possible the behaviors to be modified; they have also suggested methods to achieve modification (4, 15, 27, 32).

Modification Procedures

An illustration of the interaction of behavior and consequence is contained in a report by Krop (14). He specified three general classes of behavior as most antagonistic to sustaining attention: locomotion, communicative or quasi-communicative activity interfering with a task assignment, and distraction. Operant-conditioning procedures were employed successfully to modify these behaviors; the child was rewarded with either praise and/or candy when the behaviors did not occur, and ignored when any one of them did. Follow-up four weeks after the last conditioning session indicated that the obtained reduction in hyperactivity was being maintained.

Operant conditioning is perhaps the most frequently employed behavioral method in treating hyperkinesis. Prout (26) reviews the literature and cites many studies in which the technique was used to shape new behaviors and extinguish undesirable ones with token systems and systematic programming of social reinforcement by adults important to the patient. A significant feature of this and almost all behavioral intervention is the use of parents as surrogate therapists. They become cotherapists with the primary therapist, extending the training procedures in time and place.

Effective brief treatment in about six sessions by operant conditioning for a child showing hyperactivity and short attention span, in which the parents, siblings, and teachers are mobilized as therapists, is reported by Phillips and Mordock (25). In their procedure, sessions with the parents avoid discussion of the parents' problems and emphasize eliciting a description of the child's major problems. Parents help plan the therapeutic program and are instructed in the use of positive reinforcements and the withholding of negative ones. The involvement of parents in this way also tends to counteract the feelings of impotence and pessimism so many parents feel when there is nothing they seem able to do to help their child. The goal in positive reinforcement is seen by Feighner and Feighner (9) as the provision of a consistent environmental control that facilitates internalization; their technique uses positive reinforcements that exploit the child's assets.

The training and use of parents as surrogate behavioral therapists is widely accepted. One study cited in a national report (11) describes how parents were trained to reward desired behavior with praise and punish undesired behavior with isolation. Of eight hyperactive boys, two improved enough to be withdrawn from stimulant medication; reductions of medication by 25 to 50 percent were possible for four others. An important behavioral technique used in this study is the "contract," an agreement specified between patient and therapist—in this study the parents—as to the effort to be made, the methods to be used, and the consequences. Results of a related study (8) also supported training parents to be "primary" reinforcement therapists with their hyperactive children. Ross (29) states that behavioral-modification principles, being logical and straightforward, can be taught readily to parents. Systematic training of teachers as well as parents to serve as surrogate therapists is also practiced (24, 34).

The literature has also been excellently reviewed by Bower and Mercer (1). In addition to environmental manipulation and medication, they cite successes in reducing hyperkinesis by operant conditioning, contingent reinforcement, payment for improved grades in reading and arithmetic, shaping procedures, and combinations of reinforcement and extinction. They also describe a technique of verbal mediation in which the child is conditioned to "stop, listen, look, and think" before responding. And they comment upon the power of so-called "observational models" (quiet, reflective teachers or peers) to reduce impulsivity (19, 21, 23), a form of conditioning called learning by identification in psychoanalytic terminology.

It is still unclear whether reinforcement should be negative or positive. All the methods described above are primarily positive. Other studies used negative consequences. Loss of marbles for incorrect responses did more than winning marbles for correct responses in modifying the behaviors of 48 hyperactive and 48 normal boys on a discrimination-learning task (7). In a related project, withdrawal of TV privileges reduced hyperactivity, measured by a stabil-metric chair in a four-year-old boy (22). These two reports are in contrast to the finding that positive rewards (food and praise) reduced the number of play activities by a hyperactive boy. Stimulant medication was noted to increase attention but was accompanied by decreased intelligibility of speech and responsiveness to demands (30). And dramatic improvement in a nine-year-old hyperkinetic girl in response to token and verbal rewards is recorded (5). Moreover the improvement was sustained at a follow-up two months later.

Another important behavioral approach is an effort to test the relative effect of reinforcers. Bugental *et al.* (4) found that interventions focused on self-control were more effective than social reinforcements. The former resulted in better perception of personal control over academic behavior; the latter resulted in improved ratings of impulsivity by teachers. Reinforcement procedures are judged by Zentall (35) to be successful in modifying hyperactive behavior because they increase stimulation in the child whose impulsive erratic behavior is caused by a state of stimulus hunger or sensory deprivation.

Recently, biofeedback procedures have come into prominence. Braud and his colleagues (2, 3) used electromyographic (EMG) biofeedback to reduce hyperactivity in a six-and-a-half-year-old boy in eleven sessions. Concomitant improvements are reported in general behavior, psychological- and achievement-test scores, self-esteem, and psychosomatic symptoms. Some deterioration (erratic behavior) observed seven months after the last training session was attributed to a lack of reinforcement by parents and teachers. This observation was coordinated by Lupin *et al.* (18) with the notion that the hyperkinetic child is also tense, and that tension can produce the very symptoms identified as hyperkinesis. Since EMG is a laboratory procedure, they developed a relaxation technique that would permit treatment at home under the direction of the parents. The method is Edmund Jacobson's "progressive relaxation," first developed in 1934, in which various muscle groups are alternately tensed and relaxed. Tapes of instruction were produced individually for parents and child. The parents' tapes described behavior-modification techniques, and gave directions for helping the child and for aiding the parents in their own relaxation. The child's tapes provided instruction accompanied by relaxing imagery. Putre *et al.* (27) studied 20 hyperactive boys to compare the effectiveness of a tape that instructed in Jacobson's progressive relaxation with a control tape that recounted boy's-level adventure stories. Both tapes produced similar effects (a 34-percent decrease in forehead muscle tension); no significant differences between effects of the two tapes were obtained. Reduction of tension through progressive relaxation and large-muscle exercise for impulsive boys correlated with improved cognitive performance on the *Matching Familiar Figures Test* (12).

An illuminating study of the comparative effectiveness of reinforcers was conducted by Clement *et al.* (6), specifically examining self-reinforcement versus self-observation in modifying hyperactivity. Their subjects, children, were given the status of "employees," not clients or patients. Research staff members were designated "employers." Employees—the children—had an opportunity in the employment situation to earn money and other privileges (e.g., participation in an outing). The employment task was for the child, with instruction from the employer, to get what he wanted in school without making teachers and other students unhappy about the way he did it. When the child accepted the terms, his parents were informed of them and their acceptance obtained. A written contract with the child was executed. The child was then trained in use of the equipment he would use in his self-regulatory efforts in the classroom: (1) a timing device to measure and signal the end of a designated period; (2) a counting device to record success or failure in obtaining the desired (target) behaviors.

Of great importance is the researchers' effort to evaluate some of the factors within the concept of reinforcement. They report that self-reinforcement is superior to self-observation in modifying the impulsive behavior of these children, and that to strengthen a weak (desired) behavior is easier than to weaken a strong (undesired) behavior. Compliance with the details of the contract was greater with self-regulation efforts than with self-observation procedures, and the more compliance with the self-regulation contract, the more change was effected in the target behavior. Finally, the strategy used—the employee and employer relationship—was highly effective in maintaining the contact of the child with the therapist. At least three aspects of behavioral therapy are reflected in these conclusions: the choice of reinforcers, the choice of target behaviors, and the nature of the relationship between patient and therapist.

The study report is valuable as well in postulating some other general guidelines to behavioral modification. The therapeutic agent, Clement and his colleagues state, may be, but need not be, a professional. The therapist may otherwise be a parent, a teacher, a symptom-free peer, a peer with problems similar to the child, or the child may treat himself. The effectiveness of therapy is enhanced, they found, when the stimuli emphasized in the therapy are similar to stimuli in circumstances outside therapy, and where therapy takes place in situations in which the child will ultimately be involved, not in the relatively isolated office situation. Finally, avoidance of negative feelings and responses in favor of concentration upon positive aspects proved more effective than the opposite.

Comment

Behavioral modification theory, thus, emphasizes clarity and economy of design in defining and isolating "target" behaviors and strategies for altering them; it renounces any potential benefit from designing therapy from prior determination of etiology. Yet statements of theory and intent do not always coincide with actual therapeutic efforts reported. Nirk et al. (24), while critical of medication alone, are willing to incorporate its use, as they are to combine "psychoanalytic and cognitive developmental principles," with their behavioral-modification designs. Obviously, these incorporations "contaminate" the purity of design, but they should not obscure the valuable role of behavioral-modification therapy.

Behavioral techniques prove effective in ameliorating certain aspects of the MBD syndrome. Symptoms of hyperkinesis are particularly amenable to the method, and the improved control of these has sometimes contributed to an increased learning capability. Application of behavioral techniques may reduce or eliminate the need for stimulant medication; they offer success for the child in tasks levelled so as to not overwhelm him. The techniques have reached hyperactive children otherwise responsive only when medicated, among them some who when medicated react with side effects that impair the seeming accessibility induced.

Because behavior techniques and prescriptions cut through the often vague terminology of diagnosis and the mystique of therapy, and set "target" behaviors that parents, teachers, and patient can comprehend and observe for change, the method encourages the use of parents and teachers as therapists, secondary or primary. The benefits are many. The therapeutic locale becomes the real-life situation rather than the professional office. Needed gains are made directly in relationships with parents, siblings, teachers, peers. Transfer attenuation of gains is thus minimized. Treatment time is increased vastly over what is usually possible in scheduled office therapy, and therefore the frequency of reinforcement is much higher.

Because of their training and participation as surrogate therapists, parents and teachers are less vulnerable to feelings of confusion and impotence that often arise when the child's treatment is strictly in the hands of the relatively isolated professional. The mutual effort does much to counteract the divisive impact of hyperkinesis upon a family.

Apart from criticisms that claims of clarity tend to be honored in the breech, a bloc of resistance to behavioral modification arises from questions about its impact on human and civil rights (17). These critics hold that the behavioral approach does not allow for freedom of choice, that the participation of professionals in such programs is unethical, and that participation of teachers and parents extends a "fascistic" treatment environment. Defenders counter that the behavioral approaches seek to encourage spontaneity and creativity, not to produce mindless automatons (10). One author believes that the debate probably arises from the insistence of some behaviorists that the identification of abnormal behaviors is a social judgment, and from their insistence that the behaviors require social, environmental change (17).

All sides in this controversy appear to overlook the central matter of the quality of the working or therapeutic relationship between patient and therapist. Pro-modifiers seem guilty of this oversight in their zest for stressing the scientific in their approach. Herbert (10), for example, acknowledges some value in a therapeutic relationship of confidence and trust, but states that the value is minimal and the quality not essential. To extend this argument into an absurdity is all too easy, but nothing would be gained. As one speaks with behavioral therapists and reads their literature, one can be sure that they do seek to create cooperative relations with their patients. The value of behavioral methods should not be overlooked, despite the attempt to impose simplicity upon extremely complex sets of behavior, and to minimize both the patient-therapist relationship and any concept of underlying causation found among their advocates.

Those who wish to pursue behavior-modification procedures in more detail will be interested in the book edited by Quay and Werry (28) on the diagnosis and therapy of childhood disorders, in which Ross reviews behavioral methods. Among other recent books of value are an edited volume by Lahey (16) on the application of behavioral therapy to hyperactive and learning-disabled children, and Herbert's impressive work (10) on the behavioral approach to conduct disorders.

Here as elsewhere, the clinician should remember the complexity of MBD and the innumerable variations of personality, social, cultural, familial, and economic situations in which the dysfunctions occur. There is no panacea for this complexity, no single theory, intervention, or profession capable of explaining and successfully treating all of its victims. Help and elucidation from all sources are welcome, as is the evidence of increasing rapprochement between behavioral and insight therapies (20).

Chapter 16

Parents in the Treatment Process

PARENTING, MUSE FROSTIG AND PASCALE (13), is the most difficult of professions. With an MBD child the difficulty of parenting is enormously increased, and parental roles multiply. The father and mother must examine their reactions and those of their other children and relatives to the victim; they must try to modify reactions damaging to the already damaged child; often they must become part of the actual treatment process; and, they will discover, they can foster their child's welfare by public social and political actions that help all MBD children. They have all the usual chores and pains of parenting, plus the extra burden and disappointment of a learning-disabled, dyslexic, or hyperactive family member, often with emotional and personality difficulties (2). They can help or damage their MBD child directly and indirectly. They need much information, training, guidance, and many contacts. Sometimes parents need psychotherapy, to avoid the extreme reactions of overprotection or rejection that minimal brain dysfunction in one's child makes all too probable.

Parental Reactions to the Child's Symptoms

Parents often struggle against accepting their child's condition or against recognizing the family pathology that may aggravate that condition; they may even cause some seriously disturbing aspects of it.

The infant destined to become a hyperactive child may manifest vegetative difficulties from birth: irritability, crying, lethargy, hyperkinesis, feeding problems (29). Parents are found to recognize learning problems in their children earlier than do their teachers, but the parents are notably and perhaps understandably slower than the teachers in asking for evaluation and help (28).

Low "need for achievement" on the *Thematic Apperception Test* was identified at a significant level for 16 MBD children *and their mothers,* in contrast with an equal number of normal children and their parents (35). The fathers of the MBD children, nine of them college graduates, also produced lower, but not significantly lower, levels of the need than did fathers of the normal children, of whom eight were college graduates. Parents, of course, may denigrate school achievement actively or by implication. By identification the child is discouraged from making efforts to overcome disabilities. Severe intra-family psychopathology may block or minimize the motivation of the vulnerable child and keep him from the very experiences he needs, the researchers comment.

Dependency in a child may be fostered by some parents who, unconsciously or otherwise, seek to enhance their own sense of power. Excessive caretaking can impede a child's will and ability to develop mastery and competence, to explore, ultimately to individuate and separate (36). Even a child's favorable responsivity to medication has been found correlated with the lower degrees of maternal anger and paternal hostility (38). The symptomatic behaviors of MBD children may distress their parents to the point where their reactions are harmful. Intellectually oriented parents with high goals may not be able to tolerate their child's low academic achievement and may react in a way that seriously attacks the child's self-esteem. They may become upset by a series of difficult manifestations: the ceaseless repetition of a question; the expression of a wish for some activity seemingly dangerous for that child, such as automobile driving; a developing sexuality; negativism, especially during adolescence; anger; or inaccessible depression. The rejecting sentiments and actions of the child's siblings often add to the distress of parents.

Yet the quality of parental management influences the self-esteem of the MBD child, probably more than that of the less vulnerable normal child. Good parent management is defined by Loney *et al.* (24) as supplying both support and controls to the MBD sufferer. Parents in this group are described as "firm, consistent, predictable, sensitive, alert to subtle clues, sensible and/or reliable...placid, easy-going, warm, affectionate." Poor managers are "rejecting, neglectful, overprotective, or overindulgent." Among those rated poor, the "most consistent thing they had done in trying to manage the child was to lose their temper." The children of poor managers experienced frequent changes of sitters or foster homes.

Several helpful guides to the management of children with MBD problems are offered by Brown (4). Like all children, they need the feeling of being loved and secure, discipline that is firm yet loving. But more than other children, at all times they need the feeling of being accepted *despite* academic failures and misbehaviors that may make them feel they are disappointing the parents. They need more encouragement than normal children. When the time comes, they need a more gradual movement to separation and independence. Like any child, the MBD child evokes punishment, and in the management of this aspect of the parents' responsibility, Brown is especially helpful. He reminds us that facial expressions, body English, and other silent behaviors convey parental attitudes to the child that may contradict the parents' oral professions. By the same token, prolonged silent unresponsiveness to the child is perhaps the cruelest of punishments. The MBD child should not be punished for behavior he cannot control, his hyperactivity, impulsiveness, inattention. Physical punishment should be avoided; spanking usually arouses so much excitement that the purpose of the punishment may be lost. Withholding of privileges and brief quiet isolation are preferrable. Similar reasoning favors prompt punishment; delay results in the child being confused about his misbehavior and prolongs and intensifies his anxiety to a degree disproportionate to the original offense. Punishment should be appropriate to the offense; it should not vary in nature or degree at different times for the same offense. Discipline should be applied directly and simply, avoiding sermons, long logical speeches, requests for assurance from the child that he will not repeat the offense, bribes, threats, harangues, harsh criticisms. Invoke any punishments threatened, but especially do not threaten severe punishments that are never administered; parents should be alert to the danger that their frustration and resulting anger will distort the situation beyond its real dimensions. The child should clearly understand that what the parents dislike is some aspect of his behavior, not himself. Parents should also strive for a consistent attitude, one that avoids extremes of anger and forgiveness. The child's bed should never by used as the site for punishment; the bed should be respected as the child's sanctuary, a place for rest. Brown's final point is a reminder that punishment for misbehavior is reinforced by consistent rewards for good behavior.

Brown's guidelines illuminate the possibility that parental reactions can either ameliorate an MBD child's behavior or intensify and fix its pathology; their reactions may help the child build self-esteem or lose it. The etiological role of the family in hyperactivity is uncertain, but its role in diminishing or intensifying the syndrome is indisputable (32).

Parents often forget that each family and each child differ in significant ways from other families and other children, so that individual judgments and evaluations should often be sought. Generalizations are immensely helpful, but only when they are checked for appropriateness in the specific family context. Moreover, the attitudes and values within a family are not necessarily homogeneous. The parents seldom present a monolithic front to their children, a fact that has both good and bad consequences for the MBD child. Differences between the mother's level of understanding of the child's limitations and his reactions and the father's may lead to differences in their expectations. The differences may complicate anxiety, guilt, and anger in relationship to the child. A child may benefit from these differences because one parent's understanding and patience may offset the other's anger and disappointment. But in other instances of marked difference in understanding the child may be made more bewildered and more conflicted, more uncertain that he himself is acceptable. Parents do well to examine their differences honestly and try to evaluate whether their differences are confusing or helpful to their child.

Parental Roles

First-time parents are usually anxious about the behavior and well-being of their newborn infant. Discomforts in the child, feeding and sleep problems, protracted crying, developmental lags, all intensify that anxiety and send the parents in search of help, understanding, and guidance to experienced parents, to pediatricians, and to published parent guides. And so it is with the parents of MBD children. Becoming knowledgeable about MBD and its ramifications becomes an early and major responsibility; it is primary among the several responsibilities their child's syndrome places upon them.

Parents' Knowledgeability

The symptoms of MBD are baffling to most parents. There is no definitive neurological disorder; a lovely, responsive child may become suddenly eruptively impulsive; a bright, intellectually competent child may prove to be unable to read effectively. What do the symptoms mean? Where have they come from? What causes them? What can make them go away? Perplexed and confused parents simply cannot meet the special needs that are inescapable in their MBD child. The first job imposed upon them is to get the information they need. Essentially they must come to understand their child's symptoms realistically and fully; and they must become acquainted with resources for help. Later they must understand the nature and prospects of the treatment or treatments their child receives, and they must try to keep in touch with developments about MBD.

Parents need help in understanding realistically the present status of their child's limitations and in tolerating them. They need help in evaluating the degree of change likely in the future, in estimating what they reasonably may and may not expect for the child now and later. Discouragement and over-expectation are both harmful to the child. Parents may need help with their feelings to prevent fostering overdependence or to avoid brutalization, to counteract guilt and anxiety in themselves and in the child. Parents are helped by being informed that while intensive positive investment in the MBD child may not produce great immediate gains, it is likely to forestall negative acting-out and delinquent behaviors, to open the child to future amelioration, and to improve his later response to developmental changes as he matures.

Many special publications are available that, like the classic works of Spock and Gesell, provide basic definitions, explanations, and prospects. An introductory guide for both the parents and the child with a handicap is provided by Gordon (17). The New Hope Guild Center in Brooklyn, N.Y. distributes a lively, illustrated explanation of learning disabilities, their causes, associated school problems, effects on parents, actions parents can take, and the special aids that are available to them (39). The special psychology of the learning-disabled adolescent is described by Kronick (22). A handbook for the parents of a dyslexic child has been edited by Hamilton (19). Crook, a pediatrician, offers some cogent data, especially about drugs and diets, for the parents of the hyperactive learning-disabled child (7). Much useful and stabilizing information can be found in the personal accounts of individuals who have "survived" MBD to grow into effective, competent adults (6, 31). The task of confronting the reality of learning disabilities is described by Hayes (21).

Where to get advice about diagnostic and treatment resources within their community is a major need. Ideally, pediatricians, day-care and nursery-school personnel, and first-grade teachers would be trained in the early detection of the vulnerable child and in how to move parents and child toward appropriate professional and educational resources. But such early-detection sensitivity and resources are not always available. The parents who somehow sense certain of those "soft" neurological signs in their child may have to pursue actively the help they need. Following are some possible steps: visiting the local school and superintendent's office; checking with accessible hospitals, social agencies, and universities, to ask about special-education programs and clinics; and writing to the Education, the Health and/or the Rehabilitation Departments of the state government. Also, the federal government, fortunately, has in recent years joined the effort to help parents find services needed for a handicapped child. The Office of Education (of the former U.S. Department of Health, Education, and Welfare) regularly uses television and radio to advertise its newsletter, *Closer Look,* [1] to keep parents informed about resources, laws, and developments. One article, for example, was about a respite service for parents that would allow them recreative time away from the demanding care of their child; another directed parents to sources of information about summer camps; a third described recent developments in federal laws affecting handicapped children; a fourth reviewed a book instructing parents in the role of teacher.

National and state membership organizations available to parents include: the Association for Children with Learning Disabilities (ACLD)[2]; the Orton Society[3]; the California Association for Neurologically Handicapped Children (CANHC)[4]; the New York Association for Brain Injured Children and its related Association for Children with Learning Disabilities. [5]

[1] Box 1492, Washington, DC 20013, or at regional offices throughout the country.
[2] 5225 Grace Street, Pittsburgh, PA 15236.
[3] 8415 Bellona Lane, Townson, MD 21204.
[4] P.O. Box 4088, Los Angeles, CA 90051.
[5] P.O. Box 710, Grand Central Station, New York, NY 10017.

These organizations publish newsletters, list resources for special education, list and review new books, print special articles, advise on sources of financial aid through state governments, announce and interpret changes in law, issue directories of special services, sell informative pamphlets and books, hold meetings, conferences, and workshops. The parents of the MBD child are well advised to join one or more, in order to stay informed and to learn about journals and publishers such as *The Exceptional Parent* and Academic Therapy Publishers. Recent articles in ACLD *Newsbriefs* guide parents in how to evaluate the Individual Education Plan (called the IEP) that new laws require be designed by his school for their child who has MBD (25). Another explains provisions of Medicaid and Supplemental Security Income (SSI) programs possibly helpful to MBD persons not able to earn enough to support themselves (9). Both membership in and information available from these organizations can do much to counteract parents' feelings of isolation and helplessness in the face of a complex problem.

Exploration may also turn up local groups of parents of MBD children who are working together to obtain improved services, more constructive state and federal laws, to act as advocates for the MBD population and for individual children, and to provide the mutual support and understanding they all need. Where these groups do not exist, parents can make no better contribution to the treatment of their child than to find other parents with an MBD child and form such a group. These children are all about us everywhere. A moderate estimate is that about 10 percent of all children have MBD. Gaines (14) urges parents of "perceptually deprived" children to participate in "Parent Reality Groups" to combine overall treatment with better understanding by parents of the "needs and also the person for whom they are caring." Gaines sees the groups as places for training sessions in reinforcement procedures based upon analyzing tasks into steps and levels, so that the parent is better equipped to carry out at-home extension of training with behavior modification.

Some parents, especially those whose children are hyperkinetic, must decide whether to initiate medication, or to continue medication should undesirable side effects appear. Among parents in a group are likely to be some whose past experience with these choice-making processes will be helpful in rounding out the information available. Such groups also provide peer associations for MBD children, both individually and as a group. They can extend horizons otherwise drastically limited, increase the child's sense of mobility, and do much to restore self-esteem lowered by social isolation or ostracism, and feelings of being bizarre and unique.

Parents, we see, do most when intimately involved in the treatment of their child. They should know enough about the child's condition to put meaningful questions to any professional, whether educator, psychotherapist, or physician, about whatever may perplex them (3). To do everything possible, parents need valid information about every aspect of their child's dysfunctions. The MBD child benefits from the active participation of his parents, provided their efforts are not overprotective or felt to be so. Parental input as the child matures can make the difference between schizoid isolation in the MBD victim grown to adulthood and his effective social and occupational activity.

Parents as Patients

Some parents and some families clearly and directly exacerbate their child's MBD symptoms, rejecting the child as "bad," "inferior," "disappointing." In other families, a fear of and/or disparagement of learning deprives the child of motivation to make the extra effort to mitigate a dysfunction. Any parental indifference or harshness must be converted into a constructive orientation if the child is to progress rather than regress. And those parents who develop severe emotional problems in response to their child's symptoms must be helped if the child is to be helped.

The symptoms of some children, though resembling MBD, may arise directly from the emotional disturbance of a parent. Some hyperkinetic children, Ney (27) reports, are conditioned into their behavior by the depression of their parents, usually a single mother. The child seeks the attention of the depressed parent that he gets only when he is hyperactive. Ney uses a behavioral approach to treating the mother, not the child, in these cases. She is taught to recognize and respond to the child's efforts to please her and to ignore him when he is hyperactive, as well as how to reinforce his quiet behavior. The method is designed to help her see improvement by concentration upon one behavior at a time, thus coming in a short time to enjoy her child and to feel that she is a good mother. Ney's approach would seem to assume that the mother's depression is reactive to the child's hyperkinesis, not the other way around, as his hypothesis states. Presumably, other factors may be contributing to her depression, factors that might best benefit from psychotherapy, financial aid, or a stabilized adult relationship, for example.

When parents or whole families with psychopathology are accessible to the idea, either family therapy or individual psychotherapy for the parents may be indicated. Videotape feedback is used in such therapy by Feighner and Feighner (11). The recorded examples of parent-child interaction are edited to shorten and focus them, and played back. Parents are then counseled about desirable changes. For some families, a psychiatric nurse visits the home to instruct parents there. Where severe psychopathology characterizes either or both parents, individual psychotherapy is indicated. Generally, however, group therapy with the focus on helping their child is helpful in ventilating guilt, anger, and anxiety, and enables the parents to act more benignly. Parents who collapse emotionally under the impact of their child's difficulties, who are unable to cope or function, obviously need psychotherapy oriented toward ego strengthening. Some parents can make their greatest contribution to their child's treatment by themselves becoming patients.

Parents as Educators and Therapists

Parents may be mobilized to serve as cotherapists in behavioral-modification programs (8) under the direction of the professional therapist. As adjunct remediation teachers under the direction of an education specialist, they supervise homework according to the prescribed plan for their child. They can be trained to apply the principles of special education to the many tasks in home and social life that are outside the province of the specialists. Parents can be trained to make discipline short, firm, non-negotiable. The effect of these activities by parents goes far beyond the immediate task; they provide the quality of understanding, support, and recognition that can sustain the child's motivation and self-esteem during many difficult years.

Parental strategies identified as psychotherapeutic are promoted by Berlin (1). He advises their intervention during very early months with hyperactive infants. The mother is instructed in techniques of singing, gently talking, and light body massage that are reported to quiet the restless child. Parents participate at weekly meetings with professionals who assess the changes reported and reinforce their efforts. During the preschool years, the parent is encouraged to help the child hear and obey the word "No." Parents meet with other parents and professionals. They are instructed in operant-conditioning procedures and helped to perceive their often extremely ambivalent feelings about their children. These efforts to establish and maintain parental authority within a loving and respectful context are continued during the school years, to curb the damage of hyperactivity to the child's learning ability.

Frostig and Pascale (13) advocate a remediation approach by parents in which tasks are broken down into small steps, each progressively within the child's ability, each promising success. They illustrate the practical devices within the home that can be used in special kinds of deficit remediation: spring clothespins to practice finger-thumb opposition; pullover shirts; a jacket with fewer and larger-than-usual buttons, from which the child gradually progresses to more and smaller buttons. They also recommend: verbalizing about each activity while the child is doing it; maintaining consistency in approach to the child; listening with the child to television programs with a learning content, such as Sesame Street and The Electric Company, and using the suggestions in guide books provided by the programs; applying reinforcement strategies to encourage desired behaviors; and showing the child recognition, understanding, and acceptance of his feelings.

Gordon (18) urges the structuring of a child's activities to give him a sense of the future, to combat feelings of disorganization, and to encourage a sense of stable environment. Where this is needed, he advises parents not to fear that they are robbing the child of his independence; these children have trouble making and keeping friends, and benefit from having their social experiences outside the classroom organized for them. Indicated for them are associations with other MBD children, special camps, clubs, play groups, or activities with normal children where the MBD child's dysfunctions are not differentiating and isolating. Also advised is teaching the child social skills and leisure activities, again with step-level methods: shopping, eating at restaurants, using public transportation, sports, theatre, museums, cooking, and sewing. Guide books and pamphlets are available that offer both general principles and specific exercises to help parents. Their focus is upon special-education and remedial programs (10, 16, 20, 26, 30, 33, 34, 37).

Some professionals would direct more effort to modifying the parent-child relationship and somewhat less to specific behaviors of the child, observes Cantwell (5). He cites the work of G. Paterson of the University of Oregon, where parents are offered courses of ten to twelve weeks that require mastery of one level of parenting before proceeding to the next, a standard behavioral approach. But the course is taught by two group leaders, one of whom concentrates on psychodynamic, interpersonal issues, the other on parent training of the step-level kind.

Obviously, these programs can quickly overburden parents who have other heavy demands and responsibilities such as other children, elderly parents, personal illness, an ailing spouse, or job and financial worries, or those with emotional problems. More slowly, perhaps, attempts to complete such programs can overburden any parents, even those without additional problems. Parents cannot be expected to do what is beyond them, but they can often be encouraged to find out what they can learn to do, with satisfaction, for their child burdened with MBD.

Parents as Political Activists

Facilities for helping the MBD child, and public willingness to do so, still vary among communities and states, despite the present federal laws mandating the earliest possible detection and most comprehensive treatment of the MBD syndrome. "School districts have different criteria for identifying the handicapped (learning disabled); some are having difficulty preparing educational curriculums and others are trying to determine how to finance a staff and acquire proper equipment" (15). As New York City schools prepared to open in September 1981, more than 12,000 children, entitled by law to special-education programs had either not been evaluated for placement or had not been placed. A thousand more special-education teachers remained unhired, millions of dollars of new construction were required, school districts had to be convinced to provide space and welcome for these children, and the 442 evaluating teams (each with a psychologist, social worker, and educational evaluator) had to be increased in number and their efficiency improved (21A).

Financial problems plague school districts. In New York State many districts serve less than 10 percent of their learning-disabled population at a cost of at least 10 percent of their entire budget. And budgets for the learning disabled are reported to be increasing at twice the rate recorded for other school costs (12). New York defines the child eligible for special education as one whose actual achievement is 50 percent less than what would be expected from the child's intellectual level. What needed special services are available, then, for the child whose discrepancy between actual and expected achievement is 49 percent? And should that discrepancy of 49 percent be allowed to continue throughout the formative years, until ineffectiveness has become the hallmark of the adult?

Actual designation of the handicapped child is done by a committee within each district, composed of a multidisciplinary group of school staff that interprets the state regulations. The committee evaluates the status of each child and recommends a special-education program for him. Committee standards or interpretations vary from district to district, depending upon complex interacting factors of money, staff, facilities, number of dysfunctional children, biases, and politics. The committees are mandated by national Public Law 94-142, *Education for All Handicapped Children*. This mandate, with the complex variables listed, often leads to serious differences between professional practice and administrative decision. The parents seek the earliest and best help for their child and the administrator strives to coordinate or juggle law and fact. Too often the result is ''mainstreaming'' (thereby mislabeling) a child who is not suited for a regular classroom.

Meanwhile, having enacted P.L. 94-142, the Congress is not now contributing and is not expected to contribute an increasing share of state and community costs for special education. Even the present 12 percent federal contribution is vulnerable to decreases under the present administration, which has pledged to eliminate the U.S. Department of Education altogether. If support shrinks through federal withdrawal and the debilitating effects of inflation, special-education services will suffer drastically.

The implication for parents of MBD children is clear. To assure the best possible treatment for their child they must now become actively involved with both the professional and legal aspects of special education:

1. Parents should review the required IEP, that is, the diagnostic findings and treatment plan evolved for their child by the local school district committee. They may challenge the committee's report and request a hearing, for which they will need some professional and legal advice. This expertise can be obtained through membership in the organizations described and through a local group of parents (organized for the purpose if it does not already exist). *Closer Look* regularly publishes articles explaining the operation of the federal special-education laws; a 1980 article on the financial aspects of the laws is especially useful (23). On Long Island in New York State, Monica Callies, president of the Coordinating Council of 31 Special-Education P.T.A.s, is reported to have accompanied 800 parents to committee hearings (15). The New York State Education Department distributes a guide for parents of

handicapped children, *Your Child's Right to an Education,* and county offices of the Board of Cooperative Educational Services (BOCES) may be approached for answers to specific questions. A useful manual (28A) helps parents of handicapped children deal with school officials and professionals in obtaining an appropriate educational program.

2. Parents should make sure that their representatives in the entire political structure—community, county, state, national—are thoroughly acquainted with the needs of the learning-disabled child and that these representatives are regularly reminded of the need for support of current legislation with appropriation of funds.

3. Finally, parents should actively lobby for laws that will both improve current services for their MBD child and later help the adult he will become to be trained for and find suitable employment. Services to the adult limited by a history of MBD should encompass college-level and graduate programs, vocational training, and special vocational habilitation programs for the more severely dysfunctional among the MBD population. In short, parents of these numerous afflicted citizens should monitor how immediate, short-term needs of their children are being met and look ahead to needs that will acquire increased importance as this generation matures through adolescence into adulthood.

Chapter 17

Psychotherapy

MBD IS ALMOST ALWAYS emotionally disruptive and frequently damaging. And often, psychotherapy is indicated as a corollary to other treatments. By reducing the inhibiting effects of pathological defenses, psychotherapy can improve the MBD child's responses to any remediation undertaken. Without doubt, improvement in a learning disability is also psychotherapeutic in itself. Nonetheless, a child's inner emotional experience of his dysfunctions and limitations and his awareness of the interpersonal reactions they evoke may hamper or even block the effect of any remediation. The emotional burdens remain as he grows into adolescence and adulthood. The MBD victim is a feeling person as well as an overly active or a learning-disabled one. The quality of his learning, his social and vocational adjustment, his very life is inextricably involved with an emotional state affected adversely by his dysfunctions.

Not all of the many professional specialists treating MBD support this view that psychotherapy can foster the patient's personal, familial, social, educational, and vocational adjustment.

The pragmatic drug therapist—Wender (29) is an outspoken advocate of that approach—asserts that psychotherapy is of no value. The often quick and dramatic reduction of hyperactivity by the stimulant medications has led many professionals to believe that psychotherapy is not needed in these disorders. Acknowledging that the "biological risks of psychotherapy are virtually nonexistant," Winsberg and Camp (31) move from damning with that faint praise to a vigorous attack. Psychotherapy, they remind us, is time-consuming, expensive, frequently stigmatizing; they also state that it is ineffective in diminishing "behavioral deviance."

Some moderate this opposition by limiting their interdiction to the use of psychotherapy with younger children, accepting it for those older children, adolescents primarily, where maladaptive behavior has been long-established (8) or where lessened hyperactivity makes them consider an adolescent more accessible to psychotherapy. Even some who view hyperkinesis as a disorder of heterogeneous etiology, like Ney (22), regard psychotherapy as useful only in special circumstances. He would recommend it for those parents whose depression is believed to elicit hyperactivity in the child as an effort to obtain attention, or for a child who must be removed from a chaotic home while the parents also undergo psychotherapy. Gardner, who has written extensively and positively on psychotherapy in MBD (11, 12, 13, 14, 15), nonetheless ranks it at the bottom of his list of therapeutic modalities, giving first position to medication. Overall, the moderate view is that psychotherapy for the younger child is at best adjunctive, but may move to a position of central emphasis in adolescence and adulthood.

Both moderates and the more rigidly pragmatic either ignore psychodynamics or consider them negligible in MBD whatever its syndrome manifestations, as if to disclaim the interaction of organic deficits with the psychological and emotional aspects of personality development. Their focus is upon the most prominent of the symptoms: a motor dysfunction, learning disability, hyperactivity. If any recognition is given to psychological concomitants, it usually accompanies the secure belief that these will disappear if the "primary symptom" is treated. Some may consider that their neglect of the psychological is justified by the relative ineffectiveness in MBD of treatment solely on the classical psychoanalytic model: uncovering of unconscious material, resolution of the Oedipal and other conflicts, the unfolding of a transference neurosis. But in my view there is no justification for neglecting the emotional components of MBD, factors that cause damage and impede development in so many sufferers.

The Complex Interaction of Emotional Causes and Consequences

The neglect of psychotherapy in MBD is grave; it goes beyond a downgrading of the ability of psychoanalysis to help the MBD child. The opposition ignores the specific psychodynamics set in motion by dysfunctions in the developing child. These dynamics produce symptoms similar to those in another child whose disturbance has a cause purely emotional, but which has a different evolution and requires a different kind of psychotherapeutic intervention. Delaying work with the emotional interactions until adolescence often allows psychopathology to encroach upon many aspects of the personality. Defenses, denial particularly, can become so firmly fixed that the MBD adolescent or young adult is not only more difficult to treat but even likely to reject treatment altogether.

Psychotherapy's importance with children cannot be stressed too much. The MBD victim as a child is as amenable as he will ever be, and a process started when he is young promises to help him through the years ahead as he lives with his limitations and/or their effects.

Psychological effects and complications are prominent in MBD for at least two reasons. Most compelling, perhaps, are the effects that arise as direct responses to the cognitive and social dysfunctions the child experiences, and that multiply and rigidify to oppress him as he grows older. There are children whose emotional difficulties appear to originate specifically in identifiable central-nervous-system disorders. And then there are children in whom emotional conflicts and disturbance appear to exacerbate a most minimal brain dysfunction, one otherwise insignificant and likely to escape detection because its impact on cognitive skills would be so small. This section discusses both the effects of the dysfunctions on the emotions and the effects of the emotions on the appearance of MBD symptoms.

Emotional Consequences of MBD

The child whose MBD arises from genetic, perinatal causes rooted in early infancy and childhood is coping simultaneously with the tasks of normal psychological development and the burdens of integrative dysfunctions. He is saddled with adverse effects on early ego development and on early and later individuation (19). Perception and cognition may be distorted, with consequent distortion of body image and/or the image of the external world. Sensory input may be subliminal or excessive. Object relations can readily become disordered and even pathological, with the MBD victim's early language and other behavior evoking rejection, distancing, crippling over-protection, and other disruptive reactions from parents. Superego development may be fostered by some parents of hyperactive and impulsive children, at the expense of ego functions. Sharp fear of abandonment may develop early, and may combine later with cognitive difficulties to produce a school phobia marked by panic-level anxiety or decathexsis and aversiveness that may approach the schizoid. Defenses are likely to become pathological in both nature and degree. Self-esteem is likely to be damaged in a way that limits motivation, increases isolation, and intensifies an ever-present depression. Other mood disorders are possible: hypomanic behavior in the service of denial, anger as a consequence of anxiety. MBD interacts with the normally developing emotional processes to intensify vicissitudes of intrapsychic, interpersonal, and family dynamics (20, 21).

The major sources of anxiety and of personality distortion in children with central-nervous-system dysfunction described by Silver (presented in Chapter

5) should be recalled here. First, the distorted perceptions cause frustration, confusion, learning difficulties, pressures at home and at school. The emotional reactions to repeated failure vary with the resources of the individual child, the nature of the dysfunction, and the quality of home and school support. The child may give up effort and withdraw into a state resembling autism. Or he may stagger along academically, socially, emotionally, perhaps clowning defensively at school while acting depressed, demanding, and rigid at home. At best the child will keep on trying, burdened with a pervasive sense of inadequacy, feeling his world of parents, school, and peers is harsh and demands the impossible from him.

A second source of disturbance from neurological dysfunction described by Silver is the Moro Startle Reaction, apparent in the earliest months of life, to a sudden, unexpected stimulus. The infant reacts with abduction of the limbs, then adduction, extension, and flexion. This becomes the protypical pattern of response to sudden stimuli throughout life. The normal person reacts and then restores equilibrium, but with a certain neurological dysfunction, waves of physiological reactions continue: increase of heart contractions, sweating, gastrointestinal disturbances, dilation of the pupils, muscle tension, metabolic upset. As these persist, anxiety increases; the individual is reactively flooded by uncontrollable stimuli. The original stimulus may arise either endogeneously or exogenously, from causes ranging from the reflexive and autonomic to more complex psychic elements. Maintenance of both physiological and emotional homeostasis becomes increasingly difficult. Impulse control is weakened. Superego pressures mount. Anxiety and guilt intensify, often generating phobias and/or hypochondriasis. Rigid, obsessional defenses are likely to develop in the effort to mitigate anxiety and guilt.

A third neurodysfunction contributing to anxiety and subsequent personality disruption observed by Silver is an abnormal reaction to anti-gravity play. The infant with a physiological difficulty in sustaining muscle tone and spatial orientation experiences no delight in being held upside down, swung, tossed, or balanced. "Survival anxiety" makes him cling; physical dependency leads to emotional dependency. In some, dependency needs become so great that they cannot be met realistically; the child's need for support, presence, guidance, and availability become constant. We can see in Silver's perceptive description a physical cause for some severe patterns of abandonment panic in MBD children.

A condition of "object inconsistency" has been observed in the MBD child by Schechter (25), who relates it to the physical disruption of perception. The perceptual disruption prevents the formation and mainenance of a "constant immutable internal image" of a stimulus. Auditory, visual, and haptic stimuli and kinesthetic perception of their bodies in space are registered by such children in an inconsistent manner that creates distortion. These distortions are then projected into the external world upon people, things, and situations. The child so afflicted does not relate to parents and other people in a usual way, because his inner images of these others are variable, inconsistent. A significant result is the development of superego lacunae, that permit impulsivity, cruelty, disobedience, and anti-social behaviors. These very behaviors in turn cause people to treat the MBD child inconsistently, adding to the disruption of the child's control of affect, thoughts, and impulses. His inner language doesn't make sense, doesn't "add up."

More specifically, Schechter finds that early difficulties in processing auditory information result in a deficiency in the "internal language" necessary for self-control and for the maturational development from primary-process to secondary-process thinking, as well as for the development of adequate reality perception and testing. Similarly, he sees difficulties in encoding visual stimuli as resulting not only in reading problems and geographic and proprioceptive dysfunctions but also in an inadequate self-image. The child with this limitation develops little sense of place in space or how clothes should look or fit; he continues to make errors in personal, social, and academic matters. Then, degraded by others, he degrades himself in ceaseless negative engramming. He becomes—in his own view—bad, the klutz, the goof-off, the oddball. These dynamics, Schechter finds, are frequently a prelude to suicide.

Many professionals consider a negative self-image the major psychological damage of MBD. The development of low self-esteem in reaction to early perceptual deficits is traced by Palombo (24). His model corresponds with Niederland's (23) observation that when physical impairment comes after a period of health, the body area impaired may be excluded from perception and treated as if nonexistent. Palombo modifies this somewhat in applying the model to children with perceptual deficits from birth; in them the impaired area is never experienced. Never contributing to experience, the impairment results in an incomplete, distorted body image. Seldom directly perceived by the child, the deficit distorts his perception of reality and of social relations. The child early gains his sense of self from seeing himself mirrored in the responses of others, particularly his mother. A sensitive, perceptive mother who reacts protectively to compensate for the child's deficits may convince the child that he can never learn to do the things that she can do. Thus dependency is prolonged and individuation delayed. The less sensitive mother may demand reaction and response from the child, that he perform like other children. This child all the more rapidly becomes aware that something is wrong with him. He is likely to withdraw or to overcompensate narcissistically with notions of grandiosity, in both cases isolating himself.

Defects in the body aspects of self-image create a sense of physical vulnerability and susceptibility to regression when anxious, physically ill, or encountering a maturational change, such as loss of first teeth, a sharp increase in height, or sexual development. These children are poorly equipped for the ongoing need, throughout life, to adapt to changes in body image. They are first unable to develop the early idealized image of themselves with which the normal child begins his series of self-perceptions, one that in the normal child becomes tempered by reality. Overlooking successes, the dysfunctional child is aware only of failures. The end result is either a lack of ambition and self-confidence, or a regressive emphasis upon false grandiosity. Uppermost in psychotherapy is less likely to be rage at the parents, the classical oedipal conflict, with castration or homosexual anxiety, and rather rage at the perceptual deficits and their impact upon the child's self-image and self-regard.

To these considerations should be added other often conspicuous emotional reactions and defenses.

Daydreaming is the symptom most frequently observed by Schechter (25), a habitual pattern probably related to the regressive grandiosity in Palombo's model, or to the depressed withdrawal he also finds possible for the impaired child.

Anxiety levels are high. This may arise from feelings of special physical vulnerability and appear in psychosomatic complaints. Separation anxiety is also prominent; it often expresses a fear of abandonment by the parents, who are perceived as disappointed by the child's inadequacies. The anxiety sometimes takes the form of frank phobias of school, the dark, insects, among others, or the more disguised forms of stubborn school refusal, or sleep and appetite disturbances. Tics are also frequent, motor expressions of the child's tension and anxiety.

Protracted eneuresis is also reported (25). Gardner (15) views this as a sign of failure to progress in maturation, that is, a fixation or a regression. Other signs of these developmental abnormalities are clowning, clinging, avoiding age-appropriate responsibilities about dressing and home chores, or preferring to associate with younger children. A boy with minimal aggressiveness may prefer play with girls, finding them less competitive. Parental overprotectiveness promotes these tendencies to fixation or regressions, Gardner found.

Anxiety often evokes anger, and the MBD child may feel ceaselessly pressured to confront fear-arousing and frustrating situations. With poor inner controls, the child is likely to react impulsively and inappropriately, further impairing his relations with others and intensifying his feelings of humiliation. The child, already inhibited because of inadequate conflict-free energy to apply to learning, is also blocked in learning by impulsiveness (6).

Negativism also impedes growth and learning in some MBD children. The negativistic child rejects opportunities out of fear of failure, or rejects relationships out of distrust of others, expecting rejection and denigration. Negativism may appear as a rejection of the values, judgments, requests, demands, and expectations of all elders, including teachers and employers, arising from the MBD child's feeling that he has been deceived in a significant way by his parents.

Little wonder that depression is so often observed in the MBD victim. With low self-esteem, an extremely negative self-image, a persistent sense of denial of respect and love, the inward deflection of anger and depression increases, as does its overt manifestations, when the child moves into adolescence and adulthood.

Depression and anxiety without impulsivity and hyperactivity are remarked as major symptoms in adults with MBD by Mann and Greenspan (18). They believe that this shift reflects ego maturation with age, resulting in a somewhat better capacity for self-perception and internalized control. With less impulsive externalization of anger comes more inward deflection; with increased self-perception comes more realistic acceptance of the negative self-image and less resort to grandiosity.

At all ages, emotional crises are likely in the MBD person: severe depression, intensified withdrawal, acting out of aggression and antisocial behavior, episodes of increased hyperactivity, refusals to cooperate or to try. These crises may reflect internal or external pressures: a long series of failures; a transitional life-stage confrontation; a reaction from a parent, teacher, or employer that is sadistic or chaos-producing.

Adolescence, a crisis well recognized in normal development, is painfully intensified in the MBD child. The major tasks of adolescence (increased individuation and separation from parents, sexual maturation, and vocational choice) carry double burdens of anxiety and conflict for him. The usual emotional freight in adolescence, the revival of the oedipal conflict and its ultimate resolution, must be carried, along with the traces of those earlier ceaseless failures, self-doubts, humiliations, and a pervasively negative self-image (3). Many dysfunctions do not become manifest in the MBD child until the age-appropriate demands of a higher level of development are reached. Where an MBD child's social aversiveness may have been only a minor problem before, the internal and external pressures for dating and sexual exploration are so enormous, persistent, and ubiquitous in the adolescent that they cannot be glossed over.

Where the MBD child's behavior and personality have alienated his peers and made them mocking, threatening, or remote, the child moving into and through adolescence is without their support and the peer experiences that enable the normal child to separate, individuate, and move on to an adult self. The avoidance of this normal adolescent task is likely to be recognized by everyone including the adolescent as seriously pathological. In similar fashion, the MBD child whose moderate cognitive deficits have allowed him to scrape by in the intermediate grades now faces a series of challenges: the increasing level of difficulty in high-school courses and the spectre of college or employment beyond. Adolescence is a time of threatening crisis to which the MBD adolescent most often responds with intensification of the pathological defenses he has exercised throughout his life.

Denial is a major defense in MBD: there are no deficits, there is no problem, so there is no need for worry, for anxiety. Where concern is grudgingly admitted, the need for long, hard work to overcome the problem may be denied. Faith, in many instances, is now placed in tomorrow and the magic cure: new glasses, eye exercises, macromolecular diet.

A revealing account of the self-frustrating use of denial in a nine-year-old nonreader is presented by Vail (28). The girl, "proud and very stubborn," tried to bluff her way in class, turning the pages of her book while watching the pace of her neighbors, and calling out that she was finished while they were still reading. Knowing that they knew, she became fearful and distrustful. When remedial help was initiated, her fears only intensified, and was masked by further bluffs, professions of her generosity to others or of the grandeur of her family. So much energy went into her defenses that little was available for education. Vail discovered that as the professional she also to some extent participated in the child's valiant but fruitless denial efforts, or was fearful of confronting her with them.

Denial is often initiated or fostered by the parents, who themselves need to believe all is well, or fear that recognition of the problem and its diagnosis will traumatize the child. It can be fostered by teachers or pediatricians who assure parents that the problem is transient and the child will grow out of it. Many children, aware of their dysfunctions, want and welcome help, but are unable to penetrate a parent's denial with their concern. "Something is wrong with my brain. I don't know what it is. I can't put my finger on it. I can't tie my shoelaces as good as other kids." Or "my eyes don't work right." Among these sufferers, some, alarmed by the anxiety their concern evokes in their parents, are forced into the conspiracy of denial. The child reacts to parental denial or secretiveness with distrust and negativism, with feelings of being deceived, or the fear that his disability is too terrible to talk about. He may come to fear that he is psychotic, mentally retarded, or beyond help, and so pick up the denial and with it weave other defenses as well. Gardner (15) relates two especially poignant accounts of his work with MBD children. One lad obsessively used dinosaurs in his drawings and stories, animals with large bodies but very small brains. Another told of X-ray machines that did not work; in short, that no one could or would tell him what was wrong with him. Denial by parents and/or the child deprives the victim of the opportunity to work toward remediation of his disabilities and development of his intact functions.

Rationalization often emerges when the child, being forced into recognition of a problem, denies its cause and cure: "I could do it if I wanted to, but I don't want to." Wanting to try not only means long, hard work, with gratification delayed, but also threatens failure and disappointment, after all. So the child is likely to develop a passive-aggressive stance.

The MBD child may resort to displacement. Feelings generated in the school or social arenas—anger over failure or rejection, for example—may be brought home to be wreaked upon relatives less threatening to him. Or the anger may be acted out in antisocial destructiveness, or stealing. Or the child who keeps up a cheerful facade at school may sink into a slough of depression as soon as he is home.

The frequency of escape into daydreaming has been noted. With severely damaged self-esteem, the child readily regresses into overcompensating grandiosity. But not all fantasies are grandiose. The child may be searching for an explanation, an understanding of his difficulties. Or masochism may have developed around a combination of his anger and negative self-image, so that his fantasy time is spent with images of failure, of being abused and debased. With some, the masochism may merge into a mild paranoia: "I'm no good" easily becomes "You believe I'm no good and you want to hurt me."

Obsessional qualities develop in some MBD children, particularly those who recognize their problem but seek to control it rather than correct it through remediation and psychotherapy. To protect themselves against the fear of cognitive failure, these children may become so over-inclusive when they consider alternatives that they are unable to progress to a solution. Or the premium placed on control of affects and impulses may become so great, so ego alien, that classical compulsive and obsessional behaviors emerge in the effort at control.

Another major defense is aversiveness and withdrawal into social isolation. Seeking to avoid repetition of failure and shame, the child withdraws from confrontation of tasks and from association with peers. Tending to generalize his inadequacies, he avoids many tasks and situations in which he is actually equipped to do well. Extremely sensitive to criticism, the child has little tolerance for normal bantering and teasing of peers. This child is likely to move from being a passive observer to being a schizoid personality as an adult.

Psychologically, the child with brain dysfunctions, however minimal, is subject to proliferating vicissitudes in the development of competence. These damage self-esteem, impede or prevent separation, and distort individuation as an adolescent and then as an adult. Cerebral dysfunction blocks the acquisition of skills, physical, social, academic. Failures in many important life tasks result, social isolation and dependency upon family increase, and pessimism about the future intensifies. Maturational progress is reversed, halted, or at best slowed down (7, 30). A most poignant example of this corrosion of self-worth recently came to my attention. A childless couple, about 35 years old, asked for artificial insemination in order to have a child, after the husband had been declared sterile by one rather simple test. He refused the further investigation suggested and insisted on donor semination, explaining, "I can't read and I can't write. I don't want to pass that onto a child."

Emotional Causes of MBD-Like Symptoms

Another danger in diagnosing and treating the MBD child is to ignore a basic disruption in psychosexual development that can make for cognitive disability, social pathology, and perceptual or motor disorders. Early disturbance of object relations, for example, may create a schizoid aversiveness in the child with very mild neurological dysfunction who could learn successfully if motivated to try. Too much or too little, too punitive or too accepting a superego can curb a desired degree of assertiveness or promote an antisocial degree of acting out.

Early emotional trauma may interrupt or impede the progression from primary-process thinking to the secondary-process thinking necessary for abstraction, concept formation, and propositional thinking, leaving a child of high initial endowment able to understand and express only in concrete terms and details.

Identification with parents may be positive or negative, depending upon a host of factors in them and in the child. A bright child may avoid academic success for fear of humiliating uneducated parents, or of evoking their anger and retaliation. Or a bright, responsive child may diminish his own intellectual responsivity and expression because the parents are anti-intellectual. Another highly endowed child with minimal dysfunction may eschew an all-out effort to learn because he fears he cannot achieve the level of an over-idealized and high-achieving parent, or because he associates learning achievement with parents he has come for some reason to despise.

Anna Freud (9) has analyzed the influence of anxiety upon the ego of the child, tracing how fear of ego-alien impulses such as competitiveness, anger, or inadequacy in expressing these impulses before a superior adult can lead to an ego restriction in which the child avoids assertion, competition, or the acquisition or manifestation of skill. Ego-alien aggressive impulses in a child can develop into pathological degrees of defensive reaction formation, to appear as excessive passivity, altruism, displacement, or obsessive-compulsiveness. Any of these may find expression in a learning inhibition.

Disorders of motility—hypokinesis or hyperkinesis—can be purely emotional. The hypokinetic child may be professing helpless, impotent dependency and a terror of self-assertion. The hyperkinetic child, the reader will recall, may be clamoring desperately for the attention and caring of a detached or depressed mother.

Fear of separation or of abandonment promotes any proneness to MBD symptomatology rooted in other causes. Courage and the wish to individuate are essential components of learning. To acquire a skill is to be able to do a task alone, a major step to independence. The child deeply fearful of separation may cling to dependency through failure to learn or through a need for extra help in learning. Such a child may remain fixed at a regressed level in both psychological and cognitive development.

Finally, we must comprehend the psychosexual symbolism an emotionally disturbed child may project upon cognitive functions, avoiding the development of skill lest it express a forbidden sexual excitement in him. Reading is readily associated with the gratification of curiosity, which in the susceptible child may arouse overly excited states related to voyeurism. These states are sometimes expressed in enuresis, sometimes in a denial of the wish to know, hence to read. In another child, arithmetic processes may be found to be associated with genital processes, addition and multiplication with reproduction or with dangers, subtraction and division with castration and bodily harm. These psychodynamic reactions are among those observable in neurotic children who show many of the symptoms associated with MBD. They are observed also in children with clear MBD, in a complex interaction that makes sorting out of cause and consequence often difficult, sometimes impossible. This probable interaction increases the likelihood that psychotherapy is an intervention of necessity.

Elements of Psychotherapy in MBD

No effort is made here to present the process and progress of psychotherapy in MBD. These vary so widely among individuals, from child to adolescent to adult, from syndrome to syndrome, from therapist to therapist, that a useful description is virtually impossible. More possible is a survey of some major elements in the psychotherapy of the MBD patient, and some issues in current discussion.

Transference

The immediate and principal task in psychotherapy with an MBD patient is the establishment of a positive transference, something even more pressing for him than for other patients. Always there is therapeutic benefit for the child who feels understood by at least one adult, but for the MBD child it is often his major yearning. Most other important adults in his world find the MBD child irascible and incomprehensible. Such a kernel of understanding may prevent an abysmal pessimism and keep alive the thread of hope for change, for realistic improvement.

With positive transference the therapist can evolve a "working alliance" or a "therapeutic alliance" (27) with the MBD patient of any age that is essential to breaking through denial to motivate him to confront his situation and the ardors of remediation. In agreeing to a therapeutic alliance with specific provisions the patient is able to counteract his isolating tendencies. He can borrow enough ego from the therapist he trusts to admit the impact of failures and rejection. The therapist offers him support and encouragement to carry on through remedial efforts, and understanding—without license, however—during periods of acting out. Experience with the "working alliance" counteracts the negativism that has developed from distrust of elders. The patient himself is enlisted in a cooperative effort to sort through the various etiological, diagnostic, and treatment possibilities for him in his long effort.

In trying to establish such an alliance the therapist must come across as an understanding person who has ways of helping not usually possible from parents, teachers, or physicians. The consistent personal availability of the therapist to help the patient at times of special need or crisis is stressed. The working alliance that succeeds requires empathy, honesty, sincerity, confidence, and advocacy of the therapist. The alliance at some rare critical moment may approach over-protectiveness in its determined advocacy, but that only in an effort to give the patient a chance, long denied him, to make another effort. Usually advocacy of the patient's cause is directed toward reversing negative attitudes in parents and teacher, or forestalling their development. The therapist may have to counter an unfavorable reaction to all adults as authoritative, demanding, demeaning figures by demonstrating in a realistic way his benevolence and reasonableness.

A transference neurosis in the classical psychoanalytic sense is not allowed to develop; the ego of the MBD patient—child, adolescent, or adult—is not usually strong enough to tolerate it. Negative transference features are brought immediately to the surface and discussed. The therapist must be quick to recognize, even predict, the emergence of negative transference manifestations intended to measure his concern and good will: testing, provocative behavior, efforts to evoke manifestations of disapproval and disparagement in a counter-phobic way, attempts to establish the therapist as a mechanism of external control who replicates an unempathic, overprotective, or overly-demanding parent. With some children the positive transference may foster modeling behavior, learning through positive identification. With many it permits the therapist to employ a mirroring technique (24) that enables the patient to see and correct his tendencies, for example, to grandiosity, or to over-idealize parents and parental figures.

Maintaining positive transference does not impose upon the therapist the need to gratify the patient's wish for admiration or dependency, but rather it allows the therapist to reflect empathically the patient's need for them, to understand their derivation, and to move into positive programs of correction.

With some MBD patients the positive transference is difficult to achieve or to maintain. The factor of "object inconsistency" (25) may be so great that the child is unable to attach to anyone, parent, teacher, or therapist, in the usual way. Such a patient seems unable to see the therapist consistently as a helping person. Palombo (24) describes his feelings with an especially difficult adolescent patient as "...hanging in, trying to maintain some sense of alliance with him." Unusual perseverance is needed in such cases, and success may require remaining accessible after being rejected by the patient, should he want to return to therapy.

Countertransference must be examined carefully. These feelings in the therapist may include impatience with slow and limited progress, alienation from aggressive antisocial acting out, irritation with the repetition often necessary. A therapist who greatly values verbal skills may tend to devalue the MBD patient with difficulties in verbal expression or comprehension. The therapist must be alert to the possible presence of these feelings in himself and others, work them through in himself, and keep them from influencing his attitude to his patient.

Parameters and Flexibility

The therapist must guard also against the tendency to view the dynamics of the behavior of the MBD patient only in the ways that he has seen operative in nonorganic patients. For example, traditional psychoanalysis often sees failure in a patient as a fear of success or a wish to fail. Obviously, these may exist in an MBD patient, but he also has real limitations, and thus also may need a very reasonable setting of attainable limits to help him feel an improvement, a step-by-step movement. The therapist's wish, like that of the parent, to see the child succeed may lead him to expect more than the child can do. Palombo (24) thought he saw significance in a patient's consistently coming in second in foot races, but never first. On interpreting this to the lad, he realized at once that he had robbed him of pride in his achievement in being among the winners, and that the therapist had repeated what the parents had often done. When such errors occur, the therapist must be quick to acknowledge them and to interpret their impact upon the patient.

The therapist's willingness and ability to depart from the usual strictures of traditional insight psychotherapy allows him to draw upon therapeutic modalities of a wide variety. As we have seen above, these include the pursuit of a positive transference and an active working, therapeutic alliance. At times with one patient, or regularly with another, the therapist may use joint family-child conferences, recommendations for individual parent or family therapy, home-management counseling with a social worker, conferences with the child's teacher. He may try to promote educational programs about MBD in the community and among the patient's peers. When in an ideal circumstance the therapist undertakes the role of case manager of a team of professionals, the recommendation and even administration of these interventions are more likely to become his responsibility than when he serves only as psychotherapist. But even as psychotherapist he often will find it necessary to advise these interventions. The therapist must be receptive to the possibility that a different kind of intervention, or an intervention in the family structure other than with the child alone, is indicated for the patient's benefit and progress.

The therapist must also monitor the patient's response to medication if it is being administered elsewhere through the treatment team, and work cooperatively with the administering physician, reporting changes and questioning doses or continuation when indicated.

An established positive transference allows the therapist to become a teacher at times without risking rejection of the instruction. The therapist puts himself in the patient's place, with a sharing of the ego: "If I were in your place, I'd feel like this and I would do this and that to make a change." The didactic approach is helpful with the hyperactive, compulsive patient where a "stop and think" brake on certain acts to prevent predictably costly consequences should be acquired by the patient. It is helpful also in helping the patient behave in a desired way when he has believed the behavior was not available to him, or because it has never occurred to him that the solution to a painful problem might be found in a change in his own behavior. The therapist takes care not to overpower the patient with suggestions too far beyond his competency. Steps toward progress are graduated. Achievement is reinforced by congratulation for effort and success. Failure is shared by empathy, and followed by encouragement for another try.

Interpretation

Interpretation is moderated by two important considerations:

1. Many MBD patients suffer a complicated set of dynamics that often combines anger, anxiety, masochism, negativism, acting out, and avoidance. When these are developed in the context of impulsivity and emotional lability, the danger that direct interpretation will further weaken impulse control must be evaluated.

2. Some MBD patients have deficits in spoken language; essentially they are dysphasic, with difficulties in comprehending as well as expressing symbolic or abstract concepts. They may find interpretations hard to understand.

For the first consideration, the successful therapist adopts that all-important titrating or step-by-step, focusing approach to interpretations. He puts out partial interpretations and tests the patient's reactions before proceeding further, or waits for the patient to make the leap himself. At any point in this process where some insight appears, he may shift the emphasis to a didactic one in which the patient is helped to become aware of and responsive to the many clues that guide social exchange. The insight alone should not be pursued to its ultimate. Insight, at whatever depth, must for the MBD patient be linked with practical, achievable steps for some correction or control. Otherwise an insight may overwhelm the patient, perhaps reinforcing what he has been told repeatedly, and may further convince him of his unworthiness.

When the patient is dysphasic, a condition usually determinable early in the diagnostic interviewing and testing, simple, concrete terms should be used and repeated if necessary. Verbal illustrations that evoke visual images or very simple auditory ones are helpful, the crowing cock, for example, or the player who hits a home run and basks in the roar of the crowd. Visual thematic material may be used as well: a comic-strip character who tells a story or makes a point without using words, for example. Sessions may be tape-recorded and important ones replayed by the patient alone or with the psychotherapist. Clear understanding by the MBD patient must be pursued carefully and tested regularly; it cannot be assumed.

Engaging Denial

Acceptance by the patient of his dysfunction and of what it means for him is a prerequisite. This full understanding is avoided only in those rare instances where the diagnosis indicates that the patient's ego cannot tolerate the confrontation, and that only supportive counseling is possible.

Enabling the patient to confront and understand his deficits is likely to require that much denial be penetrated. The child must learn that he has a learning *disability,* not necessarily an *inability.* He should be helped to understand the likely causes of his disability. The burdensome task of remediation is spelled out, along with its importance for him, and the way he can take it step by step. His social problems are identified and related to his disability. Concrete, simple illustrations and examples are used, with care that the child's capacity for comprehension and logical connection is not overloaded. In effect, all the cautions necessary with the interpretation are practiced here.

Dissolution of denial ultimately improves the patient's reality perception and reality testing. In the beginning, the patient's willingness and ability—that is, his ego strength—to tolerate this process without undue intensification of anxiety and possible regression, both of which will increase resistance, are probed carefully. This exploration may be done with a graduated series of interpretations allowing the therapist to move forward toward and back away from a threatening confrontation.

Where the parents foster the denial, work with them is a necessary prelude or accompaniment to the therapy, and may require some sessions with the parents alone, and then together with the child. Or the parents may require individual treatment by other therapists. Some parents experience such elevation in anxiety and so strongly resist frank discussion that careful and sometimes extensive work with them is necessary to prevent their sabotage of the psychotherapy of their child.

Work toward improved reality perception and reality testing primarily focuses upon the many steps the patient can take to circumvent or remedy his dysfunctions and upon the assets he has available to help him in the effort. Chess (4) recommends giving the child a clear concept of his handicap, in age-specific terms. The child is helped to identify those situations in which he competes on an equal basis with peers and those in which he can participate only partially. For some children some activities are best avoided all together. Gaddes (10) recommends that the diagnosis itemize the patient's strong points and present his weak ones objectively. Many of the dysfunctions of MBD may be to a degree "defended" emotionally to their victim by analogy to tone deafness, with which a person cannot become a musician but could possibly be a mathematician, or to color blindness, with which a person can never become an airplane pilot, but can drive a car. Gaddes believes that the terms "organic" and "brain dysfunction" should be avoided in these confrontations for fear of misinterpretation. This danger, however, is minimized to the extent that a good therapeutic alliance is established. Moreover, the patient of all but the earliest years may well be entertaining notions and fears that "something is wrong with my brain," so that avoiding may allow distortion to take hold, anxiety to increase, and feelings of deception to intrude, possibly damaging the positive transference beyond repair. Therapists generally have found that in most situations it is better for the patient's ego functioning to use the facts and explain their relation to age-specific capabilities in terms understandable to the patient. To face the known with anxiety is more constructive than to continue to struggle with the unknown with both anxiety and distortion.

Vail (28) has published an important personal finding: she had to confront her own use of denial before she could help her dyslexic, resistant pupil accept remediation, instead of pretending that she could read.

Improvements in perception and testing of reality make the patient more accessible and responsive to the further help available. They remove the dysfunction itself as a rationalization for not trying, and open the door to therapeutic work with other pathological symptoms. The aversive, withdrawn patient can be helped to see his retreat as an effort to escape repetition of the humiliation of failure, and how in extending this expectation he also avoids those many situations where he could be successful and enhance his self-esteem.

Tolerance for anxiety can also be increased again through step-by-step procedures, and by the explanation of "vestibule" anxiety as a feeling always present for a person on the threshold of a new situation that eases when he enters into and engages the new experience.

Most important to therapy is the fact that improved reality perception and testing allows the use of didactic interventions as the patient becomes willing to make efforts to improve. The therapist can promote more impulse control by teaching a "stop-think-wait" guideline. This instruction by the therapist can be most effective when a similar program is used simultaneously in remedial instruction, where the benefits of the "pause on the threshold" can be made immediately evident by the teacher. A child can be helped, by making this pause a habit, to recognize the difference between his "feelings" and "actions" and ultimately to control the actions. In similar fashion, the parents can be acquainted with stimulus avoidance and tolerance, and sometimes trained in its application.

As the patient's ego strengthens through the combination of remediation and improved reality testing, more attention to the effects of affect-experience becomes possible, within the framework of the therapeutic alliance. Ventilation and catharsis can then be encouraged with lessened danger of acting out. Self-assertiveness can be fostered as self-esteem improves. Fantasies can be explored at greater depth to expose feelings such as the common ones among MBD patients, bizarre uniqueness and insurmountable inadequacy.

The gains derived from realistic confrontation with one's dysfunction may be summed up by a comparison with the person who suddenly, after a healthy life, becomes handicapped by illness or injury. Most people, for example, fantasy what being blind is like and see themselves as utterly helpless, with recourse only to suicide. But most of those who become blind recover from the trauma, the despair of impotence, and begin to learn the new skills necessary to cope, to reconstruct their lives, to find satisfactions and rewards. Being blind, of course, does not preclude the operation of denial, but the ability of the blind person to learn explains why parents and therapist must ask the MBD person to look frankly at his dysfunctions. In his fantasy these are equated with severe physical and mental disabilities, with grotesqueness and disfigurement. And this distortion is exactly what must be exposed to the light of reality to release him to use what he has.

Crises

Naturally, psychotherapy gains are seldom achieved in smooth linear fashion. Crises are to be expected as the patient is asked to give up his essentially phobic defenses. And often, before reality testing can begin to improve, the MBD patient is impelled to encounter a depression he has been warding off for years. He often makes use of the therapeutic alliance and its support to grieve for himself, to live out affectively the despair he has felt, to expose his wounded self-esteem, to ventilate the anger with which he has flagellated himself, or to allow to erupt those paroxysms of anxiety he has struggled to contain. The crisis, so used by both parties to the therapeutic alliance, becomes a milestone in progress.

Working Through

Working through in MBD is a long process, and a termination of psychotherapy is less likely than a discontinuance (24). Very common is a series of interruptions, brought about by summer vacations and camp stays, by the preferability of a real-life experience—for example, employment—over psychotherapy at a certain stage, or the completion of high school, with the happy result that the MBD patient can go away to college and return for brief therapeutic contacts on holidays.

Two Models of Child Therapy

Gardner has specialized in the psychotherapy of children; his somewhat redundant publications (11, 12, 13, 14, 15) emphasize the techniques he has developed or adapted for exposing and then combatting fantasy in these children, in order to develop inner controls. He seeks to build superego rather than to encourage insight, and provides the child with a model that with directive guidance he expects the child will follow.

His sessions with children are structured, not open-ended; he reasons that the MBD child needs organization, that open-endedness evokes anxiety and counteracts the development of controls. As much as possible he has a parent (usually the mother, presumably) sit in on sessions, maintaining that confidentiality is irrelevant to the preadolescent, a presumption that many therapists would challenge. His rationale is that the arrangement avoids the we-they schism, and guides the parent in handling the child.

He tape-records and videotapes sessions to provide the reinforcement through which many MBD children best learn. This concept of intersensory stimulation is also used in the pictures, toys, and games Gardner has developed and adapted. These are designed to contribute to the structure of the therapeutic sessions, to evoke associations, and thus to allow the therapist to communicate meaningfully with the child, perhaps in order to develop some insight, but chiefly to structure and guide. The artifacts are not therapies in themselves, Gardner comments, but facilitators of communication between patient and therapist. They would appear to be widely useful with all child patients, especially useful with the withholding, resistant patient, and applicable as well with many adolescents (11).

In his "Mutual Storytelling Technique," Gardner (13) tries to communicate at the child's level. The method requires knowledge of psychodynamics, dream analysis, and projective techniques, coupled with skill in speaking the child's language. A story is evoked from the child and its dynamic content is assessed for pathology. The therapist, using the characters in the child's story, tells his own version of the story but with a "healthier" resolution. Sometimes he engages the child in a dramatic re-enactment of the story for heightened effect. Gardner has no reticence about letting the child know exactly how he reacts to the child's behavior in mirroring it in games and play. On hearing that a child patient has pulled the leg off a frog, Gardner rolled on the floor screaming with simulated pain, and demonstrating that such acts hurt and can kill. On double-jumping his patient in a game of checkers, he may scream as he knows the child feels like doing, and has done before. Or when the child talks of being teased by peers Gardner may pretend to cry.

Many therapists will feel that this tactic may leave the child with feelings of shame, fears of being bizarre, and more deeply humiliated than before. They would not necessarily eschew the method altogether but would mitigate it with an ego-sharing technique, in which they tell the child they, too, have had feelings like his, and point out better ways of dealing with such situations.

Emphasizing the teaching of better ways to react is precisely how Gardner attempts to make progress from these emotional confrontations, to demonstrate that there is a different way to deal with frustrations and anger; the techniques are a way for the child to learn about himself and how to make himself more comfortable as well as more acceptable to others. The confrontations seek to promote models of behavior to acquaint the child with better ways to cope. Gardner's pragmatic approach in general emphasizes a "work ethic." He also tries with those devices to help the child express his feelings before tension mounts and touches off his acting out, and at the same time to learn ways to express feelings without arousing antagonism in others.

Furthermore, Gardner functions within the context of the quality of the relationship he is able to establish with a given child, the therapeutic alliance that makes any psychotherapy possible. His manner is calculated to improve self-esteem, not to attack it; he fosters self-assertion by talking openly of commonality in feelings, thoughts, and impulses; he discourages parents from trying to mask the child's dysfunctions by doing tasks for the child; he encourages the child steadily to use his capabilities and to work hard on his deficits. His method demands much participation from the therapist.

Schechter (25) tends to work more strictly within the insight-interpretation model of psychotherapy. In one-to-one psychotherapy with an MBD child or adolescent, he explicates the unconscious processes that lead to anxiety, interprets impulsivity as a search for punishment and hence for control from the outside. He teaches ways to build better internal control by adopting a "stop-look-listen" technique before acting. Deficits are logically and clearly explained. Families are drawn into the process where their conflicts contribute to or aggravate psychopathology in the child.

Different as they are, both approaches combine some of the didactic methods of special education with some of the principles of traditional insight therapy to treat the MBD child.

Therapy with the Adolescent and Adult

For the adolescent or adult, the clinical picture for psychotherapy is considerably different. Hyperactivity is rare, but impulsivity is frequently pronounced, and depression is more likely to be frank. Need for concrete evidence of acceptance and affection often leads to sexual adventures, in which the patient is likely to be exploited and rejected. The dependence-independence conflict has often not been resolved, parents are weary and perplexed, the patient is demanding, yet easily infuriated and hurt if parents "pry" or "overprotect." Jealousy of siblings who have been successful in education, work, and marriage is prominent.

But although the clinical picture has changed, the successful psychotherapeutic approaches to adults known to have MBD are similar in some major respects to those practiced with children. They, too, benefit from stable understanding; sometimes they still require careful instruction in the consequences of behavior and control of impulse. Practical recommendations address the problems of approaching maturity. Often with girls, it is advisable to insist upon contraceptive instruction and its practice at once, even before initiating impulse-control therapy.

An adult with MBD often benefits most from success in a paid job, since it directly bolsters sagging self-esteem. Occupations recommended should emphasize physical activity and social exchange; the degree of specific verbal or spatial skill required should match the individual diagnosis. Vocational counseling and placement services, and vocational training programs developed by rehabilitation specialists, are uniquely equipped to make these careful referrals.

Many MBD patients benefit from encouragement to establish their own living quarters, away from parents and siblings, but one must be sure that the patient is mature enough to tolerate the separation. One cannot pursue indiscriminately the usual psychotherapeutic goal of fostering individuation through separate living, since the adult patient with MBD may appear more mature than is the fact.

Group Therapy

Group therapy with other adolescent and young adult MBD patients is often fruitful, especially if minimal brain dysfunction is accepted by the individual patient as a likely determinant of some of his difficulties. In such groups, goal-directed discussion fruitfully centers around exploration of the following subjects: their differences from other people because of the minimal brain dysfunction itself; differences which may arise because their emotional experiences have been and continue to be different from those of most people; the possibility that some aspects of an MBD victim's characteristically intense emotional response may be of specific value to him; and that they are not helpless to modify or restrain their emotional expressions, whatever may be the cause of their behavior. Gordon (16) advocates that group therapy focus on practical problems of living rather than on feelings. One might add, however, that feelings *are* problems of living and in many instances there are practical ways to deal with them.

Group therapy is strongly recommended by Zbuska (32) for the exceedingly hyperactive hospitalized child and for the hyperactive child in school or outpatient clinic, in either an all-MBD or a heterogeneous group. Where impulsivity prevents the child from sitting still for more than a few minutes, several adults rather than one leader may join the group to promote more calm and control. The adults, interspersed between the children, can interrupt trouble-causing behavior before it spreads. Sessions are kept short, to about 30 minutes, but are held frequently, perhaps three times weekly. Ground rules concerning sitting, asking for permission to get up or to leave, speaking one at a time, and against any hitting are enunciated and quickly and consistently enforced. Games are the therapeutic modality; they are designed to enable these exceedingly impulsive children to begin to interact with one other person first, and then to accommodate to a small-group activity. When the games have accomplished this goal, talking may be gradually introduced in their place, so that anxiety-evoking situations, such as a staff change, can be discussed instead of reacted to impulsively.

Procedures are similar for Zbuska's homogeneous outpatient group, where the child is protected from peer banter and ridicule. Because frequent sessions are more difficult for outpatients, a meeting held once a week is lengthened somewhat. In the heterogenous outpatient group, the MBD child is confronted with the dissimilarity of his problems from those of other children. But he also learns an important similarity: the fact that other children have other problems. Careful preparatory work with his therapist in individual sessions is necessary, because the MBD child will have to tell the group why he is there and spell out what his problems are. "Editorial" intercession by the therapist may be needed at first to explain hyperactivity and its effects to the group. Less structuring by the therapist is needed as the child's experience with the group increases. Participation with others is evoked in a dramatic way by "position stands," with the patient enacting a cotherapist role, or a position favoring another child's parents, friends, teachers, or siblings.

Involving Parents or Family

As we have seen, participation from parents and/or family is frequently necessary in the psychotherapy of the MBD patient to promote the growth of the patient, whether child, adolescent, or adult. The hunger of the MBD child for understanding often demands that his parents and siblings be drawn into the process. The immediate purpose may be to increase the family's tolerance for the child's behavior. Or the essential may be to counsel the parents about the realities of their child's condition, his assets and limitations in age-specific terms, what they may and may not expect from him, and what further development may bring. Or the parents may need instruction in home and educational management, such as the administration of firm, short, non-negotiable discipline. Attention to the parents' guilt and anxiety and their reduction through realistic explanation and delineation of goals can improve the child's emotional environment at home and reduce damage to his self-esteem. Often a real contribution from a parent to the child's pathology must be reversed; denial, rejection, overprotectiveness are among the attitudes of family members that burden many MBD patients.

The Resistant Patient

When the MBD patient resists individual therapy and refuses to cooperate, his cooperation may be sought gradually by involving the parents in child-parent therapy, or involving the entire family in therapy. This proposal may mitigate the patient's sense of stigma. The family's ability to tolerate the stress of family therapy is evaluated in interviews before the recommendation is made. A colleague of the MBD patient's therapist should be enlisted for either family therapy or work with the parents, since the MBD adolescent or adult with emotional problems severe enough to need psychotherapy will require the undiluted support and the unbreachable confidentiality of his own therapist once he begins.

For the adolescent resistant to psychotherapy, placement in a special school where all the students are coping with emotional and/or learning problems is often helpful to "reach" the unwilling person and turn him toward the helping potential in psychotherapy and remediation. This acceptance is especially likely if the school provides remediation facilities without pressure to use them, but where many of the students do use them. If many students are in individual or group psychotherapy and talk about their experiences, the resistant student sooner or later learns what progress is possible for others, and perhaps for him.

Finally, bibliotherapy can be a useful approach with the resistant adolescent or adult. He can be exposed to biographical accounts of children burdened with MBD handicaps in learning who have become successful adults (5, 26), newspaper accounts of famous people who are said to have had MBD (17), or a simple direct exposition of what MBD is and what can be done about it (2). Some find the easiest first step an autonomous one: simply looking over published material.

The Goal

Psychotherapy in MBD undertakes the task of restarting or accelerating developmental progression of the sense of self that has been impaired by the disorder. It works to remove emotional blocks to individuation and maturation, and toward the acquisition of competence or its improvement—cognitive, social, vocational, sexual. No easy task, but one not to be avoided, and one best engaged as early as possible.

Psychotherapy alone cannot achieve the maximum help to an MBD patient, nor can any single intervention. Only multiple, cooperating treatment modalities can do that.

Chapter 18

Vocational Counseling and Training

MATING AND WORKING have been said to be the two most important activities of life and to require its most important decisions. Apart from this rather somber view, work presents opportunities for achieving complex gratifications: economic, social, psychological, both drives and defenses against drives. Doing work and being paid for it is part of the development of competence, a step that fosters separation and individuation. The significance of this developmental process cannot be overstressed. The relationship between work, wages, and worth, between competence, recognition and compensation for that competence, and the impact on one's self-esteem make the achievement of employability a most important stage in maturation. This importance holds for all youth, but handicaps of all kinds—including MBD—increase both the internal and external difficulties of finding one's place in the world of paid work.

Parents most often, and correctly, are caught up with the immediate current concerns of an MBD handicap, concerns determined by the age and status of the child and the effects of the particular MBD symptoms on the child, themselves, and others—perhaps quieting hyperactivity, perhaps improving reading or language skills or peer relations. As the child moves into adolescence, his future moves closer, and with it looms the question of his ability to support himself in adulthood. But the economic meaning is only one of the many meanings of work. All of work's implications should impel the parents of an MBD child to begin their concern with the vocational future earlier rather than later. After immediate concerns are dealt with, thinking about the vocational future of their child is never premature. This orientation

223

requires, of course, that whatever parental denial is present be confronted, that parents not count on the future taking care of itself, or on the reassuring but unlikely hope that "this too will pass." They will need information about the relationship of their child's capabilities and dysfunctions to the requirements of different occupations, and how regular and special education and training relate to these requirements. As the years pass, they will have to learn what vocational-training possibilities are available, locally or at some distance. The societal and legal supports for such opportunities will have to be investigated, and new developments followed.

Perhaps the only developmental task for which parents have time to think and plan before the task comes pressing upon the child is his vocational direction. This time allowance permits some degree of prevention, especially of the frustrating drift in the work world that could concretize the painful negative self-image they have helped him fight so long.

Vocational thoughts in our culture begin rather early in life, with daydreams in childhood about "What I'm going to be when I grow up." Soldier, sailor, tinker, spy, these early expressions of vocational interest and choice usually contain fantasies that seek gratification of personal drives and social pressures, excited by identification with a parent, and by the stimuli of stories, TV, movies, newspapers. As the child moves into high school, vocational concerns become more realistic. Fantasy, however, is not abandoned and indeed its reasonable gratification is a prerequisite for normal job satisfaction. The danger, greater where there is handicap—physical, cognitive, emotional—is that fantasy will outweigh the realistic, with attendant psychopathological consequences (7).

With high school, vocational questions loom larger. More immediate answers are demanded in deciding on appropriate courses, academic or commercial, technical or service. What is the MBD adolescent's direction after high school? College toward a specific occupation? College just to be in college? Specialized vocational training? On-the-job training? Just a job, any job?

Many MBD youths, too many, drift seemingly aimlessly into inappropriate-for-them jobs that, while not over-taxing their dysfunctions, require too little of their capabilities. For many the drift can be prevented by early assessment, remedial education, and vocational planning (2). Vocational counseling in the high-school years can minimize the drift into inevitable frustration for many MBD youths looking for work. Regular and special education are sometimes so concerned with getting the youth through and out of high school that he may be given little knowledge of the realities of job life. Vocational educational opportunities in high school for the learning disabled are limited, and the graduates are ill-equipped to deal with employers and supervisors who are impatient and rejecting of the slow, or the careless and forgetful, which the MBD youth may appear to be.

Vocational counseling is indispensible to most MBD youth. The process includes both testing and interviewing procedures, assesses the interests of the youth, helps him look at them realistically, and assesses dysfunctions and capabilities (called aptitudes in counseling language). Finally it helps him to make a choice, usually with some alternatives, that incorporates his interests, aptitudes, the current job market, and training needs and availability. Library collections of publications on up-to-date job demands and opportunities can be helpful in this search (1), for the youth motivated and energetic enough to extend the information on which he decides.

MBD youths vary enormously in the degree to which they are both oriented toward and equipped for jobs, careers, professions, businesses. Many make it with little or no help. Their interests, gifts, talents and capabilities are so prominent and applicable, their dysfunctions so slight, that they move directly into a chosen field. Many go on to college and to higher degrees. Among the gifted and high-level MBD youth are some less fortunate, those whose dysfunctions are severe and compete with their gifts, such as a talent for mathematics coexisting with a severe dyslexia (3). Their vocational direction is clear but they need much remediation, psychotherapy, and family support to travel its path. Other MBD youth need "water-treading" time. Many of their developmental processes are slower than the norm, but they catch up in the work world as they have demonstrated before in their development.

Some youths need moderate degrees of support through specially designed training procedures, now provided by some colleges—such as Curry, Plano, and Goddard—and by post-high-school vocational training facilities. These programs have recently been increasing in number at both levels. [1]

But many need the more extended, step-by-step services in which special-education techniques are applied to vocational training, an application increasingly available through so-called habilitation services. Derived from long-established rehabilitation procedures, these help the first-time job seeker. Like numerous individuals who are returning to the work world after a permanently limiting illness or physical disability, the severely dysfunctional MBD person usually needs much help to become employable, to learn a valuable skill, to sustain the hours of a work schedule, to maintain concentration, to practice responsibility, to establish cooperative relationships with peers and supervisors, to seek work when trained, to handle himself appropriately in the job-application procedure, to acquire the techniques and habits of daily survival that most of us take for granted. Some of these tasks are structured for the learning-disabled young male in a manual that instructs in shopping, grooming, budgeting, laundering, care of clothes, and the organization of bureau drawers and closets. [2]

Services provided to the MBD adolescent and adult by the Altro Health and

---

[1] A useful recent publication details the offerings to learning-disabled students by 155 colleges, universities, technical schools, and other post-secondary institutions in the United States and Canada: *A Guide to Post-Secondary Educational Opportunities for the Learning Disabled.* The guide may be purchased from Time Out to Enjoy, Inc., 113 Garfield Street, Oak Park, Illinois 60304. $12.00 (includes postage).

[2] Bebe Antell, *Clothing and Grooming Manual for Special Young Men.* The manual may be purchased from Perceptions, P.O. Box 142, Milburn, New Jersey 07041, $2.45 (includes postage). A similar manual for young women is being prepared.

Rehabilitation Services in New York City illustrate the adaptation of rehabilitation procedures to help those in need of habilitation, that is, those whose need is not a return to a former level of employment ability but who must acquire these skills for the first time (6).

Altro provides an umbrella of diagnostic, therapeutic, vocational, and follow-up services. Social workers, psychiatrists, psychologists, vocational counselors, remedial specialists, physicians, and nurses serve diagnostic functions. Psychotherapeutic casework is provided by psychiatric social workers, in cooperation with personnel of referring social agencies, with consultation from medical, vocational, psychiatric, and psychological specialists.

Job skills are acquired and work experiences provided in real work settings, producing real products sold on the real market for real wages. Clients are assigned to work training at various levels of complexity depending upon their skills, aptitudes, dysfunctions, and physical and emotional status. The training opportunities range from the simple to the complex, from easy assembly tasks to computer programming. Workshops manufacture garments, machined pieces, printed products. Another shop produces clerical and office services, again ranging in level of complexity.

Preparatory programs are available for clients not yet ready for the demands and stimuli of a regular work setting. Here they can function at an individually comfortable pace, developing cognitive skills to a level where they can be applied to more complex tasks. Clients may move from one setting to another, from the preparatory programs to a regular work program, from a relatively simple training program to a more complex one. Program selection and movement are determined by diagnostic considerations. The goals are multiple: to help the client to achieve employable skills and habits, to tolerate and sustain demands and hours, to function socially in the work setting.

A client is in regular contact with his psychiatric social worker whose office is nearby in the workshop building. The social worker deals immediately with eruptive problems, anxieties, defensive withdrawals, and other crises that might seriously disrupt or even end the training effort. The casework service offered concurrently with paid work training engages both the problems the client brings to work and those that the work and its setting generate. Practical matters of living, matters in which the MBD youth often has little skill, are also dealt with in the casework service. Follow-up services reinforce the gains made in the workshop, to help the client find and sustain outside employment, to establish living quarters, to develop social contacts, maintain family ties, and to develop higher-level skills through further training and education.

The victim of MBD is in a special situation among the handicapped under existing law. Federal and state laws were promulgated in 1920 to promote vocational training for the physically and emotionally disabled. The national Rehabilitation Services Administration and State Offices of Vocational Rehabilitation (OVR) operate under Public Law 95-602 and the 1978 Amendments to the Rehabilitation Act to assure provision of diagnostic and vocational training for the disabled. The programs are funded by both federal (80 percent) and state (20 percent) contributions. But neither the original law nor its amendment specifically includes learning disabilities. The fate of the individual MBD victim in seeking vocational training under this legislation depends upon the regulations and definitions promulgated by the separate states and especially upon the concept and philosophy of disability entertained by state administrators. According to the 1978 Amendments, learning disabilities "in and of" themselves do not necessarily establish eligibility for vocational rehabilitation services (5).

Keeping current with the status of vocational programs is part of the responsibility of all professionals working with an MBD child as he develops. In actual operation, many rehabilitation workers in state agencies are not familiar with learning disabilities and do not understand that the diagnosis of learning disability may be considered qualifying under the regulations of a particular state. Moreover, as regulations and definitions vary from state to state, so do the extent and nature of services.

The issue of support for vocational training of the MBD victim is confused and confusing. *Closer Look* (5) suggests steps that individuals and organizations can take to help the MBD child obtain what he needs. It cannot be stated too often that getting help for one's own child is often best achieved by organizing to help other children with similar needs. Parents of MBD children and young MBD adults must recognize the need for political action bearing upon state legislatures, the Congress, and the Rehabilitation Services Administration. The latter office in 1981 was part of the new federal Department of Education, a department in 1982 slated for severe curtailment, possibly even extinction (4). The whole national effort, so full of promise, is endangered.

The MBD adult applying for a federal government job qualifies for special consideration of his specific dysfunctions in the administration of selection tests. These considerations are negotiated with the Personnel Research and Development Center of the U.S. Office of Personnel Management, Examinations Services Branch, Washington, D.C. Procedures are detailed in the *Guide for Administering Examinations to Handicapped Individuals for Employment Purposes,* by Sandra Heaton *et al.* Among the special conditions that may be provided individually are oral administrations of tests for the dyslexic applicant, extra time for special administration, checking multiple-choice answer sheets filled in by applicants with visual problems, extra care in giving oral instructions to applicants with hearing problems. Special arrangements are also provided for applicants with motor dysfunctions or dysgraphia.

Parents especially must look ahead to the future, to when their child will have grown to adulthood and is entering the job market. Their child will most benefit as an adult if the parents strive now for those services the child will need later. Increasingly, we are recognizing that much of MBD simply does not go away with the passage of time. There are all too many adults unable to function as adults because they are ill-equipped vocationally, just as they were once ill-equipped in those cognitive and social skills the parents worried about so much when they were children.

The adult MBD population has recognized that organization is critical for them by forming the new National Network of Learning Disabled Adults.[3] Also, the expressed concerns of the Association for Children with Learning Disabilities[4] have been extended to include the interests of learning-disabled adults.

Parents cannot manage and negotiate every vicissitude for their child, but their pain and their child's pain is lessened when they know realistically what can be done and do it. There is no panacea. But early recognition, early diagnosis, early treatment, and early planning help the many among us with minimal brain dysfunction.

[3] P.O. Box 3130
Richardson, Texas 75080
[4] 4156 Library Road
Pittsburgh, Pa. 15234

References

Chapter 1

1. Benton, A. L. Some conclusions about dyslexia. In A. L. Benton and D. Pearl (eds.), *Dyslexia: An Appraisal of Current Knowledge.* New York: Oxford University Press, 1978.

2. Benton, A. L. and Pearl, D. (eds.). *Dyslexia: An Appraisal of Current Knowledge.* New York: Oxford University Press, 1978.

3. Benton, A. Developmental dyslexia. *J. Ped. Psychol.,* 1:3, 1976.

4. Benton, A. L. Developmental dyslexia: Neurological aspects. In W. J. Friedlander (ed.), *Advances in Neurology.* New York: Raven Press, 1975.

5. Birch, H. G. Brain-injured children. *Rehab. Lit.,* 25, 1964.

6. Block, W. M. Cerebral dysfunctions: Clarification, delineation, classification. *Behavioral Neurol.,* 5, 1973–74.

7. Clements, S. D. and Peters, J. E. Minimal brain dysfunction in the school age child: Diagnosis and treatment. *Arch. Gen. Psychiat.,* 6, 1962.

7A. *Diagnostic and Statistical Manual of Mental Disorders* (3rd ed.)—*DSM* III. Washington, D.C.: American Psychiatric Association.

8. Kennard, M. Value of equivocal signs in neurological diagnosis. *Neurol.,* 10, 1960.

9. Lewis, M. Transitory or pseudo organicity and borderline personality in a 7-year-old child. *J. Amer. Acad. Child Psychiat.,* 15:1, 1976.

10. *Minimal Brain Dysfunction: A New Problem Area for Social Work.* National Easter Seal Society for Crippled Children and Adults. Chicago: 1968.

11. *Minimal Brain Dysfunction in Children: Educational, Medical and Health Related Services.*

Phase Two of a Three-Phase Project. U.S. Dept. of Health, Education, and Welfare. Public Health Service Publication, No. 2015, 1969.

12. Ochroch, R. A review of the minimal brain dysfunction syndrome. In R. Ochroch (ed.), *The Diagnosis and Treatment of Minimal Brain Dysfunction in Children: A Clinical Approach.* New York: Human Sciences Press, 1980.

13. Pincus, J. H. and Tucker, G. J. *Behavioral Neurology* (2nd ed.). New York: Oxford University Press, 1978.

14. Reger, R. Learning disabilities: Futile attempts at a simplistic definition. *J. Learn. Disabilities.* 12:8, 1979.

15. *Report of the Conference on the Use of Stimulant Drugs in the Treatment of Behaviorally Disturbed Young School Children.* Washington: Dept. of Health, Education, and Welfare, 1971.

16. Rie, H. E. and Rie, E. D. (eds.). *Handbook of Minimal Brain Dysfunctions: A Critical View.* New York: Wiley, 1979.

17. Schackenberg, B. C. Minimal brain dysfunction in children. *Psychiatric Forum,* 7:1, 197.

18. Schain, R. J. Minimal brain dysfunction in children: Neurological viewpoint. *Bull. Los Angeles Neurological Societies,* 33:3, 1968.

19. Smith, B. K. *Dilemma of a Dyslexic Man.* Austin, Texas: The Hogg Foundation for Mental Health, The University of Texas, 1973.

20. Werner, H. and Strauss, A. A. Pathology of figure-background relation in the child. *J. Abnormal Soc. Psychol.,* 36, 1941.

Chapter 2

1. Abrams, J. C. and Kaslow, F. W. Learning disability and family dynamics: A mutual interaction. *J. Clin. Child Psychol.,* 5:1,1976.

2. Adams, J. Visual and tactual integration and cerebral dysfunction in children with learning disabilities. *J. Learn. Disabilities,* 11:4, 1978.

3. Alley, G. R. *et al.:* Minimal cerebral dysfunction as it relates to social class. *J. Learn. Disabilities,* 4:5, 1971.

4. Anderson, C. M. Minimal brain damage. *Mental Hygiene,* 56:2, 1972.

5. Anthony, E. J. A psychodynamic model of minimal brain dysfunction. *Annals New York Acad. Sci.,* 205, 1973.

6. Arnold, L. E. Causes of hyperactivity and implications for prevention. *School Psychol. Digest,* 5:4, 1976.

7. Badran, N. A. and Wolff, P. H. Manual asymmetrics of motor sequences in boys with reading disability. *Cortex,* 13:4, 1977.

8. Bannatyne, A. *Language, Reading and Learning Disabilities.* Springfield, Ill.: Charles C. Thomas, 1971.

9. Barlow, B. *et al.* Perinatal events as precursors of reading disability. *Reading Res. Quart.,* 11:1, 1975–76.

10. Bauer, R. and Kenny, T. An ego disturbance model of MBD. *Child Psychiat. Human Devel.,* 4:4, 1974.

11. Bax, M. The active and the over-active school child. *Devel. Med. Child Neurol.,* 14:1, 1972.

12. Benton, A. L. and Pearl, D. (eds.). *Dyslexia: An Appraisal of Current Knowledge.* New York: Oxford University Press, 1978.

13. Benton, A. L. Some conclusions about dyslexia. In A. L. Benton and D. Pearl (eds.), *Dyslexia: An Appraisal of Current Knowledge.* New York: Oxford University Press, 1978.

14. Benton, A. Developmental dyslexia. *J. Ped. Psychol.,* 1:3, 1976.

15. Benton, A. L. Developmental dyslexia: Neurological aspects. In W. J. Friedlander (ed.), *Advances in Neurology,* vol. 7. New York: Raven Press, 1975.

16. Benton, A. L. Minimal brain dysfunction from a neuropsychological point of view. *Annals New York Acad. Sci,* 205, 1973.

17. Birch, H. G. and Belmont, L. Auditory-visual integration in normal and retarded readers. *Amer. J. Orthopsychiat.,* 34, 1964.

18. Birch, H. G. Brain-injured children. *Rehab. Lit.,* 25, 1964.

19. Block, W. M. Cerebral dysfunctions: Clarification, delineation, classification. *Behavioral Neurol.,* 5, 1973–74.

20. Bogen, J. E. Some educational aspects of hemispheric speculations. *UCLA Educator,* 17, 1975.

21. Brody, J. E. Raised level of lead is linked to hyperactivity. *New York Times,* November 9, 1972.

22. Buckley, R. Hyperkinetic aggravation of learning disturbance. *Acad. Ther.,* 13:2, 1977.

23. Buckley, R. E. A neurophysiologic proposal for the amphetamine response in hyperkinetic children. *Psychosomatics,* 13:2, 1972.

24. Cantwell, D. P. Genetic factors in the hyperkinetic syndrome. *J. Amer. Acad. Child Psychiat.,* 15:2, 1976.

25. Cantwell, D. P. Genetics of hyperactivity. *J. Child Psychol. Psychiat. Applied Disciplines,* 16:3, 1975.

26. Chaiklin, H.: The treadmill of lead. *Amer. J. Orthopsychiat.,* 49:4, 1979.

27. Checklist for teachers: CANHCgram. 8:11, 1974.

28. Collete-Harris, M. and Minke, K. A. A behavioral experimental analysis of dyslexia. *Behav. Res. Therapy,* 16:4, 1978.

29. Colletti, L. F. Relationship between pregnancy and birth complications and the later development of learning disabilities. *J. Learn. Disabilities,* 12:10, 1979.

30. Conners, C. K. *Food Additives and Hyperactive Children.* New York: Plenum, 1980.

31. Conners, C. K. *et al.* Food additives and hyperkinesis: A controlled double-blind experiment. *Pediatrics,* 58:2, 1976.

32. Cott, A. Treatment of learning disabilities. *J. Orthomolecular Psychiat.,* 3:4, 1974.

33. Dargassies, S. S-A. Neurodevelopmental symptoms during the first year of life. *Devel. Med. Child Neurol.,* 14, 1977.

34. Davidson, E. M. and Prior, M. R. Laterality and selective attention in hyperactive children. *J. Abnorm. Child Psychol.,* 6:4, 1978.

35. Defries, J. C. *et al.* Familial nature of reading disability. *Brit. J. Psychiat.,* 132, 1978.

36. Doehring, D. G. The tangled web of behavioral research on developmental dyslexia. In A. L. Benton and D. Pearl (eds.), *Dyslexia: An Appraisal of Current Knowledge.* New York: Oxford University Press, 1978.

37. Dubey, D. R. Organic factors in hyperkinesis: A critical review. *Amer. J. Orthopsychiat.,* 46:2, 1976.

38. Eskenazi, B. and Diamond, S. An analysis of visual scanning strategies in dyslexic children. *Abstract in International Neuropsychology Society Bulletin,* 1979.

39. Feingold, B. F. Hyperkinesis and learning disabilities linked to the ingestion of artificial colors and flavors. *J. Learn. Disabilities,* 9:9, 1976.

40. Frank, J. and Levinson, H. Seasickness mechanism and medications in dysmetric dyslexia and dyspraxia. *Acad. Ther.,* 12:2, 1976–77.

41. Frank, J. and Levinson, H. Dysmetric dyslexia and dyspraxia: Hypothesis and study. *J. Amer. Acad. Child Psychiat.,* 12:4, 1973.

42. Frank, L. F.D.A. in shift, tests pediatrician's diet for hyperactive children. *New York Times,* February 9, 1975.

43. Gaddes, W. H. Neurological implications for learning. In W. Cruickshank and D. Hallahan (eds.), *Perceptual and Learning Disorders in Children,* vol. 1. Syracuse, N.Y.: Syracuse University Press, 1975.

44. Galaburda, A. M. and Kemper, T. L.: Cytoarchitectonic abnormalities in developmental dyslexia: A case study. *Annals Neurol.,* 6:2, 1979.

45. Gazzaniga, M. S. Educational policy and brain science. In L. Oettinger, Jr. and L. V. Majorski (eds.), *The Psychologist, the School, and the Child with MBD/LD.* New York: Grune and Stratton, 1978.

46. Gazzaniga, M. S. Brain theory and minimal brain dysfunctions. *Annals New York Acad. Sci.,* 205, 1973.

47. Gearhart, B. R. *Learning Disabilities: Educational Strategies.* St. Louis: C. V. Mosby, 1973.

48. Goldberg, H. K. and Schiffman, G. B. *Dyslexia: Problems of Reading Disabilities.* New York: Grune and Stratton, 1972.

49. Gross, K. and Rothenberg, S. An examination of methods used to test the visual perceptual deficit hypothesis of dyslexia. *J. Learn. Disabilities.,* 12:10, 1979.

50. Gross, K. *et al.* Developmental dyslexia: Research methods and inference. *Sci.,* 203:4387, 1979.

51. Gross, M. D. Improvement with L-dopa in a hyperkinetic child. *Dis. Nerv. Syst.,* 38:7, 1977.

52. Haggerty, R. and Stamm, J. S. Dichotic auditory fusion levels in children with learning disabilities. *Neuropsychologia,* 16:3, 1978.

53. Hagin, R. A. and Silver, A. A. Learning disability: Definitions, diagnosis and preventions. *New York University Education Quarterly,* Summer, 1977.

54. Hallgren, B. Specific dyslexia (congenital work blindness). *Acta Psychiat. Scand. Suppl.,* 65, 1950.

55. Harris, A. Lateral dominance, directional confusion, and reading disability. *J. Psychol.,* 44, 1957.

56. Hartlage, L. C. Differential diagnosis of dyslexia, minimal brain damage and emotional disturbance in children. *Psychol. in the Schools,* 7:4, 1970.

57. Hersher, L. and Presser, S. E. Cacography in the mothers of hyperactive children with learning disorders. *Percept. Motor Skills,* 46:3, (Part 2), 1978.

58. Hersher, L. Minimal brain dysfunction and otitis media. *Percept. Motor Skills,* 47:3, 1978.

59. Jayasekara, R. and Street, J. Parental age and parity in dyslexic boys. *J. Biosocial Sci.,* 10:3, 1978.

60. Kalat, J. W. Minimal brain dysfunction: Dopamine depletion? *Sci.,* 194, 1976.

61. Kinsbourne, M. and Caplan, P. J. *Children's Learning and Attention Problems.* Boston: Little, Brown, 1979.

61A. Knabel, N. Psychopharmacology for the hyperkinetic child. *Arch. Gen. Psychiat.,* 6, 1962.

62. Lambert, N. M. *et al.* Prevalence of hyperactivity in elementary school children as a function of social system definers. *Amer. J. Orthopsychiat.,* 48:3, 1978.

63. Lambert, N. M. *et al.* Hyperactive children and the efficacy of psychoactive drugs as a treatment intervention. *Amer. J. Orthopsychiat.,* 46:2, 1976.

64. Leisman, G. and Schwartz, J. Aetiological factors in dyslexia: I. Scaccadic eye movement control. *Percept. Motor Skills,* 47:2, 1978.

65. Leisman, G. *et al.* Aetiological factors in dyslexia: II. Ocular-motor programming. *Percept. Motor Skills,* 47:2, 1978.

66. Leisman, G. Aetiological factors in dyslexia: III. Ocular-motor factors in visual perceptual response efficiency. *Percept. Motor Skills,* 47:2, 1978.

67. Lieberman, L. M. LD adolescent: When do you stop? *ACLD Newsbriefs,* 136, 1981.

68. Loney, J. *et al.* Parental management, self-concept, and drug response in minimal brain dysfunction. *J. Learn. Disabilities.* 8:3, 1975.

69. McGlannan, F. K. Familial characteristics of genetic dyslexia. Preliminary report from a pilot study. *J. Learn. Disabilities.* 1:3, 1968.

70. McLennand, W. Hyperactive children. *Amer. Psychol.* April, 1980.

71. Marceca, A. The problem of hyperactivity. *Acad. Ther.,* 13:3, 1978.

72. Masters, L. and Marsh, G. E. Middle ear pathology as a factor in learning disabilities. *J. Learn. Disabilities,* 11:2, 1978.

73. Mattes, J. and Gittelman-Klein, R. A crossover study of artificial food colorings in a hyperkinetic child. *Amer. J. Psychiat.,* 135:8, 1978.

74. Mattis, S. Dyslexia syndromes: A working hypothesis that works. In A. L. Benton and D. Pearl (eds.), *Dyslexia: An Appraisal of Current Knowledge.* New York: Oxford University Press, 1978.

75. May, J. G. Minimal brain dysfunction: Dopamine depletion? *Sci.,* 194, 1976.

76. Meacham, M. L. Reading disability and identification: A case study. *J. School Psychol.,* 7:1, 1968–69.

77. Merrill, A. J. The role of vision in learning disorders. *J. Learn. Disabilities,* 10:7, 1977.

78. Minimal brain dysfunction. In D. N. Holvey (ed.), *The Merck Manual.* 12th edition. Rahway, N.J.: Merck & Co., 1972.

79. Morgan, S. R. The learning disabilities population: Why more boys than girls? A hot area for research. *J. Clin. Child Psychol.,* 8:3, 1979.

80. Morrison, J. R. and Stewart, M. A. The psychiatric status of the legal families of adopted hyperactive children. *Arch. Gen. Psychiat.,* 28:6, 1973.

81. Morrison, J. R. and Stewart, M. A. A family study of the hyperactive child syndrome. *Biological Psychiat.,* 3:3, 1971.

82. Myklebust, H. R. (ed.). *Progress in Learning Disabilities.* New York: Grune and Stratton, 1978.

83. Naylor, H. Reading disability and lateral asymmetry: An information-processing analysis. *Psychological Bull.,* 87:3, 1980.

84. Needleman, H. L. *et al.* Deficits in psychologic and classroom performance of children with elevated dentine lead levels. *New England J. Med.,* 300:3, 1979.

85. Ney, P. G. Four types of hyperkinesis. *Can. Psychiat. Assoc. J.,* 19, 1974.

86. Oettinger, L. *et al.* Bone age in children with minimal brain dysfunction. *Percept. Motor Skills,* 39:3, 1974.

87. Owen, F. W. Dyslexia—genetic aspects. In A. L. Benton and D. Pearl (eds.), *Dyslexia: An Appraisal of Current Knowledge.* New York: Oxford University Press, 1978.

88. Pappas, B. *et al.* Minimal brain dysfunction: Dopamine depletion? *Sci.,* 194, 1976.

89. Parr, V. E. Auditory word discrimination in male children diagnosed as having minimal brain dysfunction. *J. Clin. Psychol.,* 33:4, 1977.

90. Parsons, O. A. and Klein, H. P. Concept identification and practice in brain-damaged and process-reactive schizophrenic groups. *J. Consult. Clin. Psychol.* 35:3, 1970.

91. Peters, J. E. Minimal brain dysfunction in children. *A.F.P.,* July, 1974.

92. *Physical Trauma as an Etiological Agent in Mental Retardation.* Bethesda, Md.: U.S. Dept. of Health, Education and Welfare, 1970.

93. Pike, R. O. and Parkes, M. Hair element content in learning disabled children. *Sci.,* 198:4313, 1977.

94. Pontius, A. A. Discussion of conceptual models. *Annals New York Acad. Sci.,* 205, 1973.

95. Quiros, J. and Schrager, O. *Neuropsychological Fundamentals in Learning Disabilities.* San Rafael, Calif.: Academic Therapy Press, 1978.

96. Rapaport, H. G. and Flint, S. H. Is there a relationship between allergy and learning disabilities? *J. School Health,* 46:3, 1976.

97. Ravenette, A. T. Specific reading difficulties: Appearance and reality. *A.E.P. (Assoc. Ed. Psychologists) J.,* 4:10, 1979.

98. Reimberr, F. W. *et al.* An open clinical trial of L-dopa and carbidopa in adults with minimal brain dysfunction. *Amer. J. Psychiat.,* 137:1, 1980.

99. Reinhold, R. Experts view dyslexia, a little understood learning disability. *New York Times,* February 5, 1968.

100. Reitan, R. M. Psychological effects of cerebral lesions in children of early school age. In R. M. Reitan and L. A. Davison (eds.), *Clinical Neuropsychology: Current Status and Applications.* Washington, D.C.: Winston, 1974.

101. Rie, H. E. and Rie, E. D. (eds.). *Handbook of Minimal Brain Dysfunctions: A Critical View.* New York: Wiley, 1979.

102. Rose, T. The functional relationship between artificial food colors and hyperactivity. *J. App. Behav. Anal.,* 11:4, 1978.

103. Ross, A. O. *Learning Disability: The Unrealized Potential.* New York: McGraw-Hill, 1977.

104. Rossi, A. O. Genetics of learning abilities. *J. Learn. Disabilities,* 5:8, 1972.

105. Rourke, B. P. Neuropsychological research in reading retardation: A review. In A. L. Benton and D. Pearl (eds.), *Dyslexia: An Appraisal of Current Knowledge.* New York: Oxford University Press, 1978.

106. Rourke, B. P. Brain-behavior relationships in children with learning disabilities: A research program. *Amer. Psychol.,* September, 1975.

107. Rubenstein, B. and Levitt, M. Learning disabilities as related to a special form of mothering. *Int. J. Psycho-Anal.,* 58:1, 1977.

108. Safer, D. J. A familial factor in minimal brain dysfunction. *Behav. Genetics,* 3:2, 1973.

109. Satterfield, J. H. *et al.* Pathophysiology of the hyperactive child syndrome. *Arch. Gen. Psychiat.,* 31:6, 1974.

110. Satterfield, J. H. *et al.* Physiological studies of the hyperkinetic child: 1. *Amer. J. Psychiat.,* 128:11, 1972.

111. Schackenberg, B. C. Minimal brain dysfunction in children. *Psychiatric Forum,* 7:1, 1976.

112. Schain, R. J. Minimal brain dysfunction in children: A neurological viewpoint. *Bull. Los Angeles Neurological Societies,* 33:3, 1968.

113. Schlager, G. *et al.* Bone age in children with minimal brain dysfunction. *Develop. Med. Child Neurol.,* 21:1, 1979.

114. Schwartz, N. H. and Dean, R. S. Laterality preference patterns of learning disabled children. *Percept. Motor Skills,* 47:3, 1978.

115. Shaffer, D. and Greenhill, L. A critical note on the predictive validity of the hyperkinetic syndrome. *J. Child Psychol. Psychiat. Allied Disciplines,* 20:1, 1979.

116. Shaywitz, B. A. *et al.* Selective brain dopamine depletion in developing rats: An experimental model of minimal brain dysfunction. *Sci.,* 19, 1976.

117. Siegel, L. Perinatal factors related to cognitive deficits, specific language delay and hyperactivity. *Int. Neuropsychol. Soc. Bull.,* 1979.

118. Siggers, D. C. Human behavioural genetics. *Devel. Med. Child Neurol.,* 19:6, 1977.

119. Silin, M. W. Why many placid children have learning difficulties. *Child Welfare,* 57:4, 1978.

120. Silver, L. A proposed view on the etiology of the neurological learning disability syndrome. *J. Learn. Disabilities,* 4:3, 1971.

121. Solomons, G. Guidelines on the use and medical effects of psychostimulant drugs in therapy. *J. Learn. Disabilities,* 4:9, 1971.

122. Sperry, R. W. Lateral specialization of cerebral function in the surgically separated hemispheres. In F. J. McGuigan (ed.), *The Psychophysiology of Thinking.* New York: Academic Press, 1973.

123. Spreen, O. The dyslexias: A discussion of neurobehavioral research. In A. L.

Benton and D. Pearl (eds.), *Dyslexia: An Appraisal of Current Knowledge*. New York: Oxford University Press, 1978.

124. Spring, C. and Sandoval, J. Food additives and hyperkinesis: A critical evaluation of the evidence. *J. Learn. Disabilities*, 9:9, 1976.

125. Springer, S. P. and Eisenson, J. Hemispheric specialization for speech in language disordered children. *Neuropsychologia*, 15:2, 1977.

126. Stevens, D. A. *et al.* Reaction time, impulsivity, and autonomic lability in children with minimal brain dysfunction. *Proc. 76th Annual Convention, Amer. Psychol. Assoc.*, 1968.

127. Strain, P. S. and Shores, R. E. Social interaction development among behaviorally handicapped preschool children: Research and educational implications. *Psychol. in the Schools*, 14:4, 1977.

128. Strauss, A. and Kephart, N. *Psychopathology and Education of the Brain-Injured Child*, vol. 2. New York: Grune and Stratton, 1955.

129. Tarnpol, L. and Tarnpol, M. Motor deficits that may cause reading problems. *J. Learn. Disabilities*, 12:8, 1979.

130. Thompson, L. J. Learning disabilities: An overview. *Amer. J. Psychiat.*, 130:4, 1973.

131. Towbin, A. Cerebral dysfunctions related to perinatal organic damage: Clinical neuropathic correlations. *J. Abnormal Psychol.*, 87:6, 1978.

132. Velluntino, F. R. *et al.* Inter- versus intra-hemispheric learning in dyslexic and normal readers. *Devel. Med. Child Neurol.*, 20:1, 1978.

133. Velluntino, F. R. Toward an understanding of dyslexia: Psychological factors in specific reading disability. In A. L. Benton and D. Pearl (eds.), *Dyslexia: An Appraisal of Current Knowledge*. New York: Oxford University Press, 1978.

134. Vocational education—An idea that has met its time. *ACLD Newsbriefs: Special Supplement*, 124, 1979. Pittsburgh, Pa.: Association of Children with Learning Disabilities.

134A. Walker, S. Drugging the American child: We're too cavalier about hyperactivity. *Psychol. Today*, 8:7, 1974.

135. Warren, R. J. *et al.* The hyperactive child syndrome: Normal chromosome findings. *Arch. Gen. Psychiat.*, 24:2, 1971.

136. Webb, W. W. *et al.* The sequelae of acute bacterial meningitis: A possible clue to early school problems. *J. Spec. Ed.*, 2:4, 1968.

137. Weinstein, M. L.: A neuropsychological approach to math disability. *New York University Education Quarterly*, Winter, 1980.

138. Wender, P. H. Some speculations concerning a possible biochemical basis of minimal brain dysfunction. *Annals New York Acad. Sci.*, 205, 1973.

139. Wender, P. H. The minimal brain dysfunction syndrome in children: I. The syndrome and its relevance for psychiatry; II. A psychological and biochemical model for the syndrome. *J. Nerv. Mental Dis.*, 155:1, 1972.

140. Wender, P. H. *Minimal Brain Neurodysfunction in Children*. New York: Wiley-Interscience, 1971.

141. Werner, H. and Strauss, A. A. Pathology of figure-background relations in the child. *J. Abnormal Soc. Psychol.*, 36, 1941.

142. Werry, J. S. *et al.* Studies on the hyperactive child: VII. Neurological status compared with neurotic and normal children. *Amer. J. Orthopsychiat.,* 42:3, 1972.

143. Wolf, M. Dysnomia, dyslexia, and the tip of the tongue. Abstract in *Int. Neuropsychol. Soc. Bulletin,* 1978.

144. Yeni-Komshian, G. H. *et al.* Cerebral dominance and reading disability: Left visual field deficit in poor readers. *Neuropsychologia,* 13, 1975.

145. Zambelli, A. J. *et al.* Auditory evoked potential and selective attention in formerly hyperactive adolescent boys. *Amer. J. Psychiat.,* 134:7, 1977.

146. Zangwill, O. L. Dyslexia and cerebral dominance: A reassessment. In L. Oettinger, Jr. and L. V. Majorski (eds.), *The Psychologist, the School, and the Child with MBD/LD.* New York: Grune and Stratton, 1978.

147. Zangwill, O. L. Dyslexia in relation to cerebral dominance. In J. Money (ed.), *Reading Disability: Progress and Research Needs in Dyslexia.* Baltimore, Md.: The Johns Hopkins Press, 1962.

148. Zentall, S. S. Specific learning disabilities, communications and language process disturbance. In R. Ochroch (ed.), *Diagnosis and Treatment of Minimal Brain Dysfunction in Children: A Clinical Approach.* New York: Human Sciences Press, 1980.

149. Zrull, J. P. *et al.* Hyperkinetic syndrome: The role of depression. *Child Psychiat. Human Devel.,* 1:1, 1970.

150. Zurif, E. B. and Carson, G. Dyslexia in relation to cerebral dominance and temporal analysis. *Neuropsychologia,* 8, 1970.

Chapter 3

1. Ackerman, P. T. *et al.* Teenage status of hyperactive and nonhyperactive learning disabled boys. *Amer. J. Orthopsychiat.,* 47:4, 1977.

2. Anderson, C. *Society Pays: The High Cost of Minimal Brain Damage in Children.* New York: Walker, 1972.

3. Battle, E. and Lacey, B. A context for hyperactivity in children, over time. *Child Devel.,* 43:3, 1972.

4. Benton, A. L. Developmental dyslexia: Neurological aspects. In W. J. Friedlander (ed.), *Advances in Neurology,* vol. 7. New York: Raven Press, 1975.

4A. Birch, H. G. *et al.* Behavioral development in brain-damaged children. *Arch. Gen. Psychiat.,* 11, 1964.

5. Buckley, R. E. A neurophysiologic proposal for the amphetamine response in hyperkinetic children. *Psychosomatics,* 13:2, 1972.

6. Butler, H. J. Attention, sensory reception, and autonomic reactivity of hyperkinetic adolescents: A follow-up study. *Psychiatric J. Univ. Ottawa,* 2:3, 1977.

6A. Chess, S. Neurological dysfunction and childhood behavioral pathology. *J. Autism Childhood Schiz.,* 2:3, 1972.

7. Clarke, L. *Can't Read, Can't Write, Can't Takl Too Good Either.* New York: Walker, 1973.

8. Cott, A. Treatment of learning disabilities. *J. Orthomolecular Psychiat.,* 3:4, 1974.

9. Court, J. H. Psychological monitoring of interventions into educational problems with psychoactive drugs. *J. Learn. Disabilities,* 4:7, 1971.

10. Dykman, R. A. *et al.* Experimental approaches to the study of minimal brain dysfunction: A follow-up study. *Annals New York Acad. Sci.,* 205, 1973.

11. Gottesman, R. L. Follow-up of learning disabled children. *Learn. Disability Quart.,* 2:1, 1979.

12. Hoy, E. *et al.* The hyperactive child at adolescence: Cognitive, emotional, and social functioning. *J. Abnorm. Child Psychol.,* 6:3, 1978.

13. Huey, L. Y. *et al.* Adult minimal brain dysfunction and schizophrenia: A case report. *Amer. J. Psychiat.,* 135:12, 1978.

14. Katz, S. *et al.* Clinical pharmacological management of hyperkinetic children. *Int. J. Mental Health,* 4:1, 1975.

15. Kinsbourne, M. and Caplan, P. J. *Children's Learning and Attention Problems.* Boston: Little, Brown, 1979.

16. Laufer, M. L. Long-term management and some follow-up findings on the use of drugs with minimal cerebral syndromes. *J. Learn. Disabilities,* 4:9, 1971.

17. Loney, J. Hyperkinesis comes of age: What do we know and where should we go? *Amer. J. Orthopsychiat.,* 50:1, 1980.

18. Mangel, C. The puzzle of learning disabilities. *New York Times,* April 25, 1976.

19. Mendelson, W. *et al.* Hyperactive children as teenagers: A follow-up study. *J. Nerv. Mental Dis.,* 153:4, 1971.

19A. Menkes, M. M. *et al.* A twenty-five year follow-up study on the hyperkinetic child with minimal brain dysfunction. *Pediatrics,* 39:3, 1967.

20. Milich, R. and Loney, J. The role of hyperactive and aggressive symptomatology in predicting outcome among hyperactive children. *J. Pediatric Psychol.,* 42:2, 1979.

21. Minimal Brain Dysfunction. In D. N. Holvey (ed.), The *Merck Manual,* 12th ed. Rahway, N.J.: Merck & Co., 1972.

22. Morrison, J. R. Diagnosis of adult psychiatric patients with childhood hyperactivity. *Amer. J. Psychiat.,* 136:7, 1979.

23. Murray, M. E. Minimal brain dysfunction and borderline personality adjustment. *Amer. J. Psychotherapy,* 33:3, 1979.

24. Padilla de Olivares, A. *et al.* Behavioral immaturity and neurological immaturity. *Zeitschrift fur Kinder- und Jugendpsychiatrie,* 5:4, 1977.

25. Pincus, J. H. and Tucker, G. J. *Behavioral Neurology* (2nd ed.). New York: Oxford University Press, 1978.

25A. Rawson, M. B. *Developmental Language Disability: Adult Accomplishment of Dyslexic Boys.* Baltimore: Johns Hopkins University Press, 1968.

26. Riddle, K. D. and Rapoport, J. L. A two year follow-up of 72 hyperactive boys. *J. Nerv. Mental Dis.,* 162:2, 1976.

27. Safer, D. J. and Allen, R. P. Simulant drug treatment of hyperactive adolescents. *Dis. Nerv. Syst.,* 36:8, 1975.

28. Satz, P. *et al.* Some developmental and predictive precursors of reading disabilities: A six year follow-up. In A. L. Benton and D. Pearl (eds.), *Dyslexia: An Appraisal of Current Knowledge.* New York: Oxford University Press, 1978.

29. Schiffman, G. and Clemmens, R. *Observations on Children With Severe Reading Problems and Learning Disorders.* Seattle, Washington: Special Child Publications, 1966.

30. Shelley, E. M. and Riester, A. Syndrome of minimal brain damage in young adults. *Dis. Nerv. Syst.,* 33:5, 1972.

31. Simpson, E. *Reversals.* Boston: Houghton Mifflin, 1979.

32. Sleator, E. K. *et al.* Hyperactive children: A continuous long-term placebo-controlled follow-up. *JAMA* 229:3. 1974.

33. Sobel, D. Hyperactive children often suffer as adults. *New York Times,* December 4, 1975.

34. Stewart, M. A. *et al.* Hyperactive children as adolescents: How they describe themselves. *Child Psychiat. Human Devel.,* 4:1, 1973.

35. Thomas, A. and Chess, S. A longitudinal study of three brain damaged children: Infancy to adolescence. *Arch. Gen. Psychiat.,* 32:4, 1975.

36. Underwood, R. Learning disability as a predisposing cause of criminality. *Canada's Mental Health,* 24:4, 1976.

37. Weiss, G. Hyperactives as young adults: School, employer and self-rating scales obtained during ten-year follow-up evaluation. *Amer. J. Orthopsychiat.,* 48:3, 1978.

38. Weiss, G. *et al.* Studies on the hyperactive child: Five-year follow-up. In S. Chess and A. Thomas (eds.), *Annual Progress in Child Psychiatry and Child Development.* New York: Brunner/Mazel, 1972.

39. Weiss, G. *et al.* Studies on the hyperactive child, VII: A five-year follow-up. *Arch. Gen. Psychiat.,* 24, 1971.

40. Wender, P. H. The minimal brain dysfunction syndrome. *Ann. Rev. Med.,* 26, 1975.

41. Wender, P. H. Some speculations concerning a possible biochemical basis of minimal brain dysfunction. *Annals New York Acad. Sci.,* 205, 1973.

42. Wender, P. H. The minimal brain dysfunction syndrome in children: I. The syndrome and its relevance for psychiatry: II. A psychological and biochemical model for the syndrome. *J. Nerv. Mental Dis.,* 155:1, 1972.

43. Zinkus, P. W. *et al.* The learning-disabled juvenile delinquent: A case for early intervention of perceptually handicapped children. *Amer. J. Occup. Therapy,* 33:3, 1979.

Chapter 4

1. Bannatyne, A. *Language, Reading and Learning Disabilities.* Springfield, Ill.: Charles C. Thomas, 1971.

2. Barkley, R. A. Recent developments in research on hyperactive children. *J. Ped. Psychol.,* 3:4, 1978.

3. Benton, A. L. Developmental dyslexia: Neurological aspects. In W. J. Friedlander (ed.), *Advances in Neurology,* vol. 7. New York: Raven Press, 1975.

4. Benton, A. L. The fiction of the "Gerstmann's Syndrome." *J. Neurol. Neurosurg. Psychiat.,* 24, 1961.

5. Block, W. M. Cerebral dysfunctions: Clarification, delineation, classification. *Behavioral Neurol.,* 5, 1973–74.

6. Brown, B. S. Foreword. In A. L. Benton and David Pearl (eds.), *Dyslexia: An Appraisal of Current Knowledge.* New York: Oxford University Press, 1978.

7. Bruschek, B. Cognitive impairments in dyslectics: An attempt at an analysis of dyslexia on the basis of models of cognitive psychology. *Zeitschrift fur Kinder- und Jugendpsychiatrie,* 5:1, 1977.

8. Bryan, T. and Bryan, J. H. The social-emotional side of learning disabilities. *Behav. Disorders,* 2:3, 1977.

9. Cruikshank, W. M. Learning disabilities: Perceptual or other? *ACLD Newsbriefs,* March/April 1979.

10. deSousa, A. and deSousa, D. A. Hyperkinesis. *Child Psychiat. Quart.,* 10:4, 1977.

11. Doehring, D. G. The tangled web of behavioral research on developmental dyslexia. In A. L. Benton and D. Pearl (eds.), *Dyslexia: An Appraisal of Current Knowledge.* New York: Oxford University Press, 1978.

12. Erickson, M. T. Reading disability in relation to performance on neurological tests for minimal brain dysfunction. *Devel. Med. Child Neurol.,* 19:6, 1977.

13. Evans, J. R. and Smith, L. J. Common behavioral SLD characteristics. *Acad. Ther.,* 12:4, 1977.

14. Farnham-Diggory, S. *Learning Disabilities: A Psychological Perspective.* Cambridge, Mass.: Harvard University Press, 1978.

15. Fiedorowicz, C. *et al.* Neuropsychological correlates of three groups of dyslexia. Abstract in *Bull. Int. Neuropsychological Soc.,* 1979.

16. Fuller, G. B. and Friedrich, D. Three diagnostic patterns of reading disabilities. *Acad. Ther.,* 10:2, 1974–75.

17. Katz, S. *et al.* Clinical pharmacological management of hyperkinetic children. *Int. J. Mental Health,* 4:1–2, 1975.

18. Knights, R. M. and Bakker, O. J. (eds.). *The Neuropsychology of Learning Disorders: Theoretical Approaches.* Baltimore: University Park Press, 1976.

19. Kron, L. *et al.* Hyperactivity in anorexia nervosa: A fundamental clinical feature. *Comprehensive Psychiat.,* 19:5, 1978.

20. Lahey, B. B. *et al.* Hyperactivity and learning disabilities as independent dimensions of child behavior problems. *J. Abnorm. Psychol.,* 87:8, 1978.

21. Loney, J. Hyperkinesis comes of age: What do we know and where should we go? *Amer. J. Orthopsychiat.,* 50:1, 1980.

22. Loney, J. *et al.* An empirical basis for subgrouping the hyperkinetic/minimal brain dysfunction syndrome. *J. Abnorm. Psychol.,* 87:4, 1978.

23. Mattis, S. *et al.* Dyslexia in children and young adults: Three independent neurological syndromes. *Devel. Med. Child Neurol.,* 17:2, 1975.

24. *Minimal Brain Dysfunction in Children: Phase One of a Three Phase Project.* U. S. Dept. of Health, Education and Welfare, Public Health Service, Washington, D. C., 1966.

25. Myklebust, H. R. (ed.). *Progress in Learning Disabilities.* New York: Grune and Stratton, 1978.

26. Myklebust, H. R. Identification and diagnosis of children with learning disabilities: An interdisciplinary study of criteria. *Seminars in Psychiat.,* 5:1, 1973.

27. Ney, P. G. Four types of hyperkinesis. *Can. Psychiat. Assoc. J.,* 19, 1974.

28. Okada, S. and Hitomi, K. A critical review on minimal brain dysfunction (MBD). *Japanese J. Child Psychiat.,* 15:4, 1974.

29. O'Malley, J. E. and Eisenberg, L. The hyperkinetic syndrome. *Seminars in Psychiat.,* 5:1, 1973.

29A. Paine, R. S. *et al.* A study of "minimal cerebral dysfunction." *Devel. Med. Child Neurol.,* 10:4, 1968.

30. Peters, J. E. Minimal brain dysfunction in children. *A. F. P.,* July, 1974.

31. Poeck, K. and Orgass, B. Gerstmann's syndrome and aphasia. *Cortex,* 2, 1966.

32. Sampson, O. C. Fifty years of dyslexia: A review of the literature, 1925–75: I. Theory. *Res. Ed.,* 14, 1975.

33. Schain, R. J. Minimal brain dysfunction in children: A neurological viewpoint. *Bull. Los Angeles Neurological Societies,* 33:3, 1968.

34. Silver, L. B. The playroom diagnostic evaluation of children with neurologically based learning disabilities. *J. Child Psychiat.,* 15:2, 1976.

35. Sobel, D. Hyperactive children often suffer as adults. *New York Times,* December 4, 1979.

36. Stewart, M. A. *et al.* Hyperactive children as adolescents: How they describe themselves. *Child Psychiat. Human Devel.,* 4:1, 1973.

37. Strub, R. and Geschwind, N. Gerstmann Syndrome without aphasia. *Cortex,* 10:4, 1974.

38. Trites, R. L. (ed.). *Hyperactivity in Children: Etiology, Measurement, and Treatment Implications.* Baltimore: University Park Press, 1979.

39. Wender, P. H. Some speculations concerning a possible biochemical basis of minimal brain dysfunction. *Annals New York Acad. Sci.,* 205, 1973.

40. Zambelli, A. J. *et al.* Auditory evoked potential and selective attention in formerly hyperactive adolescent boys. *Amer. J. Psychiat.,* 134:7, 1977.

41. Zangwill, O. L. Dyslexia and cerebral dominance: A reassessment. In L. Oettinger, Jr. and L. V. Majovski (eds.), *The Psychologist, the School, and the Child with MBD/LD.* New York: Grune and Stratton, 1978.

42. Zentall, S. S. Specific learning disabilities, communication and language process disturbance. In R. Ochroch (ed.), *Minimal Brain Dysfunction in Children: A Clinical Approach.* New York: Human Sciences Press, 1980.

Chapter 5

1. Aaron, P. G. Dyslexia, an imbalance in cerebral information-processing strategies. *Percept. Motor Skills,* 47:3, 1978.

2. Aaronson, L. J. Mea culpa: A confession about minimal brain dysfunction. *The Clin. Psychol.,* Spring, 1968.

3. Abrams, J. C. and Kaslow, F. W. Learning disability and family dynamics: A mutual interaction. *J. Clin. Child Psychol,* 5:1, 1976.

4. Berman, A. Neurological dysfunction in juvenile delinquents: Implications for early intervention. *Child Care Quart.,* 1:4, 1972.

5. Birch, H. G. and Belmont, L. Auditory-visual integration in normal and retarded readers. *Amer. J. Orthopsychiat.,* 34, 1964.

6. Bryan, T. and Pearl, R. Self concepts and locus of control of learning disabled children. *J. Clin. Child Psychol.,* 8:3, 1979.

7. Campbell, P. A. Sustained attention in brain damaged children. *Exceptional Children,* 36:5, 1970.

8. Chess, S. *An Introduction to Child Psychiatry* (2nd ed.). New York: Grune and Stratton, 1969.

9. Crow, G. A. *Children at Risk: A Handbook of the Signs and Symptoms of Early Childhood Difficulties.* New York: Schocken, 1978.

10. Cunningham, C. F. and Barkley, R. A. The interaction of normal and hyperactive children with their mothers in free play and structured tasks. *Child Devel.,* 50:1, 1979.

11. Fisher, L. Attention deficit in brain damaged children. *Amer. J. Ment. Def.,* 74:4, 1970.

12. Gazzaniga, M. S. and Hillyard, S. A. *Attention Mechanisms Following Brain Bisection. Attention and Performance IV.* New York: Academic Press, 1973.

13. Gillis, J. S. and Sidlauskas, A. I. The influence of differential auditory feedback upon the reading of dyslexic children. *Neuropsychologia,* 16:4, 1978.

14. Goldberg, H. K. and Schiffman, G. B. *Dyslexia: Problems of Reading Disabilities.* New York: Grune and Stratton, 1972.

15. Haggerty, R. and Stamm, J. S. Dichotic auditory fusion levels in children with learning disabilities. *Neuropsychologia,* 16:3, 1978.

16. Hardy, J. B. *et al. The First Year of Life: The Collaborative Perinatal Project of the National Institute of Neurological and Communicative Disorders and Stroke.* Baltimore: Johns Hopkins University Press, 1979.

17. Hynd, G. W. *et al.* Development of cerebral dominance: Dichotic listening asymmetry in normal and learning-disabled children. *J. Exp. Child Psychol.,* 28:3, 1979.

18. Kalat, J. W. Minimal brain dysfunction: Dopamine depletion? *Sci.,* 194, 1976.

19. Kennard, M. Value of equivocal signs in neurological diagnosis. *Neurol.,* 10, 1960.

20. Kline, C. L. Developmental dyslexia in adolescents: The emotional damage. *Bull. Orton. Soc.,* 28, 1978.

21. Mann, H. B. and Greenspan, S. I. The identification and treatment of adult brain dysfunction. *Amer. J. Psychiat.,* 133:9, 1976.

22. Masters, L. and Marsh, G. E. Middle ear pathology as a factor in learning disabilities. *J. Learn. Disabilities,* 11:2, 1978.

23. Mauser, A. J.: Learning disabilities and delinquent youth. *Acad. Ther.,* 9:6, 1974.

24. *Minimal Brain Dysfunction in Children: Educational, Medical and Health Related Services. Phase Two of a Three-Phase Project.* U. S. Dept. of Health, Education, and Welfare. Public Health Service Publication No. 2015, 1969.

25. Mordock, J. B. The separation-individuation process and developmental disabilities. *Exceptional Children,* 46:3, 1979.

26. Morrison, J. R. and Minkoff, K. Explosive personality as a sequel to the hyperactive-child syndrome. *Compreh. Psychiat.,* 16:4, 1975.

27. Morrison, J. R. and Stewart, M. A. A family study of the hyperactive child syndrome. *Biological Psychiat.,* 3:3, 1971.

28. Murray, M. E.: Minimal brain dysfunction and borderline personality adjustment. *Amer. J. Psychotherapy, 33*:3, 1979.

29. Nirk, G. *et al.* A developmental model for treatment of hyperactive children. Mimeo. Undated.

30. Novackova, J. and Dobratka, G. Diverse parental acceptance of epileptic and minimally brain damaged children. *Psychologia a Patopsychologia Dietata, 11*:2, 1976.

31. Ossofsky, H. J. Hyperactivity in some children laid to "primary depression." *Med. Trib.,* March 20, 1974.

32. Ottenbacher, K. Identifying vestibular processing dysfunction in learning-disabled children. *Amer. J. Occupational Therapy, 32*:4, 1975.

32A. Ozer, M. N. The diagnostic assessment of children with developmental problems: A therapeutic process. In R. Ochroch (ed.), *The Diagnosis and Treatment of Minimal Brain Dysfunction in Children: A Clinical Approach.* New York: Human Sciences Press, 1980.

33. Reitan, R. M. Paper presented at ACLD Convention, Seattle, 1976.

34. Rugel, R. P. *et al.* Body movement and inattention in learning-disabled and normal children. *J. Abnorm. Child Psychol., 6*:3, 1978.

35. Rutter, M. *et al.* Interrelationship between the choreiform syndrome, reading disability, and psychiatric disorder in children of 8–11 years. *Develop. Med. Child Neurol., 8,* 1966.

36. Sabatino, D. A. Auditory and visual perceptual behavioral function of neurologically impaired children. *Percept Motor Skills, 29*:10, 1969.

37. Schain, R. J. Minimal brain dysfunction in children: A neurological viewpoint. *Bull. Los Angeles Neurological Societies, 33*:3, 1968.

38. Schechter, M. D. Psychiatric aspects of learning disabilities. *Child Psychiat. Human Devel., 5*:2, 1974.

39. Schildkrout, M. S. The hyperactive/MBD child family interaction and treatment. In R. Ochroch (ed.), *The Diagnosis and Treatment of Minimal Brain Dysfunction in Children: A Clinical Approach.* New York: Human Sciences Press, 1980.

40. Silver, A. A. Anxiety defense in children with central nervous system dysfunction. *Audio Digest, 6*:10, 1977.

41. Silver, A. A. and Hagin, R. A. Profile of a first grade: A basis for preventive psychiatry. *J. Amer. Acad. Child Psychiat., 11,* 1972.

42. Silver, L. B. The playroom diagnostic evaluation of children with neurologically based learning disabilities. *J. Child Psychiat., 15*:2, 1976.

43. Small, L. *Neuropsychodiagnosis in Psychotherapy* (revised ed.). New York: Brunner/Mazel, 1980.

44. Taglianetti, T. J. Reading failure: A predictor of delinquency. *Crime Prevention Review, 2*:3, 1975, California: Attorney General's Office.

45. Tarnpol, L. Delinquency and minimal brain dysfunction. *J. Learn. Disabilities, 3*:4, 1970.

46. Tarter, R. E. *et al.* Differentiation of alcoholics: Childhood history of minimal brain dysfunction, family history, and drinking pattern. *Arch. Gen. Psychiat., 34,* 1977.

47. Thomas, E. D. Hyperactivity not associated with MBD. *J. Ped. Psychol., 1*:3, 1976.

48. Wender, P. H. *Minimal Brain Dysfunction in Children.* New York: Wiley-Interscience, 1971.

49. Werry, J. S. *et al.* Studies on the hyperactive child: VII. Neurological status compared with neurotic and normal children. *Amer. J. Orthopsychiat.*, 42:3, 1972.

50. Zentall, S. S. Specific learning disabilities, communications and language process disturbance. In R. Ochroch (ed.), *Diagnosis and Treatment of Minimal Brain Dysfunction in Children: A Clinical Approach.* New York: Human Sciences Press, 1980.

51. Zrull, J. P. *et al.* Hyperkinetic syndrome: The role of depression. *Child Psychiat. Human Devel.*, 1:1, 1970.

Chapter 6

1. Appelbaum, A. S. Diagnostic considerations in the evaluation of hyperkinetic children. *J. Ped. Psychol.*, 3:3, 1975.

2. Benoit, M. B. Minimal brain dysfunction: The psychiatric examination. In R. Ochroch (ed.), *The Diagnosis and Treatment of Minimal Brain Dysfunction in Children: A Clinical Approach.* New York: Human Sciences Press, 1980.

3. deHirsch, K. *et al. Predicting Reading Failure.* New York: Harper and Row, 1966.

4. Eaves, L. D. *et al.* The early detection of minimal brain dysfunction. *J. Learn. Disabilities*, 5:8, 1972.

5. Kappelman, M. M. *et al.* Profile of the disadvantaged child with learning problems. *Ment. Health Digest*, 1971.

6. *Minimal Brain Dysfunction in Children: Educational, Medical and Health Related Services. Phase Two of a Three-Phase Project.* U.S. Dept. of Health, Education and Welfare. Public Health Service Publication No. 2015, 1969.

7. Ochroch, R. The "case" for the "case manager." In R. Ochroch (ed.), *The Diagnosis and Treatment of Minimal Brain Dysfunction in Children: A Clinical Approach.* New York: Human Sciences Press, 1980.

8. Oettinger, J. Learning disabilities, hyperkinesis, and the use of drugs in children. *Rehab. Lit.*, 32:6, 1971.

9. Ozer, M. N. The diagnostic assessment of children with developmental problems: A therapeutic process. In R. Ochroch (ed.), *The Diagnosis and Treatment of Minimal Brain Dysfunction in Children: A Clinical Approach.* New York: Human Sciences Press, 1980.

10. Shrier, D. K. Memo to day care staff: Helping children with minimal brain dysfunction. *Child Welfare*, 54:2, 1975.

11. Silver, A. A. and Hagin, R. A. Profile of a first grade: A basis for preventive psychiatry. *J. Amer. Acad. Child Psychiat.*, 11, 1972.

12. Silver, L. B. The playroom diagnostic evaluation of children with neurologically based learning disabilities. *J. Child Psychiat.*, 15:2, 1976.

13. Small, L. *Neuropsychodiagnosis in Psychotherapy* (revised ed.) New York: Brunner/Mazel, 1980.

14. White, B. L. Early detection of educational handicaps. *Annals New York Acad. Sci.*, 205, 1973.

Chapter 7

1. Myklebust, H. R. *The Pupil Rating Scale: Screening for Learning Disabilities.* New York: Grune and Stratton, 1971.
2. Shrier, D. K. Memo to day care staff: Helping children with minimal brain dysfunction. *Child Welfare,* 54:2, 1975.
3. Valett, R. E. *Suspected Learning and Behavioral Disabilities.* Belmont, Calif.: Fearon Publishers, 1972.
4. Valett, R. E. Developmental Task Analysis. Belmont, Calif.: Fearon Publishers, 1969.

Chapter 8

1. Bellak, L. and Small, L.: *Emergency Psychotherapy and Brief Psychotherapy* (2nd ed.). New York: Grune and Stratton, 1978.
2. Bellak, L. and Hurvich, M. A systematic study of ego functions. *J. Nerv. Mental Dis.,* 148:6, 1969.
3. Bellak, L. The psychoanalytic concept of the ego and schizophrenia. In L. Bellak and P. K. Benedict (eds.), *Schizophrenia: A Review of the Syndrome.* New York: Logos Press, 1958.
4. Benoit, M. B. Minimal brain dysfunction: The psychiatric examination. In R. Ochroch (ed.), *The Diagnosis and Treatment of Minimal Brain Dysfunction in Children: A Clinical Approach.* New York: Human Sciences Press, 1980.
5. DeLeo, J. H. Early identification of minimal cerebral dysfunction. *Acad. Ther.,* 5:3, 1970.
6. Duncan, M. H. Attention deficit disorder (ADD) 1980: Unnecessary mistakes in diagnosis and treatment of learning and behavior problems of the MBD/hyperactive syndrome. *J. Clin. Child Psychol.,* 8:3, 1979.
7. Frank, J. D. The role of hope in psychotherapy. *Int. J. Psychiat.,* 5, 1968.
8. Luria, A. R. *Higher Cortical Functions in Man.* New York: Basic Books, 1966.
9. Malan, D. H. *A Study of Brief Psychotherapy.* London: Travistock Publications, 1963.
10. Menkes, M. M. *et al.:* A twenty-five year follow-up study on the hyperkinetic child with minimal brain dysfunction. *Pediatrics,* 39:3, 1967.
11. Small, L. The Briefer Psychotherapies (rev. ed.). New York: Brunner/Mazel, 1979.
12. Wender, P. H. *Minimal Brain Dysfunction in Children.* New York: Wiley-Interscience, 1971.

Chapter 9

1. Benton, A. L. Developmental dyslexia: Neurological aspects. In W. J. Friedlander (ed.), *Advances in Neurology,* vol. 7. New York: Raven Press, 1975.

2. Benton, A. L. and Joynt, R. J. Conclusion and indications for future investigative work. Presentation 21. In A. L. Benton (ed.), *Behavioral Change in Cerebrovascular Disease.* New York: Harper and Row, 1970.

3. Burg, C. *et al.* Clinical evaluation of one-year-old infants: Possible predictors of risk for the "hyperactivity syndrome." *J. Ped. Psychol.,* 3:4, 1978.

4. Camp, J. A. *et al.* Clinical usefulness of the NIMH Physical and Neurological Examination for Soft Signs. *Amer. J. Psychiat.,* 135:3, 1978.

5. Conners, C. K. Critical review of "Electroencephalographic and neurophysiological studies in dyslexia." In A. L. Benton and D. Pearl (eds.), *Dyslexia: An Appraisal of Current Knowledge.* New York: Oxford University Press, 1978.

6. Cunningham, C. F. and Barkley, R. A. The role of academic failure in hyperkinetic behavior. *J. Learn. Disabilities,* 11:5, 1978.

6A. Dargassies, S. S-A. Neurodevelopmental symptoms during the first year of life. *Devel. Med. Child Neurol.,* 14, 1972.

7. DeLeo, J. H. Early identification of minimal cerebral dysfunction. *Acad. Ther.,* 5:3, 1970.

8. Frank, J. and Levinson, H. Seasickness mechanisms and medications in dysmetric dyslexia and dyspraxia. *Acad. Ther.,* 12:2, 1976–77.

9. Frank, J. and Levinson, H. Report dyslexia due to inner ear lesion. Anon. report in *ACLD Newsbriefs,* 96, 1974.

10. Gaddes, W. H. Neurological implications for learning. In W. Cruickshank and D. Hallahan (eds.), *Perceptual and Learning Disorders in Children,* vol. 1. Syracuse, N.Y.: Syracuse University Press, 1975.

11. Gross, M. D. Violence associated with organic brain disease. In J. Fawcett (ed.), *Dynamics of Violence.* Chicago: American Medical Association, 1971.

12. Hertzig, M. E. and Birch, H. G. Neurologic organization in psychiatrically disturbed adolescents. *Arch. Gen. Psychiat.,* 19, 1968.

13. Hughes, J. R. Electroencephalographic and neurophysiological studies in dyslexia. In A. L. Benton and D. Pearl (eds.), *Dyslexia: An Appraisal of Current Knowledge.* New York: Oxford University Press, 1978.

14. Ingram T. T. S. "Soft signs." *Devel. Med. Child Neurol.,* 10:15, 1973.

15. Kennard, M. Value of equivocal signs in neurological diagnosis, *Neurol.,* 10, 1960.

16. Klatskin, E. H. *et al.* Minimal organicity in children of normal intelligence. Correspondence between psychological test results and neurologic findings. *J. Learn. Disabilities,* April, 1972.

17. Mattis, S. *et al.* Dyslexia in children and young adults: Three independent neurological syndromes. *Devel. Med. Child Neurol.,* 17:2, 1975.

18. *Minimal Brain Dysfunction in Children: Educational, Medical and Health Related Services. Phase Two of a Three-Phase Project.* U.S. Dept. of Health, Education, and Welfare. Public Health Service Publication No. 2015, 1969.

19. Mora, G. *et al.* Psychiatric syndromes and neurological findings as related to academic underachievement. Implications for education and treatment. Mimeo. Undated.

20. Mordock, J. B. and DeHaven, G. E. Interrelations among indexes of neurological "soft signs" in children with minimal cerebral dysfunction. *Proceedings 76th Annual Convention, Amer. Psychol. Assoc.,* 1968.

21. Myklebust, H. R. Identification and diagnosis of children with learning disabilities: An interdisciplinary study of criteria. *Seminars in Psychiat.*, 5:1, 1973.

22. Oettinger, L. Paper presented at ALCD convention. Seattle, 1973.

23. Peters, J. E. *et al.* A special neurological examination of children with learning disabilities. *Devel. Med. Child Neurol.*, 17:1, 1975.

24. Reitan, R. M. Objective behavioral assessment in diagnosis and prediction. Presentation 15. In A. L. Benton (ed.), *Behavioral Change in Cerebrovascular Disease.* New York: Harper and Row, 1970.

25. Rie, E. D. *et al.* An analysis of neurological soft signs in children with learning problems. *Brain and Language,* 6:1, 1978.

26. Rockford, J. M. *et al.* Neuropsychological impairments in functional psychiatric diseases. *Arch. Gen. Psychiat.*, 22, 1970.

27. Satterfield, J. H. EEG issues in children with minimal brain dysfunction. *Seminars in Psychiat.*, 5:1, 1973.

28. Schain, R. J. Minimal brain dysfunction in children: A neurological viewpoint. *Bull. Los Angeles Neurological Societies,* 33:3, 1968.

29. Schmeck, Jr., H. M. Learning disabled are studied for tell-tale brainwave pattern. *New York Times,* December 9, 1980.

30. Shaffer, D. Soft neurological signs and later psychiatric disorders. *J. Child Psychol. Psychiat. Allied Disciplines.* 19:1, 1978.

31. Sklar, B. *et al.* A computer analysis of EEG spectral signatures from normal and dyslexic children. *IGEE Transactions on Biomedical Engineering,* BME-20:1, 1973.

32. Sklar, B. *et al.* An EEG experiment aimed toward identifying dyslexic children. *Nature,* 240:5381, 1972.

33. Strub, R. L. and Black, F. W. *The Mental Status Examination in Neurology.* Philadelphia: F. A. Davis, 1977.

34. Swiercinsky, D. P. and Leigh, G. Comparison of neuropsychological data in the diagnosis of brain impairment with computerized tomography and other neurological procedures. *J. Clin. Psychol.*, 35:2, 1979.

35. Tymchuk, A. J. *et al.* The behavioral significance of differing EEG abnormalities in children with learning and/or behavior problems. *J. Learn. Disabilities,* 1970.

36. Voeller, K. A proposed extended behavioral, cognitive and sensorimotor pediatric neurological examination. In R. Ochroch (ed.), *The Diagnosis and Treatment of Minimal Brain Dysfunction in Children: A Clinical Approach.* New York: Human Sciences Press, 1980.

37. Zambelli, A. J. *et al.* Auditory evoked potential and selective attention in formerly hyperactive adolescent boys. *Amer. J. Psychiat.*, 134:7, 1977.

Chapter 10

1. Adams, J. *et al.* The efficacy of the Canter Background Interference Procedure in identifying children with cerebral dysfunction. *J. Consult. Psychol.*, 40:3, 1973.

2. Adams, J. Comparison of task-central and task-peripheral forms of the Canter BIP in diagnosing brain damage in adults. *Percept. Motor Skills,* 33:3, 1971.

3. Adams, J. Canter Background Interference Procedure applied to the diagnosis of brain damage in mentally retarded children. *Amer. J. Ment. Def.,* 75:1, 1970.

4. Anthony, E. J. A psychodynamic model of minimal brain dysfunction. *Annals New York Acad. Sci.,* 205, 1973.

5. Baker, G. Diagnosis of organic brain damage in the adult. In B. Klopfer (ed.), *Developments in the Rorschach Technique,* vol. 2. Yonkers, N.Y.: World Book, 1952.

6. Banas, N. and Wills, I. H. *WISC-R Prescriptions: How to Work Creatively with Individual Learning Styles.* Novato, Calif.: Academic Therapy Publications, 1978.

7. Belmont, I. and Birch, H. G. "Productivity" and mode of function in the Rorschach responses of brain-damaged patients. *J. Nerv. Ment. Dis.,* 134, 1962.

8. Benton, A. L. Minimal brain dysfunction from a neuropsychological point of view. *Annals New York Acad. Sci.,* 105, 1973.

9. Benton, A. L. *Benton Visual Retention Test.* New York: Psychological Corporation, 1955.

10. Birch, H. G. and Walker, H. A. Perceptual and perceptual-motor dissociation: Studies in schizophrenic and brain damaged psychotic children. *Arch. Gen. Psychiat.,* 14, 1966.

11. Birch, H. G. and Belmont, I. Functional levels of disturbance manifested by brain-damaged (hemiphasic) patients as revealed in Rorschach responses. *J. Nerv. Ment. Dis.,* 132, 1961.

12. Birch, H. G. and Diller, L. Rorschach signs of "organicity:" Physiological basis for perceptual disturbances. *J. Proj. Tech.,* 23, 1959.

13. Brown, D. *et al.* Imipramine therapy and seizures: Three children treated for hyperactive behavior disorders. *Amer. J. Psychiat.,* 130:2, 1973.

14. Burgemeister, B. B. *Psychological Techniques in Neurological Diagnosis.* New York: Hoeber Med. Div., Harper & Row, 1962.

15. Canter, A. A comparison of the background interference procedure effect in schizophrenic, non-schizophrenic and organic patients. *J. Clin. Psychol.,* 27:4, 1971.

16. Canter, A. A background interference procedure to increase sensitivity of the Bender Gestalt Test to organic brain disorder. *J. Consult. Psychol.,* 30, 1966.

16A. Christensen, A. L. *Luria's Neuropsychological Investigation.* New York: Spectrum Press, 1975.

17. Clements, S. D. and Peters, J. E. Minimal brain dysfunction in the school age child: *Arch. Gen. Psychiat.,* 6, 1962.

18. Conners, C. R. Psychological assessment of children with minimal brain dysfunction. *Annals New York Acad. Sci.,* 205, 283–302, 1973.

19. Costa, L. D. *et al.* Purdue Pegboard as a predictor of the presence and laterality of cerebral lesions. *J. Consult. Psychol.,* 27, 1963.

20. Crinella, F. M. Identification of brain dysfunction syndrome in children through profile analysis: Patterns associated with so-called "minimal brain dysfunction." *J. Abnorm. Psychol.,* 82:1, 1973.

21. Davids, A. An objective instrument for assessing hyperkinesis in children. *J. Learn. Disabilities,* 4:9, 1971.

22. Davis, W. E. *et al.* Categorization of patients with personality disorders and acute brain trauma through WAIS subtest variations. *J. Clin. Psychol.,* 27:3, 1971.

22A. de Hirsch, K. *et al. Predicting Reading Failure.* New York: Harper and Row, 1969.

23. Delay, J. *et al. Rorschach and the Epileptic Personality.* New York: Logos Press, 1958.

24. DeWolfe, A. S. Differentiation of schizophrenia and brain damage with the WAIS. *J. Clin. Psychol.,* 27:3, 1971.

25. DeWolfe, A. S. *et al.* Intellectual deficit in chronic schizophrenia and brain damage. *J. Consult. Clin. Psychol.,* 36:2, 1971.

26. Dorken, H. and Kral, V. A. The psychological differentiation of organic brain lesions and their localization by means of the Rorschach test. *Amer. J. Psychiat.,* 108, 1957.

27. Dykman, R. A. *et al.* Experimental approaches to the study of minimal brain dysfunction: A follow-up study. *Annals New York Acad. Sci.,* 205, 1973.

27A. Eaves, L. C. *et al.* The early detection of minimal brain dysfunction. *J. Learn. Disabilities,* 5, 1972.

28. Filskov, S. B. and Boll, T. J. *Handbook of Clinical Neuropsychology.* New York: Wiley-Interscience, 1981.

29. Frank, J. and Levinson, H. Dysmetric dyslexia and dyspraxia: Hypothesis and study. *J. Amer. Acad. Child Psychiat.,* 12:4, 1973.

30. Freed, E. X. Actuarial data on Bender-Gestalt Test rotations on psychiatric patients. *J. Clin. Psychol.,* 25:3, 1969.

31. Goldberg, H. K. and Schiffman, G. B. *Dyslexia: Problems of Reading Disabilities.* New York: Grune and Stratton, 1972.

31A. Golden, C. J. *et al. The Luria-Nebraska Neuropsychological Battery: A Manual for Clinical and Experimental Uses.* Lincoln, Nebraska: University of Nebraska Press, 1979.

32. Goldfried, M. R. *et al. Rorschach Handbook of Clinical and Research Applications.* Englewood Cliffs, N.J. Prentice-Hall, 1971.

33. Hagin, R. A. *et al. TEACH: Learning Tasks for the Prevention of Learning Disability.* New York: Walker, 1976.

34. Hain, J. D. The Bender Gestalt test: A scoring method for identifying brain damage. *J. Consult. Psychol.,* 28:1, 1964.

34A. Hall, L. P. and LaDriere, LaV. Patterns of performance on *WISC* similarities in emotionally disturbed and brain-damaged children. *J. Consult. Clin. Psychol.,* 33:3, 1969.

35. Hartlage, L. C.: Differential diagnosis of dyslexia, minimal brain damage and emotional disturbances in children. *Psychol. in the Schools,* 7:4, 1970.

36. Hartlage, L. Common psychological tests applied to the assessment of brain damage. *J. Proj. Tech.,* 30, 1966.

37. Hécarn, H. and Albert, M. L.: *Human Neuropsychology.* New York: John Wiley, 1978.

38. Heimburger, R. F. and Reitan, R. M. Easily administered written test for lateralizing brain lesions. *J. Neurosurg.,* 18, 1961.

39. Hughes, R. M. A factor analysis of Rorschach diagnostic signs. *J. Gen. Psychol.,* 43, 1950.

40. Hutt, M. L. (ed.). *The Hutt Adaptation of the Bender-Gestalt Test* (2nd ed.). New York: Grune and Stratton, 1969.

41. Hutt, M. L. and Briskin, G. *The Clinical Use of the Revised Bender-Gestalt Test.* New York: Grune and Stratton, 1960.

42. Jacobson, S. and Kovalinsky, T. *Educational Interpretation of the Wechsler Intelligence Scale for Children—Revised (WISC-R).* Linden, N.J.: Remediation Associates, Inc., 1976.

43. Johnson, J. E. *et al.* The relationship between intelligence, brain damage, and Hutt-Briskin errors on the Bender-Gestalt. *J. Clin. Psychol.,* 27:1, 1971.

44. Kenny, T. J. Background interference procedure: A means of assessing neurologic dysfunction in school-age children. *J. Consult. Clin. Psychol.,* 37:1, 1971.

45. Kirk, S. A. and Kirk, W. D. *Psycholinguistic Learning Disabilities: Diagnosis and Remediation.* Urbana, Ill.: University of Illinois Press, 1974.

46. Klatskin, E. H. *et al.* Minimal organicity in children of normal intelligence: Correspondence between psychological test results and neurologic findings. *J. Learn. Disabilities,* April, 1972.

47. Klebanoff, S. G. *et al.* Psychological consequences of brain lesions and ablations. *Psychol. Bull.,* 51, 1954.

48. Knights, R. M. Problems of criteria in diagnosis: A profile similarity approach. *Annals New York Acad. Sci.,* 205, 1973.

49. Koestline, W. C. and Dent, C. D. Verbal mediation in the WAIS Digit Symbol Subtest. *Psychological Reports,* 25:2, 1969.

50. Koppitz, E. M. *The Bender Gestalt Test for Younger Children.* New York: Grune and Stratton, 1963.

51. Levinger, L. and Ochroch, R. Psychodiagnostic evaluation of children with minimal brain dysfunction. In R. Ochroch (ed.), *The Diagnosis and Treatment of Minimal Brain Dysfunction in Children: A Clinical Approach.* New York: Human Sciences Press, 1980.

52. Lezak, M. *Neuropsychological Assessment.* New York: Oxford University Press, 1976.

53. Luria, A. R. *Higher Cortical Functions in Man.* New York: Basic Books, 1966.

54. McCarthy, J. J. and Kirk, S. A. *The Illinois Test of Psycholinguistic Abilities.* Urbana, Ill.: University of Illinois Press.

55. McFie, J. *Assessment of Organic Intellectual Impairment.* London: Academic Books, 1975.

56. McFie, J. and Thompson, J. A. Picture arrangement: A measure of frontal lobe function. *Brit. J. Psychiat.,* 121:564, 1972.

57. Matarazzo, J. D. *Wechsler's Measurement and Appraisal of Adult Intelligence* (5th ed.). Baltimore: Williams and Wilkins, 1972.

58. Mattis, S. *et al.* Dyslexia in children and young adults: Three independent neurological syndromes. *Devel. Med. Child Neurol.,* 17:2, 1975.

59. Mauser, A. J. *Assessing the Learning Disabled: Selected Instruments* (2nd ed.). San Rafael, Calif.: Academic Therapy Publications, 1977.

60. O'Neill, G. and Stanley, G. Visual processing of straight lines in dyslexic and normal children. *J. Educ. Psychol.,* 46, 1976.

61. Parsons, L. B. *et al.* Validity of Koppitz's Developmental Score as a measure of organicity. *Percept. Motor Skills,* 33:3, 1971.

62. Parsons, O. A. and Vega, A. Different psychological effects of lateralized brain damage. *J. Consult. Clin. Psychol.,* 33:5, 1969.

63. Pascal, G. R. and Suttell, B. J. *The Bender Gestalt Test.* New York: Grune and Stratton, 1951.

64. Piotrowski, Z. The Rorschach ink-blot method in organic disturbance of the central nervous system. *J. Nerv. Ment. Dis.,* 86, 1937.

65. Pirozzolo, F. J. *The Neuropsychology of Developmental Reading Disorders.* New York: Praeger, 1979.

66. Pontius, A. A. Discussions of conceptual models. *Annals New York Acad. Sci.,* 205, 1973.

67. Rapin, I. *et al.* Evaluation of the Purdue Pegboard as a screening test of brain damage. *Devel. Med. Child Neurol.,* 8, 1966.

68. Reed, J. C. *et al.* The influence of cerebral lesions on the psychological test performance of older children. *J. Consult. Psychol.,* 29, 1965.

69. Reitan, R. M. Paper presented at ACLD Convention, Seattle, 1976.

70. Reitan, R. M. Psychological effects of cerebral lesions in children of early school age. In R. M. Reitan and L. A. Davison (eds.), *Clinical Neuropsychology: Current Status and Applications.* Washington, D. C.: Winston, 1974.

71. Reitan, R. M. and Boll, T. J. Neuropsychological correlates of minimal brain dysfunction. *Annals New York Acad. Sci.,* 205, 1973.

72. Reitan, R. M. Psychological assessment of deficits associated with brain lesions in subjects with normal and subnormal intelligence. In J. L. Khanna (ed.), *Brain Damage and Mental Retardation: A Psychological Evaluation.* Springfield, Ill.: Charles C. Thomas, 1967.

73. Reitan, R. M. and Heineman, C. E. Interaction of neurological deficits and emotional disturbance in children with learning disorders: Methods for differential assessment. Indiana University Medical Center and Fort Wayne Guidance Clinic. Mimeo, Undated.

74. Rosencrans, C. J. and Schaffer, H. B. Bender-Gestalt time and score differences between matched groups of hospitalized psychiatric and brain-damaged patients. *J. Clin. Psychol.,* 25:4, 1969.

75. Ross, W. D. and Ross, S. Some Rorschach ratings of clinical value. *Rorschach Res. Ex.,* 8, 1944.

76. Rourke, B. P. and Finlayson, M. A. Neuropsychological significance of variations in patterns of academic performance: Verbal and visual spatial abilities. *J. Abnorm. Child Psychol.* 6:1, 1978.

77. Rourke, B. P. Issues in the neuropsychological assessment of children with learning disabilities. *Canadian Psychol. Rev.,* 17:2, 1976.

78. Russell, E. W. *et al. Assessment of Brain Damage.* New York: Wiley-Interscience, 1970.

79. Satz, P. A block rotation task: The application of multivariate and decision theory analysis for the prediction of organic brain disorder. *Psychol. Mong.,* 80:21, 1966.

80. Searls, E. F. *How to Use WISC Scores in Reading Diagnosis.* Newark, Delaware: International Reading Association, 1975.

81. Selz, M. and Reitan, R. M. Rules for neuropsychological diagnosis: Classification of brain function in older children. *J. Consult. Clin. Psychol.,* 47:2, 1979.

82. Silver, A. A. and Hagin, R. A. *SEARCH: A Scanning Instrument for the Identification of Potential Learning Disability.* New York: Walker, 1976.

83. Smith, A. Neuropsychological testing in neurological disorders. In W. J. Friedlander (ed.), *Advances in Neurology.* New York: Raven Press, 1975.

84. Smith, A. *Symbol Digit Modalities Test.* Los Angeles: Western Psychological Services, 1973.

85. Smith, A. Certain hypothesized hemispheric differences in language and visual functions in human adults. *Cortex,* 2, 1966.

86. Smith, A. Verbal and nonverbal test performance of patients with "acute" lateralized brain lesions (tumors). *J. Nerv. Ment. Dis.,* 141, 1965.

87. Tymchuk, A. J. Comparisons of Bender error and time scores for groups of epileptic, retarded, and behavior-problem children. *Percept. Motor Skills,* 38:1, 1974.

88. Valett, R. E. *An Inventory of Primary Skills.* Belmont, Calif.: Lear Siegler/Fearon, 1970.

89. Vega, Jr., A. Use of Purdue Pegboard and Finger Tapping performance as a rapid screening test for brain damage. *J. Clin. Psychol.,* 25:3, 1969.

90. Voeller, K. A proposed extended behavioral, cognitive and sensorimotor pediatric neurological examination. In R. Ochroch (ed.), *The Diagnosis and Treatment of Minimal Brain Dysfunction in Children: A Clinical Approach.* New York: Human Sciences Press, 1980.

91. Watson, C. G. Cross-validation of a WAIS sign developed to separate brain-damaged from schizophrenic patients. *J. Clin. Psychol.,* 28:1, 1972.

92. Wechsler, D. *The Measurement and Appraisal of Adult Intelligence.* Baltimore: Williams and Wilkins, 1958.

93. Witkin, H. A. *et al. Psychological Differentiation.* New York: Wiley, 1950.

94. *Woodcock-Johnson Psycho-Educational Battery.* Hungham, Mass.: Teaching Resources, no date.

Chapter 11

1. Abrams, J. C. and Kaslow, F. W. Learning disability and family dynamics: A mutual interaction. *J. Clin. Psychol.,* 5:1, 1976.

2. Benoit, M. B. Minimal brain dysfunction: The psychiatric examination. In R. Ochroch (ed.), *The Diagnosis and Treatment of Minimal Brain Dysfunction in Children: A Clinical Approach.* New York: Human Sciences Press, 1980.

3. Berman, A. Learning disabilities and juvenile delinquency: A neuropsychological approach. Mimeo, 1973.

4. Deitchman, W. S. How many case managers does it take to screw in a light bulb? *Hosp. Community Psychiat.,* 31:11, 1980.

5. Feighner, A. C. and Feighner, J. P. Multi-modality treatment of the hyperkinetic child. *Amer. J. Psychiat.,* 13:4, 1974,

6. Johnson, D. J. Adolescents with learning disabilities: Perspectives from an educational clinic. *Learn. Disability Quart.,* 1, 1978.

6A. Kenny, T. J. and Burka, A. Coordinating multiple intervention. In H. E. Rie and E. D. Rie (eds), *Handbook of Minimal Brain Dysfunctions: A Critical View.* New York: Wiley, 1980.

7. Keogh, B. K. Noncognitive aspects of learning disabilities: Another look at perceptual-motor approaches to assessment and remediation. In L. Oettinger, Jr. and L. V. Majovski (eds.), *The Psychologist, the School and the Child with MBD/LD.* New York: Grune and Stratton, 1978.

8. Lamb, H. R. Therapist-case managers: More than brokers of services. *Hosp. Community Psychiat.,* 31:11, 1980.

9. Lambert, N. M. *et al.* Prevalence of treatment regimens for children considered to be hyperactive. *Amer. J. Orthopsychiat.,* 49:3, 1979.

10. Muir, M. The consideration of emotional factors in the diagnosis and treatment of learning disabled children. *J. Ped. Psychol.,* 3:3, 1975.

11. Ney, P. G. Four types of hyperkinesis. *Can. Psychiat. Assoc. J.,* 19, 1974.

12. Ochroch, R.: The "case" for the "case manager." In R. Ochroch (ed.), *The Diagnosis and Treatment of Minimal Brain Dysfunction in Children: A Clinical Approach.* New York: Human Sciences Press, 1980.

13. Oettinger, L. Pediatric psychopharmacology: A review with special reference to dianol. *Dis. Nerv. Syst.,* 38:12-2, 1977.

14. Okada, S. and Hitoni, K. A critical review on minimal brain dysfunction (MBD). *Japanese J. Child Psychiat.,* 15:4, 1974.

15. Schackenberg, B. C. Minimal brain dysfunction in children. *Psychiatric Forum,* 7:1, 1976.

16. Smith, J. D. and Polloway, E. A. Learning disabilities: Individual needs or categorical concerns. *J. Learn. Disabilities,* 12:8, 1979.

17. van der Linden, D. Children with minimal brain dysfunction. *Nederlands Tijdschrift voor de Psychologie en har Grensgebieden,* 29:8, 1974.

Chapter 12

1. Abrams, J. C. Minimal brain dysfunction and dyslexia. *Reading World,* 14:3, 1975.

2. Adams, J. Visual and tactual integration and cerebral dysfunction in children with learning disabilities. *J. Learn. Disabilities,* 11:4, 1978.

3. Behrmann, P. *Activities for Developing Auditory Perception.* San Rafael, Calif.: Academic Therapy Publications, 1975.

4. Behrmann, P. *Activities for Developing Visual Perception.* San Rafael, Calif.: Academic Therapy Publications, 1975.

5. Belmont, I. The relation of afferent change to motor performance in the rehabilitation of cerebrally damaged patients. *Bull. New York Acad. Med.,* 42, 1966.

6. Benton, A. L. and Pearl, D. (eds.), *Dyslexia: An Appraisal of Current Knowledge.* New York: Oxford University Press, 1978.

7. Bierbauer, E. Tips for parents of a neurologically handicapped child. *Amer. Nursing,* 72:10, 1972.

8. Blank, M. Review of "Toward an understanding of dyslexia: Psychological factors in specific reading disability." In A. L. Benton and D. Pearl (eds.), *Dyslexia: An Appraisal of Current Knowledge.* New York: Oxford University Press, 1978.

9. Bogen, J. E. Some educational aspects of hemispheric specialization. *UCLA Educator,* 17, 1975.

10. Cantwell, D. P. Early intervention with hyperactive children. *J. Operational Psychiat.,* 6:1, 1974.

11. Catalog, Academic Therapy Publications. Novato, California: no date.

12. Clements, S. D. and Peters, J. E. Psychoeducational programming for children with minimal brain dysfunction. *Annals New York Acad. Sci.,* 205, 1973.

13. Clements, S. D. and Peters, J. E. Minimal brain dysfunction in the school age child: Diagnosis and treatment. *Arch. Gen. Psychiat.,* 6, 1962.

14. Cox, S. The learning-disabled adult. *Acad. Ther.,* 13:1, 1977.

15. Faas, L. A. *Learning Disabilities: Competency Based Approach.* Boston: Houghton Mifflin, 1976.

16. Flax, N. The eye and learning disabilities. *J. Amer. Optometric Assoc.,* 43:6, 1972.

16A. Fowler, E. Learning disabilities: An identity crisis. *ACLD Newsbriefs,* July/August, 1981.

17. Gibson, E. J. The ontogeny of reading. *Amer. Psychologist,* 25:2, 1970.

18. Goldberg, H. K. and Schiffman, G. B. *Dyslexia: Problems of Reading Disabilities.* New York: Grune and Stratton, 1972.

19. Gromska, J. *et al.* Musicotherapy in treatment of hyperkinetic and anxiety neurosis in children. *Psychiatria Polska,* 9:6, 1975.

20. Guthrie, J. T. Principles of instruction: A critique of Johnson's "Remedial approaches to dyslexia." In A. L. Benton and D. Pearl (eds.), *Dyslexia: An Appraisal of Current Knowledge.* New York: Oxford University Press, 1978.

21. Hagin, R. A. and Silver, A. A. Learning disability: Definition, diagnosis and prevention. *New York University Education Quarterly,* Summer 1977.

22. Hagin, R. A. *et al. TEACH: Learning Tasks for the Prevention of Learning Disability.* New York: Walker, 1976.

23. Helsinger, F. S. The psychoneurological dysfunction child: Special education center versus special class within the regular school. *Dis. Nerv. Syst.,* 32:10, 1971.

24. Jacobson, S. and Kovalinsky, T. *Educational Interpretation of the Wechsler Intelligence Scale for Children—Revised (WISC-R).* Linden, N. J.: Remediation Associates, Inc., 1976.

25. Johnson, D. J. Adolescents with learning disabilities: Perspectives from an educational clinic. *Learn. Disability Quart.,* 1, 1978.

26. Johnson, D. J. Remedial approaches to dyslexia. In A. L. Benton and D. Pearl (eds.), *Dyslexia: An Appraisal of Current Knowledge.* New York: Oxford University Press, 1978.

27. Kirk, S. A. Specific learning disabilities. *J. Clin. Child Psychol.*, Winter, 1977.

28. Levi, A. Treatment of a disorder of perception and concept formation in a case of school failure. *J. Consult. Psychol.*, 19:4, 1965.

29. Levinson, B. S. and Nissenbaum, C. D. Life after diagnosis: Schooling. In R. Ochroch (ed.), *The Diagnosis and Treatment of Minimal Brain Dysfunction in Children: A Clinical Approach.* New York: Human Sciences Press, 1980.

30. Littleton, C. and Davis, F. The mystique of brain injury. *Training School Bull.*, 68:1, 1971.

31. Luria, A. R. Psychological studies of mental deficiency in the Soviet Union. In N. R. Ellis (ed.), *Handbook of Mental Deficiency.* New York: McGraw-Hill, 1963.

32. Luria, A. R. *Restoration of Function After Brain Injury.* New York: Macmillan, 1963.

33. McCarthy, J. J. and Kirk, S. A. *The Illinois Test of Psycholinguistic Abilities.* Urbana, Ill.: University of Illinois Press.

34. Merrill, A. J. The role of vision in learning disorders. *J. Learn. Disabilities*, 10:7, 1977.

35. Norton, Y. Minimal cerebral dysfunction, Part II: Modified treatment and evaluation of movement. *Amer. J. Occupational Therapy*, 26:4, 1972.

36. O'Malley, J. E. and Eisenberg, L. The hyperkinetic syndrome. *Seminars in Psychiat.*, 5:1, 1973.

37. Ozer, M. N. The use of operant conditioning in the evaluation of children with learning problems. *Clin. Proc. Childrens Hospital*, 22:8, 1966.

38. Parr, V. E. Auditory word discrimination in male children diagnosed as having minimal brain dysfunction. *J. Clin. Psychol.*, 33:4, 1977.

39. Pontius, A. A. Discussions of conceptual models. *Annals New York Acad. Sci.*, 205, 1973.

40. Porter, J. and Holzberg, B. C. The changing role of the school psychologist in the age of PL94-142: From conducting testing to enhancing instruction. *Ed. Visually Handicapped*, 10:3, 1979.

41. Reitan, R. M. Paper presented at ACLD Convention, Seattle, 1976.

42. Schmais, C. and Orleans, F. Movement education through dance therapy with the minimally brain-damaged child. In R. Ochroch (ed.), *The Diagnosis and Treatment of Minimal Brain Dysfunction in Children: A Clinical Approach.* New York: Human Sciences Press, 1980.

43. Schrager, J. *et al.* The hyperkinetic child: An overview of the issues. *J. Amer. Acad. Child Psychiat.*, 1966.

44. Searls, E. F. *How to Use WISC Scores in Reading Diagnosis.* Newark, Delaware: International Reading Association, 1975.

45. Silver, A. A. and Hagin, R. A. *SEARCH: A Scanning Instrument for the Identification of Potential Learning Disability.* New York: Walker, 1976.

46. Spano, I. The state of the art. In R. Ochroch (ed.), *The Diagnosis and Treatment of Minimal Brain Dysfunction in Children: A Clinical Approach.* New York: Human Sciences Press, 1980.

47. Velluntino, F. R. Toward an understanding of dyslexia: Psychological factors in specific reading disability. In A. L. Benton and D. Pearl (eds.), *Dyslexia: An Appraisal of Current Knowledge.* New York: Oxford University Press, 1978.

48. Vocational education—an idea that has met its time. *ACLD Newsbriefs: Special Supplement,* 124, 1979. Pittsburgh, Pa.: Association of Children with Learning Disabilities.

49. Weinstein, M. L. A neuropsychological approach to math disability. *New York University Education Quarterly,* Winter, 1980.

49A. Werner, H. and Kaplan, B. *Symbol Formation: An Organismic-Developmental Approach to Language and Expression of Thought.* New York: Wiley, 1963.

50. Zentall, S. S. Specific learning disabilities, communication and language process disturbance. In R. Ochroch (ed.), *Diagnosis and Treatment of Minimal Brain Dysfunction in Children: A Clinical Approach.* New York: Human Sciences Press, 1980.

51. Zigmond, N. Remediation of dyslexia: A discussion. In A. L. Benton and D. Pearl (eds.), *Dyslexia: An Appraisal of Current Knowledge.* New York: Oxford University Press, 1978.

Chapter 13

1. Krauch, V. Hyperactive engineering. *Amer. Ed.,* 7:5, 1971.

2. Littleton, C. and Davis, F. The mystique of brain injury. *Training School Bull.,* 68:1, 1971.

3. Loney, J. and Ordona, T. T. Using cerebral stimulants to treat minimal brain dysfunction. *Amer. J. Orthopsychiat.,* 45:4, 1975.

4. Strauss, A. and Kephart, N. *Psychopathology and Education of the Brain-Impaired Child,* vol. 2. New York: Grune and Stratton, 1955.

5. Zentall, S. S. Specific learning disabilities, communications and language process disturbance. In R. Ochroch (ed.), *Diagnosis and Treatment of Minimal Brain Dysfunction in Children: A Clinical Approach.* New York: Human Sciences Press, 1980.

6. Zentall, S. S. Optimal stimulation as theoretical basis of hyperactivity. *Amer. J. Orthopsychiat.,* 45:4, 1975.

Chapter 14

1. Abikoff, H. Cognitive training interventions in children: Review of a new approach. *J. Learn. Disabilities,* 12:2, 1979.

2. Abrams, K. E. and Kodera, T. L. Acceptance hierarchy of handicaps: Validation of Kirk's statement, "Special education often begins where medicine stops." *J. Learn. Disabilities,* 12:1, 1979.

3. Adelman, H. S. and Compas, B. E. Stimulant drugs and learning problems. *J. Spec. Ed.,* 11:4, 1977.

4. Adler, S. Megavitamin treatment for behaviorally disturbed and learning disabled children. *J. Learn. Disabilities,* 12:10, 1979.

5. Adler, S. J. Hyperactivity controversy. Reported anon: CANHC Gram, 8:6, 1974.

6. Aman, M. G. Psychotropic drugs and learning problems: A selective review. *J. Learn. Disabilities,* 13:2, 1980.

7. Arnold, L. E. *et al.* Megavitamins for minimal brain dysfunction: A placebo-controlled study. *JAMA,* 240:24, 1978.

8. Arnold, L. E. *et al.* Methylphenidate vs. dextroamphetamine vs. caffeine in minimal brain dysfunction: Controlled comparison by placebo washout design with Bayle's analysis. *Arch. Gen. Psychiat.,* 35:4, 1978.

9. Arnold, E. L. *et al.* Levoamphetamine and dextroamphetamine: Differential effect on aggression and hyperkinesis in children and dogs. *Amer. J. Psychiat.,* 130:2, 1973.

10. Arnold, L. E. *et al.* Hyperkinetic adult: Study of the "paradoxical" amphetamine response. *JAMA,* 222:6, 1972.

11. Barcai, A. and Rabkin, L. Y. A precursor of delinquency: The hyperkinetic disorder of childhood. *Psychiat. Quart.,* 48:3, 1974.

12. Barkley, R. A. and Cunningham, C. E. Stimulant drugs and activity level in hyperactive children. *Amer. J. Orthopsychiat.,* 49:3, 1979.

13. Barkley, R. A. and Cunningham, C. E. The effects of methylphenidate on mother-child interactions of hyperactive children. *Arch. Gen. Psychiat.,* 36:2, 1979.

14. Barkley, R. A. Using stimulant drugs in the classroom. *School Psychol. Digest,* 8:4, 1979.

15. Benoit, M. B. Minimal brain dysfunction: The psychiatric examination. In R. Ochroch (ed.), *The Diagnosis and Treatment of Minimal Brain Dysfunction in Children: A Clinical Approach.* New York: Human Sciences Press, 1980.

16. Bosco, J. J. and Robin, S. S. (eds.). *The Hyperactive Child and Stimulant Drugs.* Chicago: University of Chicago Press, 1977.

17. Bradley, C. Behavior of children receiving Benzedrine. *Amer. J. Psychiat.,* 94, 1937.

18. Brodemus, J. and Swanson, J. C. The paradoxical effects of stimulants upon hyperactive children. *Drug Forum,* 6:2, 1977–78.

19. Brown, G. W. Suggestions for parents. *J. Learn. Disabilities,* 2:2, 1969.

20. Brown, R. T. Impulsivity and psychoeducational intervention in hyperactive children. *J. Learn. Disabilities,* 13:5, 1980.

21. Burnett, L. and Struve, F. A. The value of EEG study in minimal brain dysfunction. *J. Clin. Psychol.,* 30:4, 1974.

22. Cantwell, D. P. Early intervention with hyperactive children. *J. Operational Psychiat.,* 6:1, 1974.

22A. Cantwell, D. P. and Carlson, G. A. Stimulants. In J. S. Werry (ed.), *Pediatric Psychopharmacology—The Use of Behavior Modifying Drugs in Children.* New York: Brunner/Mazel, 1978.

23. Chess, S. *An Introduction to Child Psychiatry* (2nd ed.).New York: Grune and Stratton, 1969.

24. Chizeck, S. P. The orthomolecular theory of schizophrenia. *Health Soc. Work,* 3:4, 1978.

25. Clements, S. D. and Peters, J. E. Minimal brain dysfunction in the school age child: Diagnosis and treatment. *Arch. Gen. Psychiat.,* 6, 1962.

26. Comly, H. H. Cerebral stimulants for children with learning disorders. *J. Learn. Disabilities,* 4:9, 1971.

27. Conners, C. K. *et al.* Magnesium pemoline and dextroamphetamine: A controlled study in children with minimal brain dysfunction. *Psychopharmacologia,* 26, 1972.

28. Conners, C. K. The effect of stimulant drugs on Human Figure Drawings in children with minimal brain dysfunction. *Psychopharmacologia,* 19, 1971.

29. Conrad, P.: The discovery of hyperkinesis: Notes on the medicalization of deviant behavior. *Soc. Problems,* 28:1, 1975.

30. Conrad, W. G. *et al.* Effects of amphetamine therapy and prescriptive tutoring on the behavior and achievement of lower class hyperactive children. *J. Learn. Disabilities,* 4:9, 1971.

31. Cott, A. *The Orthomolecular Approach to Learning Disabilities.* San Rafael, Calif.: Academic Therapy Publications, 1977.

32. Cott, A. Treatment of learning disabilities. *J. Orthomolecular Psychiat.,* 3:4, 1974.

33. Crook, W. G. Can what a child eats make him dull, stupid or hyperactive? *J. Learn. Disabilities,* 13:5, 1980.

34. Cunningham, C. F. and Barkley, R. A. The role of academic failure in hyperkinetic behavior. *J. Learn. Disabilities,* 11:5, 1978.

35. David, O. J. *et al.* Lead and hyperactivity. Behavioral response to chelation: A pilot study. *Amer. J. Psychiat.,* 133:10, 1976.

36. Denhoff, E. *et al.* Effects of dextroamphetamine on hyperkinetic children: A controlled double blind study. *J. Learn. Disabilities,* 4:9, 1971.

37. DiMascio, A. Psychopharmacology in children: Problem areas, methodological considerations, and assessment techniques. Mimeo, 1969.

38. Douglas, V. I. Are drugs enough to treat or to train the hyperactive child? *Int. J. Mental Health,* 4:1-2, 1975.

39. Feighner, A. C. and Feighner, J. P. Multi-modality treatment of the hyperkinetic child. *Amer. J. Psychiat.,* 13:4, 1974.

40. Firestone, P. *et al.* The effects of caffeine on hyperactive children. *J. Learn. Disabilities,* 11:3, 1978.

41. Fischer, D. and Wilson, W. P. Methylphenidate and hyperkinetic state. *Dis. Nerv. Syst.,* 32, 1971.

42. Fish, B. The "one child, one drug" myth of stimulants in hyperkinesis. In S. Chess and A. Thomas (eds.), *Annual Progress in Child Psychiatry and Child Development.* New York: Brunner/Mazel, 1972.

43. Fisher, M. A. Dextroamphetamine and placebo practice effects on selective attention in hyperactive children. *J. Abnorm. Child Psychol.,* 6:1, 1978.

44. Frank, J. and Levinson, H. Seasickness mechanisms and medications in dysmetric dyslexia and dyspraxia. *Acad. Ther.,* 12:2, 1976-77.

45. Gabrys, J. B. Methylphenidate effect on attentional and cognitive behavior in six-through-twelve-year-old males. *Percept. Motor Skills,* 45:3, 1977.

46. Garfinkel, B. D. *et al.* Methylphenidate and caffeine in the treatment of children with minimal brain dysfunction. *Amer. J. Psychiat.,* 132:7, 1975.

47. Greenberg, L. M. *et al.* Clinical effects of imipramine and methylphenidate in hyperactive children. *Inter. J. Mental Health,* 14:1–2, 1975.

48. Gross, M. D. Caffeine in the treatment of children with minimal brain dysfunction or hyperkinetic syndrome. *Psychosomatics,* 16:1, 1975.

49. Harvey, D. H. and Mursh, R. W. The effects of de-caffeinated coffee versus whole coffee on hyperactive children. *Devel. Med. Child Neurol.,* 20:1, 1978.

50. Hastings, J. E. and Barkley, R. A. A review of psychophysiological research with hyperkinetic children. *J. Abnorm. Child Psychol.,* 6:4, 1978.

51. Hixson, J. R. New hope for hyperactive children. *The New York Times Magazine,* August 24, 1980.

52. Huey, L. Y. *et al.* Adult minimal brain dysfunction and schizophrenia: A case report. *Amer. J. Psychiat.,* 135:12, 1978.

53. Humphries, T. *et al.* Stimulant effects on persistence of motor performance of hyperactive children. *J. Pediat. Psychol.,* 4:1, 1979.

54. Humphries, T. *et al.* Stimulant effects on cooperation and social interaction between hyperactive children and their mothers. *J. Child Psychol. Psychiat. Allied Disciplines,* 19:1, 1978.

55. Klicpera, C. Treatment of children with stimulant drugs. *Zeitschrift fur Kinder- und Jugendpsychiatrie,* 6:2, 1978.

56. Klorman, R. *et al.* Effects of methylphenidate on hyperactive children's evoked responses during passive and active attention. *Psychophysiol.,* 16:1, 1979.

57. Knights, R. M. and Hinton, G. G. Minimal brain dysfunction: Clinical and psychological test characteristics. *Acad. Ther.,* 4, 1969.

58. Knights, R. M. and Hinton, G. G. The effects of methylphenidate (Ritalin) on the motor skills and behavior of children with learning problems. *J. Nerv. Ment. Dis.,* 148:6, 1969.

59. Krager, J. M. and Safer, D. J. Type and prevalence of medications used in the treatment of hyperactive children. *New England J. Med.,* 291, 1974.

60. Krippner, S. *et al.* A study of hyperkinetic children receiving stimulant drugs. *Acad. Ther.,* 3:3, 1973.

61. Lambert, N. M. *et al.* Hyperactive children and the efficacy of psychoactive drugs as a treatment intervention. *Amer. J. Orthopsychiat.,* 46:2, 1976.

62. Laufer, M. L. Long-term management and some follow-up findings on the use of drugs with minimal cerebral syndromes. *J. Learn. Disabilities,* 4:9, 1971.

63. Leisman, G. and Schwartz, J. Aetiological factors in dyslexia: I. Scaccadic eye movement control. *Percept. Motor Skills,* 47:2, 1978.

64. Lerer, R. J. and Lerer, P. M. Response of adolescents with minimal brain dysfunction to methylphenidate. *J. Learn. Disabilities,* 10:4, 1977.

65. Levine, E. M. *et al.* Hyperactivity among white middle-class children. *Child Psychiat. Human Devel.*

66. Levinson, B. S. and Nissenbaum, C. D. Life after diagnosis: Schooling. In R. Ochroch (ed.), *The Diagnosis and Treatment of Minimal Brain Dysfunction in Children: A Clinical Approach.* New York: Human Sciences Press, 1980.

67. Lewis, J. A. and Lewis, B. S. Dianol in minimal brain dysfunction. *Dis. Nerv. Syst.*, 38:12, 2, 1977.

68. Loney, J. *et al.* Hyperkinetic/aggressive boys in treatment: Predictors of clinical response to methylphenidate. *Amer. J. Psychiat.*, 135:12, 1978.

69. Loney, J. *et al.* Parental management, self-concept, and drug response in minimal brain dysfunction. *J. Learn. Disabilities*, 8:3, 1975.

70. Loney, J. and Ordoña, T. T. Using cerebral stimulants to treat minimal brain dysfunction. *Amer. J. Orthopsychiat.*, 45:4, 1975.

71. Ludlow, C. *et al.* Effects of dextroamphetamine on auditory perceptual skills in hyperactive boys. *Bull. Int. Neuropsychological Soc.*, 1979.

72. McManis, D. L. *et al.* Effects of a stimulant drug on extraversion level in hyperactive children. *Percept. Motor Skills*, 46:11, 1978.

73. Mackay, M. C. *et al.* Methylphenidate for adolescents with minimal brain dysfunction. *New York State J. Med.*, 73:4, 1973.

74. Mann, H. B. and Greenspan, S. I. The identification and treatment of adult brain dysfunction. *Amer. J. Psychiat.*, 133:9, 1976.

75. Monroe, R. R. *Episodic Behavioral Disorders.* Cambridge, Mass.: Harvard University Press, 1970.

76. Nash, R. J. Clinical research on psychotropic drugs and hyperactivity in children. *School Psychol. Digest*, 5:4, 1976.

77. Neisworth, J. T. *et al.* Naturalistic assessment of neurological diagnoses and pharmacological intervention. *J. Learn. Disabilities*, 9:3, 1976.

78. Oettinger, L. Pediatric psychopharmacology: A review with special reference to dianol. *Dis. Nerv. Syst.*, 38:12-2, 1977.

78A. Rapoport, J. L. *et al.* Dextroamphetamine: Its cognitive and behavioral effects in normal and hyperactive boys and normal men. *Arch. Gen. Psychiat.*, 37:8, 1980.

79. *Report of the Conference on the Use of Stimulant Drugs in the Treatment of Behaviorally Disturbed Young School Children.* Washington: Dept. of Health, Education and Welfare, 1971.

80. Rie, E. D. and Rie, H. E. Recall, retention, and Ritalin. *J. Consult. Clin. Psychol.*, 45:6, 1977.

81. Rie, H. E. *et al.* Effects of Ritalin on underachieving children: A replication. *Amer. J. Orthopsychiat.*, 46:2, 1976.

82. Safer, D. J. and Allen, R. P. Stimulant drug treatment of hyperactive adolescents. *Dis. Nerv. Syst.*, 36:8, 1975.

83. Sandoval, J. *et al.* Current medical practice and hyperactive children. *Amer. J. Orthopsychiat.*, 46:2, 1976.

84. Satterfield, J. H. *et al.* Pathophysiology of the hyperactive child syndrome. *Arch. Gen. Psychiat.*, 31:6, 1974.

85. Satterfield, J. H. EEG issues in children with minimal brain dysfunction. *Seminars in Psychiat.*, 5:1, 1973.

86. Satterfield, J. H. *et al.* Response to stimulant drug treatment in hyperactive children: Prediction from EEG and neurological findings. *J. Autism Childhood Schiz.*, 3:1, 1973.

87. Satterfield, J. H. *et al.* Physiological studies of the hyperkinetic child: 1. *Amer. J. Psychiat.*, 128:11, 1972.

88. Schain, R. J. Attentional behavior and drugs in hyperactive children. In L. Oettinger, Jr. and L. V. Majovski (eds.), *The Psychologist, the School, and the Child with MBD/LD.* New York: Grune and Stratton, 1978.

89. Schnackenberg, R. C. and Bender, E. P. The effect of methylphenidate hydrochloride on children with minimal brain dysfunction syndrome and subsequent hyperkinetic syndrome. *Psychiatric Forum,* Summer, 1971.

90. Seger, E. Y. and Hallum, G. Methylphenidate in children with minimal brain dysfunction: Effect on attention span, visual-motor skills, and behavior. *Current Therapeutic Res.,* 16:6, 1974.

91. Sobel, D. Hyperactive children often suffer as adults. *New York Times,* December 4, 1979.

92. Solomons, G. Guidelines on the use and medical effects of psychostimulant drugs in therapy. *J. Learn. Disabilities,* 4:9, 1971.

93. Sprague, R. L. Man—the most difficult laboratory animal. In L. Oettinger, Jr. and L. V. Majovski (eds.), *The Psychologist, the School, and the Child with MBD/LD.* New York: Grune and Stratton, 1978.

94. Sprague, R. L. and Sleator, E. K. Dose-related effects of methylphenidate in hyperkinetic children. *Sci.,* 198, 1977.

95. Vocational education—an idea that has met its time. *ACLD Newsbriefs: Special Supplement,* 124, 1979. Pittsburgh, Pa: Association of Children with Learning Disabilities.

96. Walker, S. Drugging the American child: We're too cavalier about hyperactivity. *Psychol. Today,* 8:7, 1974.

97. Weingartner, H. *et al.* Cognitive processes in normal and hyperactive children and their response to amphetamine treatment. *J. Abnorm. Psychol.,* 89:1, 1980.

98. Wender, P. H. The minimal brain dysfunction syndrome. *Ann. Rev. Med.,* 26, 1975.

99. Wender, P. H. *Minimal Brain Dysfunction in Children.* New York: Wiley-Interscience, 1971.

100. Whalen, C. K. *et al.* Peer interaction in a structured communication task: Comparisons of normal and hyperactive boys and of methylphenidate (Ritalin) and placebo effects. *Child Devel.,* 50:2, 1979.

100A. Whalen, C. K. and Henker, B. (eds.). *Hyperactive Children: The Social Ecology of Identification and Treatment.* New York: Academic Press, 1980.

100B. Whalen, C. K. and Henker, B. Psycho-stimulants and children: A review and analysis. *Psychol. Bull.,* 83, 1976.

101. Whaley-Klahn, M. A. and Loney, J. A multivariate study of the relationship of parental management of self-esteem and initial drug response in hyperkinetic/MDB boys. *Psychol. in the Schools,* 14:4, 1977.

102. Winsberg, B. G. and Camp, J. A. Psychostimulant therapy for behavior disorders: A status review. In R. Ochroch (ed.), *The Diagnosis and Treatment of Minimal Brain Dysfunction in Children: A Clinical Approach.* New York: Human Sciences Press, 1980.

103. Wurtman, R. J. and Wurtman, J. J. (eds.). *Nutrition and the Brain,* Vol. 3: *Disorders of Eating and Nutrients in Treatment of Brain Diseases.* New York: Raven Press, 1979.

104. Wurtman, R. J. and Wurtman, J. J. (eds.). *Nutrition and the Brain,* Vol. 4: *Toxic Effect of Food Constituents on the Brain.* New York: Raven Press, 1979.

105. Zahn, T. P. *et al.* Pupillary and heart rate reactivity in children with minimal brain dysfunction. *J. Abnorm. Child Psychol.,* 6:1, 1978.

105A. Zahn, T. P. *et al.* Autonomic and behavioral effects of dextroamphetamine and placebo in normal and hyperactive prepubertal boys. *J. Abnorm. Child Psychol.,* 8:2, 1980.

106. Zentall, S. S. Specific learning disabilities, communications, and language process disturbance. In R. Ochroch (ed.), *Diagnosis and Treatment of Minimal Brain Dysfunction in Children: A Clinical Approach.* New York: Human Sciences Press, 1980.

Chapter 15

1. Bower, K. B. and Mercer, C. D. Hyperactivity: Etiology and intervention techniques. *J. School Health,* 45:4, 1975.

2. Braud, L. W. *et al.* The use of electromyographic biofeedback in the control of hyperactivity. *J. Learn. Disabilities,* 8:7, 1975.

3. Braud, L. W. The effects of EMG biofeedback and progressive relaxation upon hyperactivity and its behavioral concomitants. Mimeo, Undated.

4. Bugental, D. P. *et al.* Attributional and behavioral changes following two behavior management interventions with hyperactive boys: A follow-up study. *Child Devel.,* 49:1, 1978.

5. Carter, E. N. and Shostak, D. Imitation in the treatment of hyperkinetic behavior syndrome. *J. Clin. Child Psychol.,* 9:1, 1980.

6. Clement, P. W. *et al.* Self-regulation training for under-controlled children. In L. Oettinger, Jr. and L. V. Majorski (eds.), *The Psychologist, the School, and the Child with MBD/LD.* New York: Grune and Stratton, 1978.

7. Cunningham, S. J. and Knights, R. The performance of hyperactive and normal boys under differing reward and punishment schedules. *J. Ped. Psychol.,* 3:4, 1978.

8. Drash, P. W.: Treatment of hyperactivity in the two-year-old child. *J. Ped. Psychol.,* 3:3, 1975.

9. Feighner, A. C. and Feighner, J. P. Multi-modality treatment of the hyperkinetic child. *Amer. J. Psychiat.,* 13:4, 1974.

9A. Fine, M. J. *Intervention with Hyperactive Children: A Case Study Approach.* New York: SP Medical and Scientific Books, 1980.

10. Herbert, M. *Conduct Disorder of Childhood and Adolescence: A Behavioral Approach to Assessment and Treatment.* Chichester, England: Wiley, 1978.

11. Hixson, J. R. New hope for hyperactive children. *The New York Times Magazine,* August, 24, 1980.

12. Klein, S. A. and Deffenbacher, J. L. Relaxation and exercise for hyperactive impulsive children. *Percept. Motor Skills,* 45:3, 1977.

13. Kline, C. L. Developmental dyslexia in adolescents: The emotional damage. *Bull. Orton. Soc.,* 28, 1978.

14. Krop, H. Modification of hyperactive behavior of a brain-damaged, emotionally disturbed child. *Training School Bull.,* 68:1, 1971.

15. laGreca, A. M. and Mesibov, G. B. Social skills intervention with learning disabled children: Selecting skills and implementing training. *J. Clin. Child Psychol.,* 8:3, 1979.

16. Lahey, B. B. (ed.). *Behavior Therapy with Hyperactive and Learning Disabled Children.* New York: Oxford Press, 1979.

17. Leung, F. L. The ethics and scope of behavior modification. *Bull. Brit. Psychological Soc.,* 28, 1975.

18. Lupin, M. *et al.* Children, parents, and relaxation tapes. *Acad. Ther.,* 12:1, 1976.

19. Margolis, H. *et al.* Modification of impulsivity: Implications for teaching. *Elem. School J.,* 77:3, 1977.

20. Marmor, J. and Woods, S. M. (eds.). *The Interface Between the Psychodynamic and Behavioral Therapies.* New York: Plenum Medical Books, 1980.

21. Moore, S. F. and Cole, S. O. Cognitive self-mediation training with hyperactive children. *Bull. Psychonomic Soc.,* 12:1, 1978.

22. Moreland, K. L. Stimulus control of hyperactivity. *Percept. Motor Skills,* 45:3, 1, 1977.

23. Nagle, R. J. and Thwaite, B. C. Modelling effects on impulsivity with learning disabled children. *J. Learn. Disabilities,* 12:5, 1979.

24. Nirk, G. *et al.* A developmental model for treatment of hyperactive children. Mimeo, Undated.

25. Phillips, D. and Mordock, J. B. Parents' aid enhances operant therapy for hyperactivity. Reported anon: *Frontiers Psychiat.,* March, 1971.

26. Prout, H. T. Behavioral intervention with hyperactive children. *J. Learn. Disabilities.,* 10:3, 1977.

27. Putre, W. *et al.* An effectiveness study of a relaxation training tape with hyperactive children. *Behav. Ther.,* 8:3, 1977.

28. Quay, H. C. and Werry, J. S. *Psychopathological Disorders of Childhood.* New York: Wiley, 1972.

29. Ross, A. O. *Learning Disability: The Unrealized Potential.* New York: McGraw-Hill, 1977.

30. Shafto, F. and Sulzbacher, S. Comparing treatment tactics with a hyperactive preschool child: Stimulant medication and programmed teacher intervention. *J. App. Behav. Anal.,* 10:1, 1977.

31. Strain, P. S. and Shores, R. E. Social interaction development among behaviorally handicapped preschool children: Research and education implications. *Psychol. in the School,* 14:4, 1977.

32. Strub, R. L. and Black, F. W. *The Mental Status Examination in Neurology.* Philadelphia: F. A. Davis, 1977.

33. Strupp, H. H. A psychodynamicist looks at modern behavior therapy. *Psychotherapy Theory Res. Practice,* 16:2, 1979.

33A. Whalen, C. K. and Henker, B. (eds.). *Hyperactive Children: The Social Ecology of Identification and Treatment.* New York: Academic Press, 1980.

34. Winsberg, B. G. and Camp, J. A. Psychostimulant therapy for behavior disorders: A status review. In R. Ochroch (ed.), *The Diagnosis and Treatment of Minimal Brain Dysfunction in Children: A Clinical Approach.* New York: Human Sciences Press, 1980.

35. Zentall, S. S. Optimal stimulation as theoretical basis of hyperactivity. *Amer. J. Orthopsychiat.,* 45:4, 1975.

Chapter 16

1. Berlin, I. N. Psychotherapy with M.B.D. children and their parents. In R. Ochroch (ed.), *The Diagnosis and Treatment of Minimal Brain Dysfunction in Children: A Clinical Approach.* New York: Human Sciences Press, 1980.

2. Berman, A. Parenting learning-disabled children. *J. Clin. Child Psychol.,* 8:3, 1979.

3. Brehm, S. S. *Help for Your Child: A Parent's Guide to Mental Health Services.* Englewood Cliffs, N.J.: Prentice-Hall, 1978.

4. Brown, G. W. Suggestions for parents. *J. Learn. Disabilities,* 2:2, 1969.

5. Cantwell, D. P. Early intervention with hyperactive children *J. Operational Psychiat.,* 6:1, 1974.

6. Clarke, L. *Can't Read, Can't Write, Can't Takl Too Good Either.* New York: Walker, 1973.

7. Crook, W. G. *Can Your Child Read? Is He Hyperactive?* Jackson, Tenn.: Pedicenter Press, Undated.

8. Diament, C. and Colletti, G. Evaluation of behavioral group counseling for parents of learning-disabled children. *J. Abnorm. Child Psychol.,* 6:3, 1978.

9. Disability and financial assistance: Some questions and answers on SSI and Medicaid. *ACLD Newsbriefs,* March/April, 1980.

10. Ellingson, C. *Speaking of Children: Their Learning Abilities/Disabilities.* New York: Harper and Row, 1975.

11. Feighner, A. C. and Feighner, J. P. Multi-modality treatment of the hyperkinetic child. *Amer. J. Psychiat.,* 13:4, 1974.

12. Foltz, D. APA enters case of fired psychologist. *APA Monitor,* November., 1980.

13. Frostig, M. and Pascale, M. A. Children with learning difficulties. Los Angeles: Marianne Frostig Center of Educational Therapy *Newsletter,* Fall, 1974.

14. Gaines, R. Experiencing the perceptually-deprived child. *J. Learn. Disabilities,* 2:11, 1969.

15. Glass, J. New efforts to assist learning disabled debated across L.I. *New York Times,* November 23, 1980.

16. Golick, M. *Deal Me In!* New York: Jeffrey Norton, 1973.

17. Gordon, S. (ed.). *Living Fully.* New York: John Day, 1975.

18. Gordon, S. The "brain-injured" adolescent. *New York Association for Brain Injured Children.* March, 1966.

19. Hamilton, E. B. (ed.). *My Child Can't Read: A Parent Handbook.* Silver Spring, Md.: The Citizen Committee for Reading, 1972.

20. Hayes, M. L. *Oh, Dear, Somebody Said "Learning Disabilities": A Book for Teacher and Parents.* San Rafael, Calif.: Academic Therapy Press, 1975.

21. Hayes, M. L. *The Tuned-In, Turned-On Book.* Novato, Calif.: Academic Therapy Publications, 1974.

21A. Kleiman, D. Many disabled still not placed by city schools. *New York Times,* August 3, 1981.

22. Kronick, D. *What About Me? The LD Adolescent.* San Rafael, Calif.: Academic Therapy Press, 1975.

23. Learning disabled consumers call for change in vocational rehabilitation. *Closer Look,* Spring, 1980.

24. Loney, J. *et al.* Parental management, self-concept, and drug response in minimal brain dysfunction. *J. Learn. Disabilities,* 8:3, 1975.

25. Martin, R. You and the Law. *ACLD Newsbriefs,* January/February, 1980.

26. Mitler, J. *Helping Your Child at Home.* San Rafael, Calif.: Academic Therapy Publications, 1973.

27. Ney, P. G. Four types of hyperkinesis. *Can. Psychiat. Assoc. J.,* 19, 1974.

28. Neyhus, A. I. and Neyhus, M. Relationship of parents and teachers in the identification of children with suspected learning disabilities. *J. Learn. Disabilities,* 12:6, 1979.

28A. *Parents Are to be Seen and Heard: Assertiveness in Educational Planning for Handicapped Children.* San Luis Obispo, Calif., Box 1094: Impact Publications, Undated.

29. Schildkrout, M. S. The hyperactive/MBD child—family interaction and treatment. In R. Ochroch (ed.), *The Diagnosis and Treatment of Minimal Brain Dysfunction in Children: A Clinical Approach.* New York: Human Sciences Press, 1980.

30. Siegel, E. *The Exceptional Child Grows Up.* New York: E. P. Dutton, 1974.

31. Simpson, E. *Reversals.* Boston: Houghton Mifflin, 1979.

32. Sobel, D. Hyperactive children often suffer as adults. *New York Times,* December 4, 1979.

33. Stott, D. H. *The Parent as Teacher.* Belmont, Calif. Lear Siegler/Fearon, 1974.

34. Strother, C. *et al. The Educator's Enigma: The Adolescent with Learning Disabilities.* San Rafael, Calif.: Academic Therapy Publications, 1971.

35. Touliatos, J. and Lindholm, B. W. TAT need achievement and need affiliation in minimally brain-injured and normal children and their parents. *J. Psychol.,* 89:1, 1975.

36. Van Kaan, A. The dynamics of hope and despondency in the parents of handicapped children. *Humanitas,* 13:3, 1977.

37. Weiss, H. G. and Weiss, M. S. *Home Is A Learning Place.* Boston: Little, Brown, 1976.

38. Whaley-Klahn, M. A. and Loney, J. A multivariate study of the relationship

of parental management to self-esteem and initial drug response in hyperkinetic/MBD boys. *Psychol. in the Schools,* 14:4, 1977.

39. *What Every Parent Should Know About Learning Disabilities.* Brooklyn, N.Y.: New Hope Guild Center, 1979.

Chapter 17

1. Aaron, P. B. A neuropsychological approach to diagnosis and remediation of learning disabilities. *J. Clin. Psychol.,* 35:2, 1979.

2. Anderson, C. M. Minimal brain damage. *Mental Hygiene,* 56:2, 1972.

3. Blos, P. The second individuation of adolescence. In R. S. Eissler *et al.* (eds.), *Psychoanalytic Study of the Child.* New York: International Universities Press, 1967.

4. Chess, S. *An Introduction to Child Psychiatry* (2nd ed.). New York: Grune and Stratton, 1969.

5. Clarke, L. *Can't Read, Can't Write, Can't Takl Too Good Either.* New York: Walker, 1973.

6. Day, J. R. and Moore, M. E. Individual and family psychodynamic contributions to learning disability. *J. National Assoc. Private Psychiatric Hospitals,* 8:1, 1976.

7. Erikson, E. *Identity, Youth, and Crisis.* New York: Norton, 1968.

8. Feighner, A. C. and Feighner, J. P. Multi-modality treatment of the hyperkinetic child. *Amer. J. Psychiat.,* 13:4, 1974.

9. Freud, A. *The Ego and the Mechanisms of Defense.* New York: International Universities Press, 1946.

10. Gaddes, W. H. Neurological implications for learning. In C. W. Cruickshank and D. Hallahan (eds.), *Perceptual and Learning Disorders in Children,* vol. 1. Syracuse, N.Y.: Syracuse University Press, 1975.

11. Gardner, R. A. Psychotherapy in minimal brain dysfunction. In J. H. Masserman (ed.), *Current Psychiatric Therapies.* New York: Grune and Stratton, 1975.

12. Gardner, R. A. Techniques for involving the child with MBD in meaningful psychotherapy. *J. Learn. Disabilities,* 8:5, 1975.

13. Gardner, R. A. The mutual story telling technique in the treatment of psychogenic problems secondary to minimal brain dysfunctions. *J. Learn. Disabilities,* 8:3, 1975.

14. Gardner, R. A. Psychotherapy of minimal brain dysfunction. In J. H. Masserman (ed.). *Current Psychiatric Therapies.* New York: Grune and Stratton, 1974.

15. Gardner, R. A. Psychotherapy of the psychogenic problems secondary to minimal brain dysfunction. *Int. J. Child Psychotherapy.* 2:2, 1973.

16. Gordon, S. The "brain-injured" adolescent. *New York Association for Brain Injured Children,* March, 1966.

17. Mangel, C. The puzzle of learning disabilities. *New York Times,* April 25, 1976.

18. Mann, H. B. and Greenspan, S. I. The identification and treatment of adult brain dysfunction. *Amer. J. Psychiat.,* 133:9, 1976.

19. Mordock, J. B. The separation-individuation process and developmental disabilities. *Exceptional Children,* 46:3, 1979.

20. Muir, M. The consideration of emotional factors in the diagnosis and treatment of learning disabled children. *J. Ped. Psychol.,* 3:3, 1975.

21. Murray, M. E. Minimal brain dysfunction and borderline personality adjustment. *Amer. J. Psychotherapy,* 33:3, 1979.

22. Ney, P. G. Four types of hyperkinesis. *Can. Psychiat. Assoc. J.,* 19, 1974.

23. Niederland, W. G. Narcissistic ego impairment in patients with early physical malformations. In R. S. Eissler *et al.* (eds.), *Psychoanalytic Study of the Child.* New York: International Universities Press, 1965.

24. Palombo, J. Perceptual deficits and self-esteem in adolescence. *Clin. Soc. Work J.,* 7:1, 1979.

25. Schechter, M. D. Psychiatric aspects of learning disabilities. *Child Psychiat. Human Devel.,* 5:2, 1974.

26. Simpson, E. *Reversals.* Boston: Houghton Mifflin, 1979.

27. Small, L. *The Briefer Psychotherapies* (rev. ed.) New York: Brunner/Mazel, 1979.

28. Vail, P. L. Priscilla's Column. *Newsletter,* New York Branch of the Orton Society, Fall, 1980.

29. Wender, P. H. *Minimal Brain Dysfunction in Children.* New York: Wiley-Interscience, 1971.

30. White, R. W. Motivation reconsidered: The concept of competence. *Psychological Rev.,* 66, 1959.

31. Winsberg, B. G. and Camp, J. A. Psychostimulant therapy for behavior disorders: A status review. In R. Ochroch (ed.), *The Diagnosis and Treatment of Minimal Brain Dysfunction in Children: A Clinical Approach.* New York: Human Sciences Press, 1980.

32. Zbuska, B. Group treatment of the hyperactive/MBD child. In R. Ochroch (ed.), *The Diagnosis and Treatment of Minimal Brain Damage in Children: A Clinical Approach.* New York: Human Sciences Press, 1980.

Chapter 18

1. *A Guide to the Libraries of the New York Public Library,* 1977.

2. Bartlow, C. Vocational rehabilitation services for learning disabled adolescents. *J. Clin. Child Psychol.,* 8:3, 1979.

3. Clarke, L. *Can't Read, Can't Write, Can't Takl Too Good Either.* New York: Walker, 1973.

4. Governmental affairs committee report. *ACLD Newsbriefs,* 130, 1980.

5. Learning disabled consumers call for change in vocational rehabilitation. *Closer Look,* Spring, 1980.

6. Small, L. *The Briefer Psychotherapies* (rev. ed.). New York: Brunner/Mazel, 1979.

7. Small, L. Personality determinants of vocational choice. *Psychological Monographs,* 67:1, 1953.

Index